Infectious Disease Emergencies

Editors

BRADLEY W. FRAZEE
MICHAEL S. PULIA
CHRISTOPHER M. COLBERT

EMERGENCY MEDICINE CLINICS OF NORTH AMERICA

www.emed.theclinics.com

Consulting Editor
AMAL MATTU

May 2024 • Volume 42 • Number 2

ELSEVIER

1600 John F. Kennedy Boulevard • Suite 1800 • Philadelphia, Pennsylvania, 19103-2899

http://www.theclinics.com

EMERGENCY MEDICINE CLINICS OF NORTH AMERICA Volume 42, Number 2
May 2024 ISSN 0733-8627, ISBN-13: 978-0-443-13045-8

Editor: Joanna Gascoine
Developmental Editor: Varun Gopal

Emergency Medicine Clinics of North America (ISSN 0733-8627) is published quarterly by Elsevier Inc., 360 Park Avenue South, New York, NY, 10010-1710. Months of issue are February, May, August, and November. Business and Editorial Offices: 1600 John F. Kennedy Boulevard, Suite 1800, Philadelphia, PA 19103-2899. Customer Service Office: 6277 Sea Harbor Drive, Orlando, FL 32887-4800. Periodicals postage paid at New York, NY, and additional mailing offices. Subscription prices are $100.00 per year (US students), $388.00 per year (US individuals), $220.00 per year (international students), $505.00 per year (international individuals), $100.00 per year (Canadian students), $463.00 per year (Canadian individuals). For institutional access pricing please contact Customer Service via the contact information below. International air speed delivery is included in all *Clinics'* subscription prices. All prices are subject to change without notice. **POSTMASTER:** Send address changes to *Emergency Medicine Clinics of North America*, Elsevier Periodicals Customer Service, 11830 Westline Industrial Drive, St. Louis, MO 63146. Customer Service (orders, claims, online, change of address): Elsevier Periodicals **Customer Service, 11830 Westline Industrial Drive, St. Louis, MO 63146. Tel: 1-800-654-2452 (U.S. and Canada); 314-453-7041 (outside U.S. and Canada). Fax: 314-453-5170. E-mail: journalscustomerservice-usa@elsevier.com (for print support); journalsonlinesupport-usa@elsevier.com (for online support).**

Reprints. For copies of 100 or more of articles in this publication, please contact the Commercial Reprints Department, Elsevier Inc., 360 Park Avenue South, New York, NY 10010-1710. Tel.: 212-633-3874; Fax: 212-633-3820; E-mail: reprints@elsevier.com.

Emergency Medicine Clinics of North America is covered in *MEDLINE/PubMed (Index Medicus), Current Contents/Clinical Medicine, EMBASE/Excerpta Medica, BIOSIS, SciSearch, CINAHL, ISI/BIOMED,* and *Research Alert.*

Contributors

CONSULTING EDITOR

AMAL MATTU, MD
Professor and Vice Chair of Academic Affairs, Department of Emergency Medicine, University of Maryland School of Medicine, Baltimore, Maryland

EDITORS

BRADLEY W. FRAZEE, MD
Attending Physician, Department of Emergency Medicine, Alameda Health System, Wilma Chan Highland Hospital, Oakland, California

MICHAEL S. PULIA, MD, PhD
Associate Professor, BerbeeWalsh Department of Emergency Medicine, University of Wisconsin School of Medicine and Public Health, Madison, Wisconsin

CHRISTOPHER M. COLBERT, DO, FACOEP, FACEP, FAAEM
Associate Professor of Emergency Medicine, Assistant Residency Director, University of Illinois, Chicago, Illinois

AUTHORS

ARAVIND ADDEPALLI, MD
Resident Physician, Department of Emergency Medicine, Alameda Health System, Wilma Chan Highland Hospital, Oakland, California

FRITZIE S. ALBARILLO, MD, BSN
Associate Professor, Department of Medicine, Infectious Diseases Division, Loyola University Medical Center, Maywood, Illinois

ERIK S. ANDERSON, MD
Director of Addiction Consult Service, Department of Emergency Medicine, Division of Addiction Medicine, Alameda Health System, Wilma Chan Highland Hospital, Oakland, California Alameda Health System, Wilma Chan Highland Hospital, Oakland, California

NATHAN BRUMMEL, MD, MSCI
Division of Pulmonary, Critical Care, and Sleep Medicine, Associate Professor, Department of Internal Medicine, The Ohio State University, Columbus, Ohio

KIMBERLY C. CLAEYS, PharmD, PhD
Associate Professor Infectious Diseases, Department of Pharmacy Science and Health Outcomes Research, University of Maryland School of Pharmacy, Baltimore, Maryland

WESLEY EILBERT, MD
Professor of Clinical Emergency Medicine, Department of Emergency Medicine, University of Illinois Chicago, College of Medicine, Chicago, Illinois

BRADLEY W. FRAZEE, MD
Attending Physician, Department of Emergency Medicine, Alameda Health System, Wilma Chan Highland Hospital, Oakland, California

RICHARD DIEGO GONZALES Y TUCKER, MD
Assistant Professor, Department of Emergency Medicine, University of California San Francisco, San Francisco, California; Attending Physician, Department of Emergency Medicine, Alameda Health System, Wilma Chan Highland Hospital, Oakland, California

LARISSA HACKER, PharmD, BCIDP
Clinical Pharmacist Specialist, Pediatrics and Infectious Diseases, Department of Pharmacy, UW Health, Madison, Wisconsin

KATHERINE M. HUNOLD, MD, MPH
Assistant Professor, Department of Emergency Medicine, The Ohio State University, Columbus, Ohio

PHOLAPHAT CHARLES INBORIBOON, MD, MPH
Associate Professor, Department of Emergency Medicine, University of Illinois at College of Medicine, Chicago, Illinois

PIM JETANALIN, MD
Associate Professor of Clinical Medicine, Department Medicine, Division of Rheumatology, University of Illinois at College of Medicine, Chicago, Illinois

LAURA HERNANDO LÓPEZ, MD
Clinical Research Coordinator, Icahn School of Medicine at Mount Sinai Hospital, New York, New York

STEPHEN Y. LIANG, MD, MPHS
Associate Professor, Department of Emergency Medicine, Division of Infectious Diseases, John T. Milliken Department of Medicine, Washington University School of Medicine, St Louis, Missouri

PATRICIA MAE MARTINEZ, MD
Research Project Coordinator, Icahn School of Medicine at Mount Sinai Hospital, New York, New York

ANDREW MATELLA, DO
Emergency Medicine Physician, Department of Emergency Medicine, University of Illinois Chicago, College of Medicine, Chicago, Illinois

JUSTIN MOORE, MD
Director of Innovation, Department of Emergency Medicine, Alameda Health System, Wilma Chan Highland Hospital, Oakland, California

BERENICE PEREZ, MD
Vice-Chair, Department of Emergency Medicine, Alameda Health System, Wilma Chan Highland Hospital, Oakland, California

MICHAEL S. PULIA, MD, PhD
Associate Professor, BerbeeWalsh Department of Emergency Medicine, University of Wisconsin School of Medicine and Public Health, Madison, Wisconsin

YANINT RAKSADAWAN, MD
Resident, Department of Medicine, Weiss Memorial Hospital, Chicago, Illinois

ROBERT REDWOOD, MD, MPH, FACEP
Emergency Medicine Specialist, Bozeman Health, Absaroka Emergency Physicians,
Bozeman, Montana

ELIZABETH ROZYCKI, PharmD, BCPS
Specialty Practice Pharmacist, Emergency Medicine, Department of Pharmacy, The Ohio
State University, Columbus, Ohio

JULIA SAPOZHNIKOV, PharmD
Medical Science Liaison, Karius, Inc, Chicago, Illinois

RACHEL E. SOLNICK, MD, MSc
Assistant Professor of Emergency Medicine, Emergency Physician, Icahn School of
Medicine at Mount Sinai Hospital, New York, New York

DOUGLAS A.E. WHITE, MD
Associate Clinical Professor of Emergency Medicine, Volunteer UCSF, Director of
Emergency Department HIV, HCV, and Syphilis Screening, Department of Emergency
Medicine, Alameda Health System, Wilma Chan Highland Hospital, Oakland, California

CHARLOTTE PAGE WILLS, MD
Chair, Department of Emergency Medicine, Alameda Health System, Wilma Chan
Highland Hospital, Oakland, California

JULIANNE YEARY, PharmD, BCCCP, BCEMP
Clinical Pharmacy Specialist, Emergency Medicine, Department of Pharmacy, Barnes
Jewish Hospital, St Louis, Missouri

JASON E. ZUCKER, MD
Assistant Professor, Columbia University Vagelos College of Physicians and Surgeons,
New York, New York

Contents

Foreword: Infectious Disease Emergencies   xiii

Amal Mattu

Preface: Frontiers in Emergency Department Infectious Disease Management   xv

Bradley W. Frazee, Michael S. Pulia, and Christopher M. Colbert

The Diagnosis and Treatment of Adult Urinary Tract Infections in the Emergency Department   209

Robert Redwood and Kimberly C. Claeys

Emergency medicine has been called the art of "making complicated clinical decisions with limited information." This description is particularly relevant in the case of diagnosis and treatment of urinary tract infections (UTIs). Although common, UTIs are often challenging to diagnose given the presence of non-specific signs and symptoms and over-reliance on laboratory findings. This review provides an interdisciplinary interpretation of the primary literature and practice guidelines, with a focus on diagnostic and antimicrobial stewardship in the emergency department.

Optimizing Diagnosis and Management of Community-acquired Pneumonia in the Emergency Department   231

Katherine M. Hunold, Elizabeth Rozycki, and Nathan Brummel

Pneumonia is split into 3 diagnostic categories: community-acquired pneumonia (CAP), health care-associated pneumonia, and ventilator-associated pneumonia. This classification scheme is driven not only by the location of infection onset but also by the predominant associated causal microorganisms. Pneumonia is diagnosed in over 1.5 million US emergency department visits annually (1.2% of all visits), and most pneumonia diagnosed by emergency physicians is CAP.

Orthopedic Articular and Periarticular Joint Infections   249

Pim Jetanalin, Yanint Raksadawan, and Pholaphat Charles Inboriboon

Acute nontraumatic joint pain has an extensive differential. Emergency physicians must be adept at identifying limb and potentially life-threatening infection. Chief among these is septic arthritis. In addition to knowing how these joint infections typically present, clinicians need to be aware of host and pathogen factors that can lead to more insidious presentations and how these factors impact the interpretation of diagnostic tests.

Diabetic Foot Infections in the Emergency Department   267

Bradley W. Frazee

Diabetic foot infection (DFI) is among the most common diabetic complications requiring hospitalization. Prompt emergency department diagnosis and evidence-based management can prevent eventual amputation and associated disability and mortality. Underlying neuropathy, arterial occlusion, immune dysfunction, and hyperglycemia-associated dehydration and ketoacidosis can all contribute to severity and conspire to make DFI diagnosis and management difficult. Serious complications include osteomyelitis, necrotizing infection, and sepsis. Practice guidelines are designed to assist frontline providers with correct diagnosis, categorization, and treatment decisions. Management generally includes a careful lower extremity examination and plain x-ray, obtaining appropriate tissue cultures, and evidence-based antibiotic selection tailored to severity.

Tick-Borne Diseases   287

Wesley Eilbert and Andrew Matella

Ticks are responsible for the vast majority of vector-borne illnesses in the United States. The number of reported tick-borne disease (TBD) cases has more than doubled in the past 20 years. The majority of TBD cases occur in warm weather months in individuals with recent outdoor activities in wooded areas. The risk of contracting a TBD is also highly dependent on geographic location. Between 24 and 48 hours of tick attachment is required for most disease transmission to occur. Only 50% to 70% of patients with a TBD will recall being bitten by a tick, and TBDs are often initially misdiagnosed as a viral illness. Most TBDs are easily treated when diagnosed early in their course.

Fever and Rash   303

Richard Diego Gonzales Y Tucker and Aravind Addepalli

Infectious causes of fever and rash pose a diagnostic challenge for the emergency provider. It is often difficult to discern rashes associated with rapidly progressive and life-threatening infections from benign exanthems, which comprise the majority of rashes seen in the emergency department. Physicians must also consider serious noninfectious causes of fever and rash. A correct diagnosis depends on an exhaustive history and head-to-toe skin examination as most emergent causes of fever and rash remain clinical diagnoses. A provisional diagnosis and immediate treatment with antimicrobials and supportive care are usually required prior to the return of confirmatory laboratory testing.

Sexually Transmitted Infections in the Emergency Department   335

Rachel E. Solnick, Laura Hernando López, Patricia Mae Martinez, and Jason E. Zucker

As the United States faces a worsening epidemic of sexually transmitted infections (STIs), emergency departments (EDs) play a critical role in identifying and treating these infections. The growing health inequities in the distribution and disproportionate impact of STIs add to the urgency of providing high-quality sexual health care through the ED. Changes in population health are reflected in the new Centers for Disease Control recommendations on screening, diagnostic testing, and treatment of STIs. This review covers common and less common and emerging STIs, and discusses the state-of-the-art guidance on testing paradigms, extragenital sampling, and antimicrobial treatment and prevention of STIs.

Communicable Disease Screening and Human Immunodeficiency Virus Prevention in the Emergency Department 369

Douglas A.E. White and Rachel E. Solnick

Emergency departments (ED) provide care to populations with high rates of communicable diseases, like HIV, hepatitis C virus, and syphilis. For many patients, the ED is their sole entry point into the healthcare system and they do not routinely access screening and prevention services elsewhere. As such, the ED can serve an important public health role through communicable disease identification, treatment, and prevention. In this article, we examine national recommendations, peer-reviewed literature, and expert consensus to provide cutting edge strategies for implementing communicable infectious disease screening and prevention programs into routine ED care.

The Intersection of Substance Use Disorders and Infectious Diseases in the Emergency Department 391

Erik S. Anderson and Bradley W. Frazee

Substance use disorders (SUDs) intersect clinically with many infectious diseases, leading to significant morbidity and mortality if either condition is inadequately treated. In this article, we will describe commonly seen SUDs in the emergency department (ED) as well as their associated infectious diseases, discuss social drivers of patient outcomes, and introduce novel ED-based interventions for co-occurring conditions. Clinicians should come away from this article with prescriptions for both antimicrobial medications and pharmacotherapy for SUDs, as well as an appreciation for social barriers, to care for these patients.

Coronavirus Disease 2019: Past, Present, and Future 415

Charlotte Page Wills, Berenice Perez, and Justin Moore

Severe acute respiratory syndrome coronavirus 2 is one of the most impactful diseases experienced in the past century. While the official national health emergency concluded in May of 2023, coronavirus disease 2019 (COVID-19) continues to mutate. As the summer of 2023, all countries were experiencing a new surge of cases from the EG.5 Omicron variant. Additionally, a new genetically distinct Omicron descendant BA2.86 had been detected in multiple countries including the United States. This article seeks to offer lessons learned from the pandemic, summarize best evidence for current management of patients with COVID-19, and give insights into future directions with this disease.

Optimizing Antimicrobial Stewardship in the Emergency Department 443

Julia Sapozhnikov, Fritzie S. Albarillo, and Michael S. Pulia

Antibiotic stewardship is a core component of emergency department (ED) practice and impacts patient safety, clinical outcomes, and public health. The unique characteristics of ED practice, including crowding, time pressure, and diagnostic uncertainty, need to be considered when implementing antibiotic stewardship interventions in this setting. Rapid advances in pathogen detection and host response biomarkers promise to revolutionize the diagnosis of infectious diseases in the ED, but such tests are not yet considered standard of care. Presently, clinical decision support embedded in the electronic health record and pharmacist-led interventions are the most effective ways to improve antibiotic prescribing in the ED.

Managing Antimicrobial Resistance in the Emergency Department   461

Julianne Yeary, Larissa Hacker, and Stephen Y. Liang

Basic awareness and understanding of antimicrobial resistance and prevailing mechanisms can aid emergency physicians in providing appropriate care to patients with infections due to a multidrug-resistant organism (MDRO). Empiric treatment of MDRO infections should be approached with caution and guided by the most likely pathogens based on differential diagnosis, severity of the illness, suspected source of infection, patient-specific factors, and local antibiotic susceptibility patterns. Newer broad-spectrum antibiotics should be reserved for critically ill patients where there is a high likelihood of infection with an MDRO.

EMERGENCY MEDICINE
CLINICS OF NORTH AMERICA

FORTHCOMING ISSUES

August 2024
Environmental and Wilderness Medicine
Cheyenne Falat and Stephanie Lareau,
Editors

November 2024
**Clinical Ultrasound in the Emergency
Department**
Michael Gottlieb and Alexis Salerno,
Editors

February 2025
Risk Management in Emergency Medicine
Michael B. Weinstock and Gita Pensa,
Editors

RECENT ISSUES

February 2024
Psychiatric and Behavioral Emergencies
Eileen F. Baker and Catherine A. Marco,
Editors

November 2023
Endocrine and Metabolic Emergencies
George Willis and Bennett A. Myers,
Editors

August 2023
Cardiac Arrest
William Brady and Amandeep Singh,
Editors

SERIES OF RELATED INTEREST
Critical Care Clinics
https://www.criticalcare.theclinics.com/
Cardiology Clinics
https://www.cardiology.theclinics.com/

THE CLINICS ARE NOW AVAILABLE ONLINE!
Access your subscription at:
www.theclinics.com

Foreword

Infectious Disease Emergencies

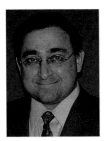

Amal Mattu, MD
Consulting Editor

"The greatest enemy we face in medicine is an enemy unseen." These words were often repeated by many clinicians and researchers during the recent COVID-19 pandemic. The words were true 6000 years ago with the birth of the first human civilization, and they remain true today, despite all the modern advances in pharmacology and immunizations. The fact that nearly 7 million people globally have died of the COVID-19 virus in just the past 4 years attests to the fact that microorganisms and viruses truly are the greatest enemy we face in modern medicine.

Infectious diseases are common in emergency medicine. Not a shift goes by when I don't see at least a handful of cases of infections, ranging anywhere from the common cold to fulminant sepsis. COVID-19 still rears its ugly head despite declarations that the pandemic has ended. "Routine" infections, such as pneumonia, urinary tract infections, and genital infections, are often anything but routine. And less common but deadly infections, such as meningococcemia, necrotizing fasciitis, and myocarditis, still keep us on our toes. Complicating our work is the fact that many of these infections do not present in classic fashion...normothermia or hypothermia may occur instead of a fever; leukocytosis may be absent; and fevers can be delayed with some infections and in some patient groups. Every prudent emergency physician needs to maintain continuous vigilance for the "unseen enemy."

Fortunately, in this issue of *Emergency Medicine Clinics of North America*, three outstanding emergency physicians with special expertise in infectious disease have teamed up as guest editors to help us "see" and treat many of these infections, which are often so challenging. Drs Bradley Frazee, Michael Pulia, and Christopher Colbert have assembled a fantastic group of additional experts to write about many types of infections that we encounter in the emergency department. These authors do a great job in addressing some of the common infections, such as diabetic foot infections, urinary tract infection, pneumonia, and sexually transmitted infections. Fever plus rash is a challenging presentation, but the article they provide on this topic will certainly clarify

Emerg Med Clin N Am 42 (2024) xiii–xiv
https://doi.org/10.1016/j.emc.2024.02.024
0733-8627/24/© 2024 Published by Elsevier Inc.

the differential diagnosis and workup. Two less-common entities are addressed, including tick-borne infections and joint infections. They also devote articles to important practice management topics, such as antibiotic stewardship and bacterial resistance, the intersection of substance abuse disorders and infections, and screening for communicable infections and HIV prevention. Finally, they address the past, present, and future of COVID-19.

This issue of *Emergency Medicine Clinics of North America* is a critically important contribution to the emergency medicine and infectious disease literature, and it represents must-learning for all of us who practice in emergency medicine. Our thanks go to Drs Frazee, Pulia, and Colbert and their colleagues for this valuable work.

Amal Mattu, MD
Department of Emergency Medicine
University of Maryland School of Medicine
Baltimore, MD, USA

E-mail address:
amattu@som.umaryland.edu

Preface

Frontiers in Emergency Department Infectious Disease Management

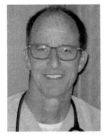

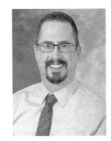

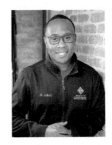

Bradley W. Frazee, MD   Michael S. Pulia, MD, PhD   Christopher M. Colbert, DO, FACOEP, FACEP, FAAEM

Editors

The diagnosis and treatment of infectious disease represents a large and very important part of emergency medicine practice. Infectious diseases account for 4 of the top 10 reasons for hospitalization from the emergency department (ED), 13% of all geriatric ED visits, and 28% of all pediatric visits.[1–3] Moreover, presentation and management of infections in the emergency setting encompass many of the twenty-first century's most pressing problems: emerging infectious diseases, pandemic management, antimicrobial resistance, and health equity in vulnerable populations.

The breadth of infectious disease challenges faced by emergency practitioners on a daily basis ranges from management of a simple skin abscess, to recognition of an unusual infection presenting as a rash in a returning traveler, to treatment of septic shock—due to any of a myriad potential sources of infection. Practitioners must obtain an appropriate history, which in the case of infection often means recognizing relevant comorbid risk factors in the past medical history or clues to potential exposure hidden in the social history. Subtle physical exam findings may be the only indication of an evolving life-threatening infection. Practitioners must select appropriate diagnostic studies from a menu of increasingly advanced imaging modalities, biomarkers, and molecular etiologic tests. Meanwhile, current treatment recommendations are always changing, reflecting both evolving antimicrobial resistance patterns and heightened attention to antimicrobial stewardship. Finally, emergency providers are increasingly called upon to act as sentinels for emerging infections and to screen for and manage communicable diseases. Given such a breadth of infectious disease topics and the amount of important information, staying current presents its own challenge.

Emerg Med Clin N Am 42 (2024) xv–xvii
https://doi.org/10.1016/j.emc.2024.02.009
0733-8627/24/© 2024 Elsevier Inc. All rights reserved.

In this issue, we and our authors have endeavored to produce a collection of 12 practical, clinically oriented reviews that cover important infectious diseases topics, while emphasizing several overlapping themes. The first of these encompasses bread-and-butter infectious disease topics where the knowledge base and recommendations are constantly changing. Our authors synthesize the latest evidence and expert guidelines in articles on pneumonia, urinary tract infection, sexually transmitted infection, and diabetic foot infection. Second is the challenge of less-common infections that often present first to the ED and are easy to miss; here our authors present articles on the notorious problems, fever plus rash, tick-borne illness, and septic arthritis. A third theme encompasses two articles covered the closely linked issues of antibiotic stewardship and antibiotic resistance in the ED. While touched on to some extent in every article, these important issues are also covered in dedicated articles written by experts on the topic. Finally, our authors turn to the increasingly important public health and safety net role played by EDs. This is the focus of the articles on COVID-19, sexually transmitted infection, ED communicable disease screening, and the intersection of substance use disorders and infection. Here again, in each case the authors are leading experts.

We wish to thank the dedicated and well-respected clinicians, educators, and clinicians who have contributed to this issue of *Emergency Medicine Clinics of North America*. We are grateful for the opportunity to have worked with this talented group of authors as well as the outstanding editorial staff at Elsevier, including Varun Gopal. We hope that this issue will prove valuable to every type of emergency practitioner that cares for patients with infectious diseases, including emergency physicians, primary care physicians, advanced practice providers, residents, and medical students.

DISCLOSURE

Dr Frazee has no relevent funding source to acknowlege. Dr Pulia has no relevent funding source to acknowlege.

Bradley W. Frazee, MD
Department of Emergency Medicine
Alameda Health System–
Wilma Chan Highland Hospital
1411 East 31st Street
Oakland CA 94602, USA

Michael S. Pulia, MD, PhD
BerbeeWalsh Department of
Emergency Medicine
University of Wisconsin School of Medicine
and Public Health
800 University Bay Drive, Suite 310
Madison WI 53705, USA

Christopher M. Colbert, DO, FACOEP, FACEP, FAAEM
University of Illinois
808 South Wood Street
Chicago, IL 60612, USA

E-mail addresses:
Bradf_98@yahoo.com (B.W. Frazee)

mspulia@medicine.wisc.edu (M.S. Pulia)
ccmp1992@gmail.com (C.M. Colbert)

REFERENCES

1. Weiss A.J., Jiang H.J., Most Frequent Reasons for Emergency Department Visits, 2018. HCUP Statistical Brief #286. 2021. Agency for Healthcare Research and Quality, Rockville, MD. Available at: www.hcup-us.ahrq.gov/reports/statbriefs/sb286-ED-Frequent-Conditions-2018.pdf.
2. Goto T, Yoshida K, Tsugawa Y, et al. Infectious Disease-Related Emergency Department Visits of Elderly Adults in the United States, 2011-2012. J Am Geriatr Soc 2016;64(1):31–6.
3. Hasegawa K, Tsugawa Y, Cohen A, Camargo CA Jr. Infectious Disease-related Emergency Department Visits Among Children in the US. Pediatr Infect Dis J 2015;34(7):681–5.

The Diagnosis and Treatment of Adult Urinary Tract Infections in the Emergency Department

Robert Redwood, MD, MPH[a], Kimberly C. Claeys, PharmD, PhD[b],*

KEYWORDS

- Antimicrobial stewardship • Asymptomatic bacteriuria • Cystitis • Diagnosis
- Diagnostic stewardship • Urinary tract infection

KEY POINTS

- Urinary tract infection (UTI) diagnosis should be made in the presence of genitourinary symptoms and signs combined with findings from urinalysis and/or urine culture. Laboratory findings alone cannot diagnose UTI.
- Empirical selection of antimicrobials for UTI should consider patient-specific risk factors for resistance as well as local community resistance patterns as determined by emergency department (ED)-specific urinary antibiograms.
- There are numerous antimicrobial stewardship interventions that can improve diagnosis and management of UTIs in the ED.
- Consideration should be given to the possibility of sexually transmitted infections and less common but potentially serious conditions such as ureterolithiasis with infection.

INTRODUCTION

Emergency medicine has been called the art of "making complicated clinical decisions with limited information." This description is particularly relevant in the case of diagnosing and treating urinary tract infections (UTIs) in the emergency department (ED).[1] Appropriate diagnosis and management of UTIs in the ED can feel like stitching together a series of probabilities, where the accuracy of the clinical decisions can only be known days later, if ever.

Are these urinary symptoms? Are these urinalysis (UA) findings caused by pathologic bacteria, colonizing bacteria, or a contaminated specimen? If pathologic, what are the offending bacterial organism and what antibiotics might have activity against

[a] Bozeman Health Emergency Department, 915 Highland Avenue, Bozeman, MT 59715, USA;
[b] Department of Pharmacy Science and Health Outcomes Research, University of Maryland School of Pharmacy, 20 N Pine Street, Baltimore, MD 21201, USA
* Corresponding author.
E-mail address: kclaeys@rx.umaryland.edu

Emerg Med Clin N Am 42 (2024) 209–230
https://doi.org/10.1016/j.emc.2024.01.001
0733-8627/24/© 2024 Elsevier Inc. All rights reserved.
emed.theclinics.com

this organism? Will the patient tolerate the effective antibiotics or have an adverse re-action? What if I am asked to "cold call" a patient whom I have not seen? Few areas of medicine blur art and science like UTIs in the ED.

The recommendations provided here represent a multidisciplinary (infectious dis-eases pharmacist, emergency medicine physician) interpretation of the primary litera-ture and current practice guidelines. Our objective is to add as much clarity as possible to an inherently unclear process of UTI diagnosis and offer a practical approach to the treatment of UTIs in the ED. We pay special attention to ED-specific conundrums, such as the approach to the elderly patient with an indwelling catheter and antibiotic stewardship considerations tailored to the ED. Whether you read this article in its entirety, to become the UTI guru of your ED, or skip to the section that is relevant to the patient in front of you, we offer guidance that is practical, evidence-based, and laser-focused on the real-world ED experience.

EPIDEMIOLOGY

Over 1 million ED visits for UTI occur annually in the United States.[2] The majority of UTIs are cases of uncomplicated cystitis occurring in women.[3,4] The exact incidence of uncomplicated cystitis varies by patient population, with a reported rate of approx-imately 0.7 cases per person year in young women.[5] It is commonly accepted that the lifetime risk of having at least one UTI is upward of 50% in women of reproductive age.[6] In addition, regardless of sex, the risk of developing UTI increases with age. The lifetime prevalence of UTI in men is 20%. The incidence of UTIs in men is approx-imately 0.9 to 2.4 cases per 1000 persons aged less than 55 years but increases to 7.7 cases per 1000 persons once age 85 is reached.[7]

MICROBIOLOGY AND ANTIMICROBIAL RESISTANCE

The most common causative organism remains *Escherichia coli,* causing over 75% of uncomplicated UTIs. Other *Enterobacterales* such as *Klebsiella pneumoniae* and *Pro-teus mirabilis,* as well as *Staphylococcus saprophyticus* are also common causes of un-complicated UTI. Complicated UTIs represent a smaller fraction of ED visits but more often result in admission to observation units or hospitalization.[4,8] Among patients with complicated UTI presenting to the ED (**Tables 1** and **2**), *Enterobacterales* species remain the primary cause of infection with *E coli* being the dominant pathogen,[9] but there is more diversity in the potential causative organisms and associated resistance patterns, including isolation of both *Pseudomonas* and *Staphylococcus aureus.*

Antibiotic resistance in the outpatient setting is on the rise, which is particularly true with respect to urinary pathogens. Variables that have been associated with increased risk of antibiotic resistance include advanced age, use of fluoroquinolones, and resi-dence in a skilled nursing facility.[10,11] When examining recent data for *E coli* urinary isolates, resistance to commonly prescribed agents such as trimethoprim/sulfameth-oxazole (TMP/SMX) often approached or exceeded 20% for cystitis and 10% for py-elonephritis—the thresholds at which empirical use of that agent should be abandoned.[12,13] In a multicenter 2019 study of ED patients with UTI caused by *E coli*, 25% were resistant to TMP/SMX.[14] Resistance of urinary isolates to fluoroquino-lones is also steeply on the rise. In a 2018 to 2020 study conducted in 15 geograph-ically diverse EDs across the United States, fluoroquinolone resistance was found in 22% of *E coli* isolates overall and exceeding 25% in several EDs.[15] Furthermore, most patients had no identifiable risk factor for resistance. Fortunately, rates of resis-tance to nitrofurantoin among uropathogens generally remain less than 10%.[12] The prescription of nitrofurantoin is associated with a decreased risk inadequate empirical

Table 1
Categorizations and definitions of urinary tract infection: categorizations of urinary tract infection

UTI Category	Patient Characteristics	Presentation	Cautions	Diagnostics	Treatment Issues
ASB	Bacteriuria, with abnormal UA or positive urine culture, absent urinary signs, symptoms, or fever. In the majority of patients, ASB is not a pathologic infectioous state. It should not be treated and should not prompt a urine culture.				
Uncomplicated cystitis	Young healthy women, nonpregnant	Dysuria, increased urinary frequency, and suprapubic tenderness	Always consider STI[a]	Consider urine culture, especially for history of recent treated UTI; consider STI testing	Nitrofurantoin is first line. Consider symptomatic treatment with NSAIDs and phenazopyridine
Complicated[b] cystitis	Men, elderly, indwelling catheter	Dysuria, increased urinary frequency, and suprapubic tenderness	Young men with voiding symptoms have an STI (not UTI) until proven otherwise; consider epididymitis and prostatitis	Urine culture advised; if catheter is present, exchange prior to UA/urine culture	Nitrofurantoin or fosfomycin is first line. Consider resistant pathogens
Prostatitis	Men of any age, especially if known enlarged prostate	Dysuria, increased urinary frequency, incontinence, hesitancy, fever	Consider prostate abscess or STI	Urine culture mandatory; consider CT for abscess and STI testing	Consider admission; Fluoroquinolones are first line for outpatient therapy. Consider resistant pathogens
Uncomplicated pyelonephritis	Young, otherwise healthy women, nonpregnant	Fever, flank pain; dysuria, and frequency may be absent; may present with sepsis	Occult obstruction (eg, ureteral stone) rare, but cannot be missed	Urine culture mandatory; POCUS for hydronephrosis advised	Consider initial parenteral antibiotics if febrile/toxic; outpatient oral treatment usually possible
Complicated pyelonephritis	Men, elderly, comorbidities, recent health care exposure	Fever, flank pain; may present with bacteremia or sepsis	Consider CT for obstruction, perinephric abscess, and so forth	Urine culture mandatory; consider blood cultures	Admission generally required; IV broad spectrum coverage

[a] Sexually transmitted infections (STIs), in the context of urinary symptoms, typically include gonorrhea, chlamydia, syphilis, and trichomonas. *Gardnerella vaginalis* may also present with urinary symptoms and is sometimes classified as an STI.
[b] See definition of Complicated UTI in Table 1B.

Table 2
Categorizations and definitions of urinary tract infection: definition of "complicated" urinary tract infection

"Complicated" refers to host factors that may confer risk for poor response to standard, narrow spectrum therapy

Class of Complication	Specific Factors
Urinary tract obstruction	Pregnancy, benign prostatic hyperplasia (older men), neurogenic bladder, urinary catheter, renal stone, ureteral stone, ureteral stricture
Immunosuppression	Diabetes, elderly, transplant, immunosuppressive medications, AIDS
Risk for multi-drug resisitance uropathogens	Previous infection or colonization with an antibiotic resistant pathogen, recent broad-spectrum antibiotics, recent or extensive health care exposure, residence in nursing home or long-term care facility, urinary catheter

therapy for lower tract UTIs.[16] In addition to increasing rates of resistance to guideline-recommended first-line oral antibiotics, resistance to beta-lactam antibiotics, which are often used to treat UTIs requiring hospitalization, is also on the rise. Among urinary isolates collected from outpatients and ED patients hospitalized for UTIs between 2010 and 2020, extended-spectrum beta-lactamase-producing Enterobacterales, such as E coli and Klebsiella, which are resistant to cephalexin and third-generation cephalosporins like ceftriaxone, were present in 7% to 17% of isolates.[13,17] Extended spectrum beta-lactamase (ESBL)-producing isolates increased 30% from 2011 to 2020. In a recent study of empirical antibiotic choices in the ED that focused on UTIs caused by Enterobacterales, among over 5000 episodes, 22% received discordant therapy, where the urinary pathogen was resistant to the initial antibiotic.[10] Discordant empirical therapy for UTIs is associated with worse downstream outcomes.[18,19] Those that received an initially ineffective agent were twice as likely to be hospitalized within the next 28 days (**Box 1**).

DIAGNOSIS AND TREATMENT OF URINARY TRACT INFECTION IN THE EMERGENCY DEPARTMENT

Focal genitourinary symptoms and signs of a UTI include urinary urgency, frequency and dysuria, and suprapubic and costovertebral angle tenderness.[22] Elderly patients without focal genitourinary symptoms are considered asymptomatic.[23,24] It is important to note that sexually transmitted infections also cause lower UTI symptoms, whereas pyelonephritis frequently presents as fever and costovertebral angle tenderness without lower genitourinary symptoms.

Box 1
Risk factors for antibiotic-resistant uropathogens[14,20,21]

Previous hospitalization in the last 30 days

IV antibiotic use in the last 90 days

Previous UTIs (especially with previously isolated resistant pathogen)

Chronic renal dialysis

Previous history of urologic procedure or urinary tract abnormality

Residence in nursing home or rehabilitation facility

Major categories of UTI are uncomplicated cystitis, complicated cystitis, prostatitis, uncomplicated pyelonephritis, complicated pyelonephritis, and severe UTI that presents as sepsis from a suspected urinary source. While asymptomatic bacteriuria (ASB) is not technically a pathologic infection state, it should be considered in the categorization scheme, as ASB is commonly encountered and is a key driver of antibiotic overprescribing. These categorizations are important because empirical antibiotic selection begins with the type of UTI being considered. They are summarized in **Tables 1** and **2** and described in detail.

Uncomplicated cystitis is the most common bacterial infection in women. Uncomplicated cystitis is classically defined as frequency and dysuria without fever occurring in an immunocompetent, nonpregnant woman who has no comorbidities or urologic abnormalities. A woman with dysuria and urinary frequency in combination with the absence of vaginal discharge or vaginal irritation has a 77% posttest probability of having uncomplicated cystitis, regardless of UA results.[25] In such cases, physical examination is often normal or just positive for suprapubic tenderness.[26] Complicated cystitis refers to a UTI that is localized to the bladder but carries a higher risk of treatment failure due to host factors such as male, pregnant, elderly, indwelling catheter, and immunocompromised (see **Tables 1** and **2**). Signs and symptoms are generally similar to uncomplicated cystitis; however, first-line antibiotic treatment recommendations may differ based on the complicating factor.

Acute prostatitis typically occurs when an organism from the urinary tract refluxes into the male prostate via the prostatic ducts.[27] Acute prostatitis can occur in healthy men at any age; however, it is more common in the context of urethral obstruction or recent urologic instrumentation. Prostatitis can present as dysuria as well as urinary retention, incontinence, and hesitancy. Fever may be present. There may be symptoms or signs related to concomitant infection in the bladder or epididymis. The onset of symptoms can be subtle, and the duration of illness may last for weeks.

Uncomplicated pyelonephritis is an upper urinary tract infection without any complicating host factors.[28] Because the infection has ascended into the ureter and kidney, voiding symptoms may be absent entirely. Symptoms and signs include flank pain, chills, nausea, vomiting, with fever and costovertebral tenderness and fever. Lower genitourinary symptoms may also be present. While patients with uncomplicated pyelonephritis may present systemically ill with abnormal vital signs, outpatient therapy is often possible if there is a good response to initial ED therapies. Complicated pyelonephritis presents with similar signs and symptoms; however, patients who are systemically ill are less likely to respond well to initial ED therapy and generally require hospital admission. In essence, complicated pyelonephritis should be investigated and treated with a high degree of suspicion for sepsis, bacteremia, and a resistant uropathogen. Empirical broad-spectrum intravenous agents may be appropriate based on the specific complicating factors.

URINE TESTING

Urine testing in the ED typically includes a UA, with or without urine culture depending on the category of UTI and patient risk factors for multidrug-resistant organisms. Point of care urine dipstick testing is used in some acute settings, such as urgent cares or low-resource EDs. As with all medical testing, ED urine testing is most effective when ordered appropriately (moderate pretest probability of disease), collected appropriately (midstream, clean catch), and interpreted appropriately (a nuanced topic). In fact, a patient with a high probability of uncomplicated cystitis after history and physical alone requires no urine testing at all (**Fig. 1**).

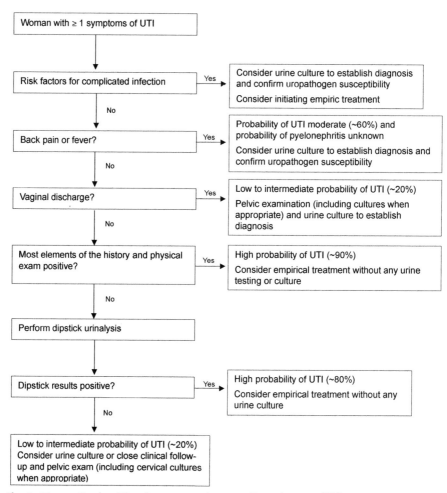

Fig. 1. Diagnostic algorithm for suspected uncomplicated cystitis.[25,30]

Dipstick, Microscopic Urinalysis, and Urine Culture

The urine specimen for UTI testing should be collected in such a way that it is as free as possible from skin and vaginal debris and contaminating bacteria, which entails a midstream clean catch or an in-and-out straight catheter sample. A urine culture is generally unnecessary in uncomplicated cystitis but is recommended if there is concern for a complicated UTI, pyelonephritis, resistant organisms, or treatment failure. Indwelling urinary catheters should be exchanged prior to obtaining the urine sample. In the case pyelonephritis or sepsis, a reasonable effort should be made to obtain a urine culture specimen prior to initiating antibiotics.

The urine dipstick is a rapid, inexpensive point of care substitute for the UA. Components tested vary by brand but typically include specific gravity, pH, protein, leukocyte esterase, nitrites, blood, ketones, glucose, bilirubin, and urobilinogen.[31] Dipstick testing does not evaluate for the presence of squamous epithelial cells or bacteria. Common causes of false positive and false negative dipstick results are shown in **Table 3**. A completely normal urine dipstick may have a negative predictive value

Table 3
Selected common pitfalls of urine dipstick testing[32]

Leukocyte Test False Positives	Leukocyte Test False Negatives	Nitrite Test False Positives	Nitrite Test False Negatives
Contamination from vagina or foreskin secretions	Increases in urine-specific gravity or glucose	Prolonged exposure of dipstick to air prior to testing	Many gram + organisms do not produce nitrites
Expired dipstick	Presence of urine ketones or protein	Expired dipstick	Urine that has not been in the bladder more than 4 hours
Improperly stored dipstick	Use of vitamin C or certain antibiotics	Medications causing reddish urine color (eg, Pyridium)	Urine pH <6, high urobilinogen or specific gravity
Discolored urine from food or medications (eg, nitrofurantoin)	Less than room temperature urine sample	Urine sample more than 4 hours old	Patients with low nitrate diet

Adapted from Eriksen, Stine Veronica, and Pia Cecilie Bing-Jonsson. "Can we trust urine dipsticks?." Nor J Clin Nurs/Sykepl Forsk 10.1 (2017): 1-14.

for UTI as high as 90% to 95%.[36] However, multiple systematic reviews and meta-analyses demonstrate that dipstick performance is nonspecific, so a "positive urine dipstick" (variably defined) does not reliably confirm the diagnosis of UTI.[37–39] As such, the dipstick analysis remains useful in certain outpatient settings as a first-level screening test (see **Tables 1** and **2**).

A complete UA includes a physical, chemical, and microscopic examination of the sample. Over time, there have been various *en vogue* aspects of the UA, held up as more sensitive or specific for diagnosing or excluding UTI. This has resulted in an inconsistent approach among clinicians, where one regards the presence of leukocyte esterase as the key to the diagnosis, whereas another may hang their hat on the presence of nitrites. Most studies have shown that leukocyte esterase and leukocytes lack specificity (can be falsely positive), whereas nitrites are more specific (fewer false positives), but lack sensitivity (can be false negative). **Table 4** demonstrates the positive likelihood ratios (which incorporate both true and false positive rates) for components of the UA.

A confirmatory urine culture is recommended, if appropriate, for formal diagnosis of a UTI. The quantitative urine culture remains the gold standard method for diagnosis of UTI. Urine cultures require up to 18 hours for bacterial growth on culture media by standard laboratory techniques, so real-time ED diagnosis based on urine culture is not feasible.[40] Cutoffs for the number of colony-forming units (CFUs) that define significant uropathogen growth vary. For example, the US Centers for Disease Control and Prevention require 100,000 CFU/mL to meet the criteria for diagnosis of UTI, while the Infectious Disease Society of America sets a lower threshold of 50,000 CFU/mL when a single, common uropathogen (ie, *E coli*) is isolated.[41] In general, young, well-hydrated women with cystitis may grow fewer colonies on culture.

Many EDs have an automatic reflex order for urine culture if pyuria is present, which runs the risk of triggering a urine culture in the absence of UTI symptoms. The prevalence of pyuria in women with ASB is estimated to be 32% overall and increases to 90% in the elderly.[42,43] This underscores the importance of testing urine only when symptoms are present, as inappropriately sent urine cultures in the elderly often leads to antibiotic treatment of ASB.

Imaging

Cross-sectional imaging is typically not warranted for UTI diagnosis or management decisions, but may be considered for patients who are septic, have suspected obstruction of the urinary tract, and have persistent clinical symptoms despite 72 hours of antimicrobial therapy. Outpatient clinicians, especially urologists, may also image patients who have recurrent infection within a month of treatment. The goal of cross-sectional imaging is to diagnose UTI complications (ie, perinephric abscess) or an anatomic feature that requires surgical intervention (ie, obstructing ureteral stone).[29] Contrast-enhanced CT, often obtained to investigate fever or abdominal

Table 4	
Positive likelihood ratios for selected urinalysis and urine culture findings[33–35]	
Bacteriuria	4.7
Leukocyte Esterase	4.2
Nitrites	4.2
Pyuria	3.3
>10^2 CFU/mL of *E coli*	6.3

pain of unclear cause, may reveal a wedge-shaped hypoattenuated region of renal parenchyma with perinephric fat stranding, indicating acute pyelonephritis. Some authors have proposed that point of care ultrasound should be performed routinely in all cases of febrile pyelonephritis or urosepsis to rule out hydronephrosis from an obstructing ureteral stone.

Urinary tract infection diagnostic algorithm

One evidence-based yet sensible way to approach the diagnosis of female UTI in the ED is to follow a stepwise algorithm, such as that proposed by Bent and colleagues (see **Fig. 1**). This approach takes into account whether or not there are signs of upper urinary tract involvement or features that would make the UTI complicated, and whether vaginitis or a sexually transmitted infection could account for the symptoms, in order to guide what urine testing is required (if any) and arrive at a likely diagnosis.[25,30]

URINARY TRACT INFECTION THERAPY

In addition to antimicrobial treatment for UTIs, it is important that emergency providers consider simultaneous treatment of associated sepsis and other symptoms and consider whether procedural source control might be required. Patients with cystitis and prominent voiding symptoms and lower abdominal discomfort should be prescribed a nonsteroidal anti-inflammatory drug and phenazopyridine (a bladder analgesic) for 2 days. Young female patients with otherwise uncomplicated pyelonephritis who initially present with fever and systemic toxicity should be treated aggressively with antipyretics, analgesics, IV crystalloids, and a single dose of parenteral antibiotics. Those with evidence of sepsis-related organ dysfunction or lactic acidosis should undergo state-of-the-art sepsis management. However, in many cases, an initially toxic but otherwise healthy young patient will "turn around" within a few hours and prove stable for discharge home to complete a course of oral antibiotic therapy. A small but critical subset of pyelonephritis cases are associated with ureteral obstruction, which can be difficult to discern by history and physical alone (hence, the recommendation abovementioned to consider routine POCUS to assess for hydronephrosis). Once identified, such cases require immediate urologic and/or interventional radiology consultation for consideration of emergent decompression, usually by percutaneous nephrostomy.

Guideline-Recommended Antimicrobial Therapy

Tables 5 and **6** shows the recommended empirical antimicrobial regimens for each category of UTI commonly encountered in the ED. The antibiotic choices presented here were derived from the 2011 IDSA UTI treatment guidelines, the Denver Health Antibiotic Guide, and the Sanford Guide.[28,44] We chose these sources because they emphasize using the narrowest spectrum agent and the shortest possible duration. It should be noted that the IDSA guidelines predate widespread emergency of resistance to commonly prescribed oral antibiotics such as TMP/SMX and fluoroquinolones. Importantly, the IDSA guidelines for uncomplicated UTIs are currently under review with new recommendations pending as of this publication. The IDSA also plans to release guidance for complicated UTIs soon as well.

Where possible, however, providers should refer to their hospital-specific empirical therapy guidelines, based on their local hospital antibiogram. In addition, patient-specific risk factors for antibiotic resistance should be taken into consideration, particularly previous isolation of a resistant uropathogen. The review of prior urine culture results should be a routine component of selecting empirical UTI treatment. Complicated patients may require consultation with infectious diseases specialist or infectious disease pharmacist.

Table 5
Empirical antibiotic choices for urinary tract infection in emergency department patients being discharged

Condition	Recommendation
Asymptomatic Patient	Do not treat
Asymptomatic bacteriuria in pregnancy	Cephalexin 500 mg PO QID for 5 days Amoxicillin–clavulanate 875/125 mg PO BID for 5 days Nitrofurantoin 100 mg PO BID for 5 days (after 1st trimester if other options are not available)
Uncomplicated cystitis	Preferred Nitrofurantoin 100 mg PO BID for 5 days *Avoid for CrCl < 30 mL/min* Alternatives Cephalexin 500 mg PO TID for 5 days Fosfomycin 3 g PO once TMP/SMX 1 160/800 mg PO BID for 3 days[a] Amoxicillin/clavulanate 875 mg PO BID for 5 days Cefadroxil 500 mg PO BID for 5 days
Pyelonephritis	Amoxicillin/clavulanic acid 875 mg PO BID for 7 days Cephalexin 1000 mg PO TID for 7 days Levofloxacin 750 mg PO daily for 5 days[b] TMP-SMX 160/800mg PO BID for 7 days[b]
Recurrent UTI	Empirical therapy based on prior cultures and susceptibilities. Obtain urinalysis and culture.

Empirical therapy recommendations based on normal renal function; dose adjustments may be necessary.

[a] If local prevalence of TMP/SMX resistance is less than 20% or confirmed susceptible by urine culture.

[b] If local prevalence of TMP/SMX or fluoroquinolone resistance < 10% or confirmed susceptibile by urine culture.

ANTIMICROBIAL STEWARDSHIP IN THE EMERGENCY DEPARTMENT
Why Stewardship in the Emergency Department Matters

Among patients presenting to the ED, 13% will leave with an antibiotic prescription, with UTIs being one of the most common indications.[45,46] Only 32.7% to 56.6% of these prescriptions are found to be appropriate.[45,47] Inappropriate drug choice, drug dose, or drug duration can all result in deleterious downstream effects, including adverse drug events that require subsequent ED visits or hospitalization.[48] Antimicrobial stewardship (AMS) programs, initially developed for inpatient setting, have begun to expand to the outpatient and ED settings. Recently, Goebel and colleagues published the "Five Ds" for outpatient AMS programs, specifically focused on the management of UTIs[48] see (**Fig. 2**). To increase its relevance to the ED, for the fifth "D," we can replace "de-escalation" with "diagnosis."[49]

Optimizing Empirical Drug Selection for Potential Drug-Resistant Urinary Tract Infections

Increasing rates of resistance to commonly recommended empirical therapy for UTIs present a challenge for ED providers. This is particularly true for complicated UTIs, where the risk of receiving inappropriate empirical therapy is highest. To reduce the risk of inappropriate empirical therapy, ED providers should refer to institution-specific antibiogram data and risk stratification tools wherever possible. These

Table 6
Empirical antibiotic choices for urinary tract infection in emergency department patients being admitted

Condition	Recommendation
Uncomplicated pyelonephritis	Low-risk for multidrug-resistant organism[a]: Ceftriaxone 1 g IV Q24H Confirmed severe PCN allergy: Levofloxacin 500 mg IV/PO Q24H
Complicated pyelonephritis ± gram-negative bacteremia	Cefepime 2 g IV Q12H OR piperacillin/tazobactam 3.375–4.5 g IV Q6H *Review recent urine culture data to guide therapy* High risk for MDRO[a]: Ertapenem 1gm IV q24H OR Meropenem 1 gm IV q8H (concern for *Pseudomonas aeruginosa*) plus vancomycin 15 - 20 mg/kg IV q8h to q 12h *Review recent urine culture data to guide therapy* Severe penicillin allergy: Levofloxacin 750 mg IV/PO Q24H plus gentamicin 3–5 mg/kg IV OR Amikacin 4–7 mg/kg IV Oral step-down therapy: TMP/SMX 160/800 mg Q12H to complete 7 total days OR Levofloxacin 750 mg PO Q24H to complete 5–7 total days OR Ciprofloxacin 500 mg Q12h to complete 5 - 7 days
Complicated UTI/CAUTI	Above, plus remove or exchange catheter

Empirical therapy recommendations based on normal renal function; dose adjustments may be necessary. These regimens represent a potential approach to empircal treatment and should be adjusted based on individual patient considerations and local antibiotic resistance patterns.
[a] Previous infection or colonization with antibiotic resistant gram-negative bacteria, residence in a nursing facility, recent broad-spectrum antibiotics, recent or extensive health care exposure.

typically combine national guideline recommendations, with local microbiology data and local drug acquisition costs. In addition, because resistance profiles differ between urinary and nonurinary gram-negative isolates and between those from inpatients and outpatients, outpatient/ED-specific antibiograms that include only urinary isolates can be developed. These can be used to guide individual empirical therapy and develop locally validated treatment guidelines.[11,50] ED AMS programs that leverage such local antibiograms and site-specific treatment algorithms have been shown to improve prescribing practices and are associated with decreased 30-day return visits.[51]

Caution Using Fluoroquinolones

Fluoroquinolones are no longer first-line agents for uncomplicated cystitis. In the 2011 IDSA uncomplicated UTI guidelines, ciprofloxacin and levofloxacin were noted to be efficacious but associated with a high risk of collateral damage and adverse drug events.[28] The Food and Drug Administration issued a black box warning in 2016 that highlighting the potentially disabling and irreversible side-effects of fluoroquinolones, such as tendon rupture, peripheral neuropathy, and central nervous system effects.[52] As recently as 2010, approximately 40% of uncomplicated UTIs were treated with fluoroquinolones.[53] Rates continued to be high even after issuance of the black box warning.[54–56] Various AMS interventions have decreased unnecessary prescribing of fluoroquinolones in the ED. Combining an uncomplicated UTI order

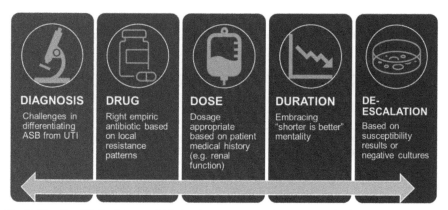

Fig. 2. The five "Ds" of stewardship in the emergency department. (*Adapted from* Goebel MC, Trautner BW, Grigoryan L. The Five Ds of Outpatient Antibiotic Stewardship for Urinary Tract Infections. *Clin Microbiol Rev.* 2021 Dec 15;34(4):e0000320.)

set for that de-emphasized fluoroquinolones with an AMS audit and feedback decreased fluoroquinolone prescriptions by 30%.[57] Guidelines, ED-specific urine antibiograms, education, and feedback improve antibiotic prescribing for UTIs and such improvements have been shown to be sustainable with recurrent education and feedback.[58]

Optimizing Drug Dose and Duration

Optimizing antimicrobial therapy for UTIs involves not only choosing the right antibiotic but also choosing the correct dose and duration. When ED patients are prescribed the right antibiotic for the indication, the dose and duration may still differ from what is recommended.[59,60] There is increasing evidence that shorter courses of therapy are associated with similar clinical cure rates compared with traditional longer courses but with lower risk of antimicrobial-related adverse events. Studies have demonstrated the efficacy of short duration therapy for women with uncomplicated cystitis and men with afebrile UTIs.[61,62] For uncomplicated cystitis in women, 5 days of nitrofurantoin, 3 days of TMP/SMX, and single dose of fosfomycin are recommended. For oral beta-lactams, such as cephalexin, the recommended duration is 5 to 7 days. For men with afebrile UTI, 7 days of antibiotics (fluoroquinolone or TMP/SMX) has been proven sufficient. However, an randomized controlled trial (RCT) involving men with febrile UTI was not able to demonstrate noninferiority of a shorter course regimen.[63] The use of indication-based antimicrobial order sets and electronic discharge prescriptions increased optimal agent selection (61% to 80%, $P < .001$), optimal dose selection (67% to 78%, $P = .036$), and optimal duration (26% to 34%, $P = .13$).[64] A multifaceted intervention combining provider education, local treatment protocols, and order sets also demonstrated significant improvements in guideline-concordant antimicrobial selection and duration (41% to 84%, $P < .001$).[65]

Diagnostic Stewardship

Since UTI diagnosis is heavily influenced by test ordering behavior and the tests are plagued by false positives, the so-called diagnostic stewardship, which takes place upstream of treatment decisions, has a high potential to improve diagnosis and thus improve downstream antimicrobial prescribing.[66] Many of the UTI diagnostic stewardship interventions studied in the inpatient setting can also be successfully applied in the ED.[67] **Table 7** shows the examples of diagnostic stewardship interventions that have been studied in the ED. Interventions aimed at urine culture orders require an interdisciplinary approach involving pharmacy, health IT, and clinical microbiology. Changing the electronic health record end user interface by adding ordering indications and clinical decision support has been shown to improve culturing.[68] Another intervention is conditional reflex urine culturing whereby urine cultures that were ordered are automatically canceled if they do not meet predefined criteria from the UA; this is the opposite practice of reflex urine cultures, which are automatically added based on the UA.[70] Conditional reflex urine culturing has been shown to improve urine culturing rates when implemented as a stand-alone intervention.[70,71,75] Least likely to impact practices in the ED are diagnostic stewardship interventions that change the way urine cultures are reported. These include changing which antimicrobial susceptibilities are reported, modifying and limiting report information, and providing nudges to reduce treatment of ASB.[73,74,76]

Asymptomatic Bacteriuria

Although true UTIs are undeniably common in the ED, the lack of specificity of both symptoms and UA results leads to significant overdiagnosis. Contributing to this overdiagnosis is the common occurrence of leukocytes and bacteria in urine without associated genitourinary symptoms, termed ASB. ASB rarely leads to subsequent infection or negative sequelae.[43,77] In populations with high rates of ASB, including spinal cord injury patients, immune compromised patients, and elderly adults with functional or cognitive impairment, the risk of antibiotic-related adverse events outweighs the potential benefits of clearing the bacteriuria. The challenge presented by ASB is particularly significant in elderly patients presenting for falls or altered mental status, where pyuria and bacteriuria in the absence of fever or genitourinary symptoms is a major driver of inappropriate antibiotic use.[78,79] Such inappropriate antibiotic use occurs across all settings, often beginning in the ED. In a 43-hospital study of adult patients with ASB, 74% received antibiotic therapy, often initiated in the ED.[80] This was associated with prolonged hospitalization and development of *C difficile* infection. Many AMS and diagnostic stewardship initiatives are directed toward deceasing the misdiagnosis of ASB as UTI and preventing unnecessary exposure to antibiotics.

COMMON URINARY TRACT INFECTION-RELATED DILEMMAS IN THE EMERGENCY DEPARTMENT
Altered Mental Status and Falls with Asymptomatic Bacteriuria

Elderly patients with chronic pyuria and bacteriuria often present to the ED with altered mental status, delirium, behavioral change, or after a fall, but without fever or specific symptoms or signs of UTI. In practice, these patients are often treated with antibiotics for a presumed UTI, especially if there is dementia or other conditions that limit the ability to communicate.[81] In response to this challenge, expert bodies like the IDSA have sought to promote a watch-and-wait strategy for admitted patients without classic UTI symptoms, particularly in the context of known chronic ASB or a competing diagnosis that explains the presentation.[42,82] Here is an example of the relevant conversation with the admitting hospitalist: "Mr. Jones is confused with asymptomatic bacteriuria and has no other clinical signs of infection, bacteremia or sepsis. I suspect the confusion is due to a new benzodiazepine prescription and recommend that we pursue a 'medication holiday' strategy. I have not started antibiotics, so we can observe and await urine culture results."

Table 7
Examples of urinary tract infection-related stewardship interventions

Strategy	Description	Challenges
Clinical indications[68]	Must select from list of evidence-based symptoms prior to ordering urine culture	Work-around possible
Clinical decision support[69]	Incorporate evidence-based guidance into EMR to guide urine culture ordering	Time-consuming to implement; need health IT resources
Reflex urine culturing[70–72]	Limit processing or urine cultures based on predefined criteria (ie, WBC on UA)	May still yield positive cultures in patients with ASB
Cascade reporting[73]	Restricting reporting of broad-spectrum antibiotics in favor of more narrow-spectrum agents for cultures growing *E coli* and *Klebsiella* spp.	Extra work for providers when specific susceptibilities needed; can be ignored
Modified reporting[74]	Report minimal results or interpretation of results in the EMR	Can be ignored

Adapted from Goebel MC, Trautner BW, Grigoryan L. The Five Ds of Outpatient Antibiotic Stewardship for Urinary Tract Infections. *Clin Microbiol Rev.* 2021 Dec 15;34(4):e0000320.

Table 8
Less common urinary infections encountered in emergency department practice

Scenario	Common Pitfall	Recommended Approach	Empirical Antibiotics
Chronic cystitis or interstitial cystitis[88]	Chronic bladder pain in the absence of other explanatory etiologies. Common in chronic regional pain syndromes.	UA and culture typically normal. Discharge with referral to urology or uro/gyn. May consider amitriptyline or pelvic floor physical therapy.	Not recommended.
Renal or perinephric abscess[89]	Easily missed diagnosis. Requires IV antibiotics and percutaneous surgical drainage	Obtain a CT scan for patients with pyelonephritis symptoms that are severe or not improving with antibiotics, especially if possibility of obstructing process.	Vancomycin 20–35 mg/kg intravenous loading dose + cefepime 1 g intravenously
Ureterolithiasis with infection[90]	Anchoring on ureterolithiasis diagnosis with checking a urinalysis.	8%–15% of kidney stones have urinary coinfection. Fever, urinary symptoms, or leukocytosis should increase suspicion. Consult urology for potential surgical intervention.	If admitted: ceftriaxone 1 g intravenously If discharged: ciprofloxacin 500 mg orally twice daily for 5–7 d
Urethritis in men[91]	Misinterpreting an STI as a UTI	Question all male dysuria patients about penile drip and sexual habits. Have a low threshold for GC/chlamydia testing.	Ceftriaxone 500 mg IM × 1 (GC) plus azithromycin 1 g PO × 1 (chlamydia)

Cloudy or Foul-Smelling Urine

Cloudy urine often results from precipitated phosphate crystals in alkaline urine, though pyuria also can be the cause. Similarly, a strong odor may be caused by urea in a concentrated specimen rather than a UTI.[83] In general, visual and olfactory inspection of urine, in the absence of UTI symptoms, is not helpful in diagnosing UTI. A study of 100 urine samples from women at a university hospital was tested for the ability to read newsprint through the sample. The sensitivity, specificity, and positive and negative predictive values of legibility, as compared to culture, were 13.3%, 96.5%, 40.0%, and 86.3%, respectively.[84] Here is an example of the relevant conversation with the ED nurse:

Registered nurse (RN): "I collected a urine sample on our patient with a migraine just in case. It looks cloudy. Should I send it for urinalysis?"

ED provider: "The patient does not have urinary symptoms and cloudy urine can be related to hydration status. Let's hold off on send the UA for now."

"Positive" Urine Culture When the Urinalysis Has Greater Than 5 Squamous Epithelial Cells per High-Powered Field

An adequate specimen has fewer than 5 epithelial cells per low-power field on UA. Urine culture results from a contaminated sample are not reliable. Contaminated specimens should be recollected either using true clean-catch methods or by in-and-out catheterization.[85]

Sterile Pyuria

Sterile pyuria refers to white blood cells on the UA without the presence of bacteria. While sterile pyuria sometimes represents a contamination of the urine sample with vaginal leukocytes from vaginal secretions, it can also be a clue to more other unusual or serious illnesses. The differential diagnosis for sterile pyuria includes intra-abdominal infections adjacent to the bladder (eg, appendicitis), sexually transmitted infections, and UTIs from atypical organisms (ie, *Ureaplasma urealyticum*).[86] There is strong evidence that STIs are commonly misdiagnosed as UTIs in women less than 25 year old.[87] The US Center for Disease Control and Prevention recommends that STI testing is obtained routinely along with a UA in this population (**Table 8**).

SUMMARY

Diagnosis and management of UTIs in the ED requires a thoughtful approach, especially given the limited amount and quality of information we are presented with, the potential for severe infection if inadequately treated, and our mandate to provide good antibiotic stewardship. Differentiating cystitis from pyelonephritis from nonurinary pathology is challenging. Emerging antibiotic resistance among uropathogens adds further complexity. Best care entails a careful history and physical examination for urinary signs and symptoms, a nuanced consideration of urine test results and their limitations, and informed judgment as to whether or not to prescribe antibiotics. Once that decision to treat has been made, empirical antibiotic selection should incorporate patient-level factors, national guidelines, and local antibiogram data.

DISCLOSURE

K.C. Claeys serves as a consultant and on the speakers' bureau for BioMérieux Inc and received grant support for the Center for Disease Control and Prevention and Veterans Health Administration.

REFERENCES

1. Kovacs G, Croskerry P. Clinical decision making: an emergency medicine perspective. Acad Emerg Med 1999;6(9):947–52.
2. Foxman B. The epidemiology of urinary tract infection. Nat Rev Urol 2010;7(12): 653–60.
3. Foxman B. Urinary tract infection syndromes: occurrence, recurrence, bacteriology, risk factors, and disease burden. Infect Dis Clin North Am 2014;28(1):1–13.
4. Zilberberg MD, Nathanson BH, Sulham K, et al. Descriptive epidemiology and outcomes of emergency department visits with complicated urinary tract infections in the United States, 2016–2018. J Am Coll Emerg Physicians Open 2022; 3(2):e12694.
5. Hooton TM, Scholes D, Hughes JP, et al. A Prospective Study of Risk Factors for Symptomatic Urinary Tract Infection in Young Women. N Engl J Med 1996. https://doi.org/10.1056/NEJM199608153350703.
6. Medina M, Castillo-Pino E. An introduction to the epidemiology and burden of urinary tract infections. Ther Adv Urol 2019;11. https://doi.org/10.1177/1756287219832172. 1756287219832172.
7. Farrell K, Tandan M, Hernandez Santiago V, et al. Treatment of uncomplicated UTI in males: a systematic review of the literature. BJGP Open 2021;5(2). https://doi.org/10.3399/bjgpopen20X101140. bjgpopen20X101140.
8. Sorensen BD, Lupton JR, Chess LE, et al. Urine culture practices for complicated urinary tract infections in an academic emergency department. Am J Emerg Med 2023;68:170–4.
9. Lodise TP, Chopra T, Nathanson BH, et al. Epidemiology of Complicated Urinary Tract Infections due to Enterobacterales Among Adult Patients Presenting in Emergency Departments Across the United States. Open Forum Infect Dis 2022;9(7):ofac315.
10. Dunne MW, Puttagunta S, Aronin SI, et al. Impact of Empirical Antibiotic Therapy on Outcomes of Outpatient Urinary Tract Infection Due to Nonsusceptible Enterobacterales. Microbiol Spectr 2022;10(1):e0235921.
11. Jorgensen S, Zurayk M, Yeung S, et al. Emergency Department Urinary Antibiograms Differ by Specific Patient Group. J Clin Microbiol 2017;55(9):2629–36.
12. Frisbie L, Weissman SJ, Kapoor H, et al. Outpatient Antibiotic Resistance Patterns of Escherichia coli Urinary Isolates Differ by Specialty Type. Microbiol Spectr 2022;10(4):e0237321.
13. Dunne MW, Aronin SI, Yu KC, et al. A multicenter analysis of trends in resistance in urinary Enterobacterales isolates from ambulatory patients in the United States: 2011-2020. BMC Infect Dis 2022;22(1):194.
14. Wesolek JL, Wu JY, Smalley CM, et al. Risk Factors for Trimethoprim and Sulfamethoxazole-Resistant Escherichia Coli in ED Patients with Urinary Tract Infections. Am J Emerg Med 2022;56:178–82.
15. Faine BA, Rech MA, Vakkalanka P, et al. High prevalence of fluoroquinolone-resistant UTI among US emergency department patients diagnosed with urinary tract infection, 2018-2020. Acad Emerg Med 2022;29(9):1096–105.
16. Rosa R, Abbo LM, Raney K, et al. Antimicrobial resistance in urinary tract infections at a large urban ED: Factors contributing to empiric treatment failure. Am J Emerg Med 2017;35(3):397–401.
17. Talan DA, Takhar SS, Krishnadasan A, et al. Emergence of Extended-Spectrum β-Lactamase Urinary Tract Infections Among Hospitalized Emergency Department Patients in the United States. Ann Emerg Med 2021;77(1):32–43.

18. Walker E, Lyman A, Gupta K, et al. Clinical Management of an Increasing Threat: Outpatient Urinary Tract Infections Due to Multidrug-Resistant Uropathogens. Clin Infect Dis 2016;63(7):960–5.
19. Mark DG, Hung YY, Salim Z, et al. Third-Generation Cephalosporin Resistance and Associated Discordant Antibiotic Treatment in Emergency Department Febrile Urinary Tract Infections. Ann Emerg Med 2021;78(3):357–69.
20. Barré SL, Weeda ER, Matuskowitz AJ, et al. Risk Factors for Antibiotic Resistant Urinary Pathogens in Patients Discharged From the Emergency Department. Hosp Pharm 2022;57(4):462–8.
21. Kratochwill L, Powers M, McGraw MA, et al. Factors associated with ciprofloxacin-resistant Escherichia coli urinary tract infections in discharged ED patients. Am J Emerg Med 2015;33(10):1473–6.
22. Loeb M, Bentley DW, Bradley S, et al. Development of minimum criteria for the initiation of antibiotics in residents of long-term-care facilities: results of a consensus conference. Infect Control Hosp Epidemiol 2001;22(2):120–4.
23. Stone ND, Ashraf MS, Calder J, et al. Surveillance Definitions of Infections in Long-Term Care Facilities: Revisiting the McGeer Criteria. Infect Control Hosp Epidemiol 2012;33(10):965–77.
24. High KP, Bradley SF, Gravenstein S, et al. Clinical practice guideline for the evaluation of fever and infection in older adult residents of long-term care facilities: 2008 update by the Infectious Diseases Society of America. J Am Geriatr Soc 2009;57(3):375–94.
25. Bent S, Nallamothu BK, Simel DL, et al. Does This Woman Have an Acute Uncomplicated Urinary Tract Infection? JAMA 2002;287(20):2701–10.
26. Colgan R, Williams M. Diagnosis and treatment of acute uncomplicated cystitis. Am Fam Physician 2011;84(7):771–6.
27. Gill BC, Shoskes DA. Bacterial prostatitis. Curr Opin Infect Dis 2016;29(1):86–91.
28. Gupta K, Hooton TM, Naber KG, et al. International clinical practice guidelines for the treatment of acute uncomplicated cystitis and pyelonephritis in women: A 2010 update by the Infectious Diseases Society of America and the European Society for Microbiology and Infectious Diseases. Clin Infect Dis 2011;52(5): e103–20.
29. Kawashima A, LeRoy AJ. Radiologic evaluation of patients with renal infections. Infect Dis Clin North Am 2003;17(2):433–56.
30. Cline D.M., Ma O., Cydulka R.K., et al., editors. Tintinalli's Emergency Medicine Manual, 7e. The McGraw-Hill Companies; 2012. Available at: https://access emergencymedicine.mhmedical.com/content.aspx?bookid=521&sectionid= 41068918. Accessed February 26, 2024.
31. Roberts JR. InFocus: Urine Dipstick Testing: Everything You Need to Know. Emerg Med News 2015;37(5):14.
32. Can we trust urine dipsticks? Published September 9. 2016. Available at: https:// sykepleien.no/en/forskning/2017/01/can-we-trust-urine-dipsticks. [Accessed 25 June 2023].
33. Little P, Turner S, Rumsby K, et al. Developing clinical rules to predict urinary tract infection in primary care settings: sensitivity and specificity of near patient tests (dipsticks) and clinical scores. Br J Gen Pract J R Coll Gen Pract 2006; 56(529):606–12.
34. Fihn SD. Clinical practice. Acute uncomplicated urinary tract infection in women. N Engl J Med 2003;349(3):259–66.
35. Stamm WE, Counts GW, Running KR, et al. Diagnosis of coliform infection in acutely dysuric women. N Engl J Med 1982;307(8):463–8.

36. Rehmani R. Accuracy of urine dipstick to predict urinary tract infections in an emergency department. J Ayub Med Coll Abbottabad JAMC 2004;16(1):4–7.

37. Devillé WL, Yzermans JC, van Duijn NP, et al. The urine dipstick test useful to rule out infections. A meta-analysis of the accuracy. BMC Urol 2004;4(1):4.

38. Williams GJ, Macaskill P, Chan SF, et al. Absolute and relative accuracy of rapid urine tests for urinary tract infection in children: a meta-analysis. Lancet Infect Dis 2010;10(4):240–50.

39. Teeuw HM, Amoakoh HB, Ellis CA, et al. Diagnostic accuracy of urine dipstick tests for proteinuria in pregnant women suspected of preeclampsia: A systematic review and meta-analysis. Pregnancy Hypertens 2022;27:123–30.

40. Najeeb S, Munir T, Rehman S, et al. Comparison of urine dipstick test with conventional urine culture in diagnosis of urinary tract infection. J Coll Physicians Surg 2015;25(2):108–10.

41. Miller JM, Binnicker MJ, Campbell S, et al. A Guide to Utilization of the Microbiology Laboratory for Diagnosis of Infectious Diseases: 2018 Update by the Infectious Diseases Society of America and the American Society for Microbiology. Clin Infect Dis 2018;67(6):e1–94.

42. Nicolle LE, Gupta K, Bradley SF, et al. Clinical Practice Guideline for the Management of Asymptomatic Bacteriuria: 2019 Update by the Infectious Diseases Society of America. Clin Infect Dis 2019. https://doi.org/10.1093/cid/ciy1121.

43. Nicolle LE. Asymptomatic bacteriuria: when to screen and when to treat. Infect Dis Clin North Am 2003;17(2):367–94.

44. Sanford Guide | Antimicrobial Stewardship. https://www.sanfordguide.com/. [Accessed 27 June 2023].

45. Denny KJ, Gartside JG, Alcorn K, et al. Appropriateness of antibiotic prescribing in the Emergency Department. J Antimicrob Chemother 2019;74(2):515–20.

46. Shively NR, Buehrle DJ, Clancy CJ, et al. Prevalence of Inappropriate Antibiotic Prescribing in Primary Care Clinics within a Veterans Affairs Health Care System. Antimicrob Agents Chemother 2018;62(8):003377, e418.

47. Kiel A, Catalano A, Clark CM, et al. Antibiotic prescribing in the emergency department versus primary care: Implications for stewardship. J Am Pharm Assoc JAPhA 2020;60(6):789–95.e2.

48. Goebel MC, Trautner BW, Grigoryan L. The Five Ds of Outpatient Antibiotic Stewardship for Urinary Tract Infections. Clin Microbiol Rev 2021;34(4):e0000320.

49. Pulia M, Redwood R, May L. Antimicrobial Stewardship in the Emergency Department. Emerg Med Clin North Am 2018;36(4):853–72.

50. Marsh KJ, Mundy L, Holter JJ, et al. Analysis of urine-specific antibiograms from veterans to guide empiric therapy for suspected urinary tract infection. Diagn Microbiol Infect Dis 2019;95(4):114874.

51. Jorgensen SCJ, Yeung SL, Zurayk M, et al. Leveraging Antimicrobial Stewardship in the Emergency Department to Improve the Quality of Urinary Tract Infection Management and Outcomes. Open Forum Infect Dis 2018;5(6):ofy101.

52. Research C for DE, FDA Drug Safety Podcast. FDA updates warnings for oral and injectable fluoroquinolone antibiotics due to disabling side effects. FDA 2022;. https://www.fda.gov/drugs/fda-drug-safety-podcasts/fda-drug-safety-podcast-fda-updates-warnings-oral-and-injectable-fluoroquinolone-antibiotics-due. [Accessed 25 June 2023].

53. May L, Mullins P, Pines J. Demographic and treatment patterns for infections in ambulatory settings in the United States, 2006-2010. Acad Emerg Med 2014; 21(1):17–24.

54. Cowart K, Worley M, Rouby NE, et al. Evaluation of FDA Boxed Warning on Prescribing Patterns of Fluoroquinolones for Uncomplicated Urinary Tract Infections. Ann Pharmacother 2019;53(12):1192–9.
55. Sankar A, Swanson KM, Zhou J, et al. Association of Fluoroquinolone Prescribing Rates With Black Box Warnings from the US Food and Drug Administration. JAMA Netw Open 2021;4(12):e2136662.
56. Bratsman A, Mathias K, Laubscher R, et al. Outpatient fluoroquinolone prescribing patterns before and after US FDA boxed warning. Pharmacoepidemiol Drug Saf 2020;29(6):701–7.
57. Hecker MT, Fox CJ, Son AH, et al. Effect of a Stewardship Intervention on Adherence to Uncomplicated Cystitis and Pyelonephritis Guidelines in an Emergency Department Setting. PLoS One 2014;9(2):e87899.
58. Nys CL, Fischer K, Funaro J, et al. Impact of Education and Data Feedback on Antibiotic Prescribing for Urinary Tract Infections in the Emergency Department: An Interrupted Time-Series Analysis. Clin Infect Dis 2022;75(7):1194–200.
59. Maddali N, Cantin A, Koshy S, et al. Antibiotic prescribing patterns for adult urinary tract infections within emergency department and urgent care settings. Am J Emerg Med 2021;45:464–71.
60. Durkin MJ, Keller M, Butler AM, et al. An Assessment of Inappropriate Antibiotic Use and Guideline Adherence for Uncomplicated Urinary Tract Infections. Open Forum Infect Dis 2018;5(9):ofy198.
61. Lutters M, Vogt-Ferrier NB. Antibiotic duration for treating uncomplicated, symptomatic lower urinary tract infections in elderly women. Cochrane Database Syst Rev 2008;3:CD001535.
62. Drekonja DM, Trautner B, Amundson C, et al. Effect of 7 vs 14 Days of Antibiotic Therapy on Resolution of Symptoms Among Afebrile Men With Urinary Tract Infection: A Randomized Clinical Trial. JAMA 2021;326(4):324–31.
63. Lafaurie M, Chevret S, Fontaine JP, et al. Antimicrobial for 7 or 14 Days for Febrile Urinary Tract Infection in Men: A Multicenter Noninferiority Double-Blind, Placebo-Controlled, Randomized Clinical Trial. Clin Infect 2023;76(12):2154–62.
64. Vuong L, Kenney RM, Thomson JM, et al. Implementation of indication-based antibiotic order sentences improves antibiotic use in emergency departments. Am J Emerg Med 2023;69:5–10.
65. Zalmanovich A, Katzir M, Chowers M, et al. Improving urinary tract infection treatment through a multifaceted antimicrobial stewardship intervention in the emergency department. Am J Emerg Med 2021;49:10–3.
66. Vaughn V, Gupta A, Petty LA, et al. 1592. SHEA Featured Oral Abstract: Reducing Unnecessary Antibiotic Treatment for Asymptomatic Bacteriuria: A Statewide Collaborative Quality Initiative. Open Forum Infect Dis 2022;9(Suppl 2):ofac492. https://doi.org/10.1093/ofid/ofac492.114.
67. Claeys KC, Trautner BW, Leekha S, et al. Optimal Urine Culture Diagnostic Stewardship Practice-Results from an Expert Modified-Delphi Procedure. Clin Infect Dis 2022;75(3):382–9.
68. Watson KJ, Trautner B, Russo H, et al. Using clinical decision support to improve urine culture diagnostic stewardship, antimicrobial stewardship, and financial cost: A multicenter experience. Infect Control Hosp Epidemiol 2020;41(5):564–70.
69. Munigala S, Jackups RR, Poirier RF, et al. Impact of order set design on urine culturing practices at an academic medical centre emergency department. BMJ Qual Saf 2018;27(8):587–92.
70. Claeys KC, Zhan M, Pineles L, et al. Conditional reflex to urine culture: Evaluation of a diagnostic stewardship intervention within the Veterans' Affairs and Centers

for Disease Control and Prevention Practice-Based Research Network. Infect Control Hosp Epidemiol 2021;42(2):176–81.

71. Lynch CS, Appleby-Sigler A, Bork JT, et al. Effect of urine reflex culturing on rates of cultures and infections in acute and long-term care. Antimicrob Resist Infect Control 2020;9(1):96.

72. Coughlin RF, Peaper D, Rothenberg C, et al. Electronic Health Record-Assisted Reflex Urine Culture Testing Improves Emergency Department Diagnostic Efficiency. Am J Med Qual 2020;35(3):252–7.

73. Vissichelli NC, Orndahl CM, Cecil JA, et al. Impact of cascade reporting of antimicrobial susceptibility on fluoroquinolone and meropenem consumption at a Veterans' Affairs medical center. Infect Control Hosp Epidemiol 2022;43(2):199–204.

74. Daley P, Garcia D, Inayatullah R, et al. Modified Reporting of Positive Urine Cultures to Reduce Inappropriate Treatment of Asymptomatic Bacteriuria Among Nonpregnant, Noncatheterized Inpatients: A Randomized Controlled Trial. Infect Control Hosp Epidemiol 2018;39(7):814–9.

75. Penney JA, Rodday AM, Sebastiani P, et al. Effecting the culture: Impact of changing urinalysis with reflex to culture criteria on culture rates and outcomes. Infect Control Hosp Epidemiol 2022;1–6. https://doi.org/10.1017/ice.2022.178.

76. Langford BJ, Seah J, Chan A, et al. Antimicrobial Stewardship in the Microbiology Laboratory: Impact of Selective Susceptibility Reporting on Ciprofloxacin Utilization and Susceptibility of Gram-Negative Isolates to Ciprofloxacin in a Hospital Setting. J Clin Microbiol 2016;54(9):2343–7.

77. Nicolle LE. The Paradigm Shift to Non-Treatment of Asymptomatic Bacteriuria. Pathogens 2016;5(2):38.

78. Anderson CM, VanHoose JD, Burgess DR, et al. Appropriateness of antibiotic use in patients with and without altered mental status diagnosed with a urinary tract infection. Antimicrob Steward Healthc Epidemiol ASHE 2022;2(1):e198.

79. Mayne S, Bowden A, Sundvall PD, et al. The scientific evidence for a potential link between confusion and urinary tract infection in the elderly is still confusing - a systematic literature review. BMC Geriatr 2019;19(1):32.

80. Petty LA, Vaughn VM, Flanders SA, et al. Assessment of Testing and Treatment of Asymptomatic Bacteriuria Initiated in the Emergency Department. Open Forum Infect Dis 2020;7(12):ofaa537.

81. D'Agata E, Loeb MB, Mitchell SL. Challenges in assessing nursing home residents with advanced dementia for suspected urinary tract infections. J Am Geriatr Soc 2013;61(1):62–6.

82. Shimoni Z, Levinger U, Dubin I, et al. Decreasing urine culture rates in hospitalized internal medicine patients. Am J Infect Control 2020;48(11):1361–4.

83. Simerville JA, Maxted WC, Pahira JJ. Urinalysis: a comprehensive review. Am Fam Physician 2005;71(6):1153–62.

84. Foley A, French L. Urine clarity inaccurate to rule out urinary tract infection in women. J Am Board Fam Med JABFM 2011;24(4):474–5.

85. Pappas PG. Laboratory in the diagnosis and management of urinary tract infections. Med Clin North Am 1991;75(2):313–25.

86. Wise GJ, Schlegel PN. Sterile pyuria. N Engl J Med 2015;372(11):1048–54.

87. Tomas ME, Getman D, Donskey CJ, et al. Overdiagnosis of Urinary Tract Infection and Underdiagnosis of Sexually Transmitted Infection in Adult Women Presenting to an Emergency Department. J Clin Microbiol 2015;53(8):2686–92.

88. Hanno PM, Burks DA, Clemens JQ, et al. AUA guideline for the diagnosis and treatment of interstitial cystitis/bladder pain syndrome. J Urol 2011;185(6):2162–70.

89. Yen DH, Hu SC, Tsai J, et al. Renal abscess: early diagnosis and treatment. Am J Emerg Med 1999;17(2):192–7.
90. Abrahamian FM, Krishnadasan A, Mower WR, et al. Association of pyuria and clinical characteristics with the presence of urinary tract infection among patients with acute nephrolithiasis. Ann Emerg Med 2013;62(5):526–33.
91. Pfennig CL. Sexually Transmitted Diseases in the Emergency Department. Emerg Med Clin North Am 2019;37(2):165–92.

Optimizing Diagnosis and Management of Community-acquired Pneumonia in the Emergency Department

Katherine M. Hunold, MD, MPH[a],*, Elizabeth Rozycki, PharmD, BCPS[b],
Nathan Brummel, MD, MSCI[c]

KEYWORDS

- Pneumonia • Community-acquired pneumonia • Diagnosis and management
- Emergency medicine

KEY POINTS

- Community-acquired pneumonia (CAP) is a common cause of emergency department (ED) visit with higher mortality in the youngest and oldest patients.
- ED-specific guidelines do not recommend the routine use of polymerase-chain reaction pathogen assays or other biomarkers to guide antibiotic initiation.
- Recommend empiric treatment for low-risk outpatients with no comorbidities is amoxicillin or doxycycline. In patients with comorbidities and/or risk factors for resistant organisms, this should be escalated to combination therapy with a beta-lactam and beta-lactamase inhibitor plus doxycycline or a macrolide.
- Blood and sputum cultures should be obtained in patients with severe CAP and those initiated on broad-spectrum antibiotics.

INTRODUCTION

Pneumonia is split into 3 diagnostic categories: community-acquired pneumonia (CAP), health care-associated pneumonia, and ventilator-associated pneumonia. This classification scheme is driven not only by the location of infection onset but also by the predominant associated causal microorganisms. Pneumonia is diagnosed in over 1.5 million US emergency department (ED) visits annually (1.2% of all visits),[1]

[a] Department of Emergency Medicine, The Ohio State University, 376 W 10th Avenue, 760 Prior Hall, Columbus, OH 43220, USA; [b] Emergency Medicine, Department of Pharmacy, The Ohio State University, 376 W 10th Avenue, 760 Prior Hall, Columbus, OH 43220, USA; [c] Division of Pulmonary, Critical Care, and Sleep Medicine, Department of Internal Medicine, The Ohio State University, 376 W 10th Avenue, 760 Prior Hall, Columbus, OH 43220, USA
* Corresponding author.
E-mail address: Katherine.Buck@osumc.edu

Emerg Med Clin N Am 42 (2024) 231–247
https://doi.org/10.1016/j.emc.2024.02.001
0733-8627/24/© 2024 Elsevier Inc. All rights reserved.

emed.theclinics.com

and most pneumonia diagnosed by emergency physicians is CAP. CAP is associated with a low (1%) mortality rate in those treated as an outpatient but up to 50% mortality of intensive care unit (ICU) patients; both the youngest and oldest age groups experience higher mortality.[2] Further, it is estimated that one-third of hospitalized CAP patients die within 1 year.[3] Thus, a clear understanding of the most up-to-date diagnostic modalities and treatment recommendations is critical.

CURRENT GUIDELINES

The most current relevant guidelines for treatment of CAP in the ED are the 2019 Infectious Disease Society of American/American Thoracic Society (IDSA/ATS) CAP guidelines,[4] the 2020 American College of Emergency Physicians (ACEP) Clinical Policy,[5] and the 2011 Pediatric Infectious Diseases Society and IDSA CAP pediatric guidelines.[6] Recently published recommendations from the European Respiratory Society, the European Society of Intensive Care Medicine, and Latin America Thoracic Association provide guidelines specifically for the management of severe CAP.[7]

DIAGNOSTIC CRITERIA

Both the 2019 IDSA/ATS CAP guidelines[4] and 2020 ACEP Clinical Policy[5] define pneumonia as symptoms of pneumonia plus radiographic evidence of pneumonia. This definition was not updated from previous guidelines, and at this time, this clinical/radiographic combination definition is the diagnostic standard. However, these criteria have significant limitations that must be considered by clinicians including but not limited to their performance in certain populations and the accuracy of chest radiographs.

CAP is further classified into nonsevere or severe based on the acuity of illness. The IDSA/ATS provide specific criteria for severe CAP that include factors such as specific vital sign abnormalities and need for vasopressors or mechanical ventilation.[4] Severe CAP is defined by the presence of at least 1 major criterion or 3 minor criteria. Empiric antibiotic recommendations vary depending on whether or not the patient meets severe CAP criteria or has risk factors for infection with multidrug-resistant organisms. Populations that require special therapeutic considerations include pediatrics, geriatrics, and those with recent international travel.

PATHOPHYSIOLOGY

In the most basic terms, pneumonia is an infection of the lungs. In the majority of cases, causative organism enters through inhalation or migration from the upper respiratory tract or aspiration. While aspiration causes 5% to 15% of CAP[8] and is traditionally associated with geriatric and comorbid patients, aspirating small volumes of upper airway secretions can occur in young and healthy individuals during sleep.[9] Rarely, pneumonia is caused by hematogenous spread, such as from right-sided endocarditis.

CAUSES OF PNEUMONIA

CAPs are most commonly caused by single bacteria, virus or in rare circumstances fungal organisms. Coinfections are rare but can also occur, particularly with a virus and bacterial pathogen. The causative bacterial agents in CAP are classically identified, in order, as *Streptococcus pneumoniae, Haemophilus influenzae, Staphylococcus aureus*, and gram-negative bacilli.[10,11] Importantly, the "atypical" bacteria are also important to consider as *Mycoplasma* is identified in 4% to 11% of CAP and *Legionella* in 3% to 8%.[11] A recent study that included only hospitalized CAP patients with a "high-quality" sputum specimens identified a causative pathogen in 95.8%, with one-quarter being components of normal respiratory flora rather than the bacterial pathogens classically implicated as earlier.[12] The authors hypothesized that aspiration of oral flora may been an important yet underappreciated cause of CAP. A 2016 meta-analysis examined the use of viral polymerase chain reaction (PCR) from upper airway swabs in adults with CAP; pooled estimates identified a viral pathogen in 24.5% (95% CI 21.5%–27.5%). Only 2 studies in the review reported on viral pathogens from lower respiratory specimens, with prevalence reported at 44.2%. Of note, coinfection by bacteria and viral pathogens doubled the odds of death.[10]

Depending on the study, the most common causative pathogens identified varies, likely due to the varying types of diagnostic modalities used, quality of specimens and patient populations. For example, PCR assays may have higher diagnostic yield than traditional culture methods but may also identify colonizing pathogens.[13] This likely explains why some studies have found higher rates of viral organisms and variations based on age (see Special Populations later section).[14,15] It is important to recognize that diagnostic yield is directly related to the sample quality and consider ED-specific barriers to optimal collection.[16–19] For example, in the ED, expectorated sputum is the primary sample source, which is associated with known quality limitations.[20]

COVID-19

The COVID-19 pandemic showed the potential for devastation from a novel viral pneumonia pathogen with young children (<1 year) and older adults being at highest risk of mortality.[21] Bacterial coinfection with SARS-CoV-2 estimates vary greatly with a recent meta-analysis reporting a rate of approximately 7%.[22–24] As with non-SARS-CoV-2 infections, bacterial coinfection with SARS-CoV-2 is associated with increased risk for severe disease (ICU admission, mechanical ventilation) and death.[25] Public health measures instituted during this pandemic decreased the transmission of other common pneumonia pathogens.[26] COVID-19 is discussed in detail elsewhere in this issue.

Influenza

Prior to the COVID-19 pandemic, influenza was the most commonly identified cause of viral CAP,[10] with the young children (<5 years of age) and older adults ($\geq$65 years of age) at highest risk.[27] Peaks of influenza activity occur seasonally.[28] The 2019 IDSA/ATS guidelines recommend rapid testing for influenza during peak times.[4] Vaccination decreases influenza incidence and associated morbidity and mortality.[29] Following the release of the COVID-19 vaccine, influenza vaccination rates decreased,[30] the impact of which is yet to be determined.

DIAGNOSTIC MODALITIES

There are many potentially useful diagnostic modalities in pneumonia. Importantly, the utility of the modalities may differ between the ED and inpatient settings. For example, though frequently obtained in the ED, sputum and blood cultures take several days to result and are therefore not available to ED physicians. Similarly, laboratory markers with a single value may have limited value in the ED but may have clinical utility if trended. Therefore, the following discussion is focused primarily on strategies used in the ED. Nevertheless, we emphasize that studies that may not be useful in the ED should still be sent to assist downstream clinicians caring for the patient after ED disposition, particularly as it pertains to tailoring or de-escalation of antibiotic therapy.

Chest Imaging

One component of the current standard definition of pneumonia is a positive chest radiograph. However, a recent meta-analysis estimated the sensitivity and specificity of a chest radiograph for pneumonia to be 75%.[31] Debate exists in the literature among experts about whether positive chest radiography should be required.[32] Computed tomography (CT) has been proposed as a potential alternative imaging test as it is more accurate and this has a demonstrated effect on clinical management.[33–35] Nevertheless, a recent trial showed no difference in short-term functional health, hospital admissions, and length of stay, suggesting that though more pneumonias may be detected with CT imaging, these findings may not improve patient outcomes and therefore there is insufficient evidence to support a change in the standard of care.[36] Further research is needed before a definitive recommendation can be made about whether CT imaging should be used routinely to diagnose CAP.

The question remains—what should clinicians do with (1) high clinical suspicion and negative chest radiograph and (2) low clinical suspicion and a vague chest radiograph report? Based on the available evidence and current guidelines, we recommend treating empirically in both above cases. The primary driver for this recommendation is the phenomenon of delayed or initially negative chest radiograph findings[37,38] and data showed positive CT findings of pneumonia with negative chest radiographs.[33–36,39] Further, this is consistent with current IDSA/ATS guidelines that no laboratory test currently exists to reliably and rapidly differentiate viral from bacterial causes of pneumonia[5,4].

Ultrasound is another tool that emergency physicians can use to identify lung pathology, including CAP. Lung ultrasound can narrow the differential diagnosis in ED patients with dyspnea.[40] One study demonstrated good accuracy of emergency physician performed lung ultrasound compared to chest radiograph for pneumonia diagnosis.[41] However, this study enrolled a convenience sample, and ultrasounds were performed by physicians with ultrasound training and 2 or more years of experience, limiting generalizability. Another recent study failed to demonstrate an advantage of ultrasound over chest radiograph.[42] We recommend considering the use of lung ultrasound, particularly by emergency physicians with ultrasound training, particularly as a "rule in" rather than "rule out" tool, pending further studies.

Blood and Sputum Culture

Although the results of blood and sputum cultures will not be available to emergency physicians when making treatment decisions, it is important that emergency physicians understand when to send these prior to antibiotic treatment. The 2019 IDSA/ATS guidelines recommend blood and sputum cultures in "patients with severe disease as well as in all inpatients initiated on empiric therapy that includes coverage for *Methicillin-resistant Staphylococcus aureus* (MRSA) or *Pseudomonas aeruginosa*." Additionally, the IDSA/ATS guidelines provide conditional recommendations to obtain blood and sputum cultures in patients who "were previously infected with MRSA or *P aeruginosa* or were hospitalized and received parenteral antibiotics in the last 90 days." A recent observational cohort study confirms that the highest utility of blood culture is in patients with severe CAP (14.7% with bacteremia).[43] The centers for medicare & medicaid services (CMS) SEP-1[44] mandate to obtain blood cultures prior administering antibiotics in patients being admitted with signs of sepsis may further expand the group of patients requiring blood cultures.

Utility of sputum culture depends on a good quality specimen and the ability to obtain high-quality sputum specimens in EDs has been questioned. A recent study demonstrated that tracheal suction has superior quality to expiratory techniques[45] In the ED, tracheal suction can be readily performed only in intubated patients. Importantly, a recent study demonstrated that no ED empiric antibiotic choices were changed by sputum culture results when available.[46] Advances in point of care testing, such as PCR tests (see later discussion), may lead to better tools for determining CAP etiology from sputum specimens and potentially affecting ED treatment decisions.

Urine Antigen Detection

Urine antigen testing is available for *S pneumoniae* and *Legionella pneumophila*.[47] The IDSA/ATS guidelines do not recommend routinely testing for these causes except in 2 clinical scenarios: (1) based on epidemiologic factors and (2) in those with severe CAP. Epidemiologic factors include known *Legionella* outbreak or recent travel to high-risk areas.[4] Their reasoning is that testing did not change patient-centered outcomes including death, clinical relapse, ICU admission, hospital length of stay, duration of antibiotic treatment, or cost of treatment.[48,49]

In the appropriate geographic area, emergency providers should consider testing for histoplasmosis, coccidioidomycosis, or blastomycosis with urine testing or IgG/IgM depending on standard at your hospital and can assist with early detection but is not the gold standard test (identification via culture or histologic examination).[50]

The ACEP guidelines do not recommend withholding or altering initial ED antibiotic treatment based on the result of urinary antigen tests[5] due to low rates of definitive cause identification in previous literature. Of note, due to frequent colonization, urinary antigen tests are not recommended in children.[51]

Polymerase Chain Reaction Pathogen Identification

Recent guidelines agree that there is low evidence for the routine use of viral pathogen PCR assays in CAP.[4,5,7] This is because the exact meaning of positive results is unknown as it may represent only asymptomatic upper respiratory colonization, coinfection or prior infection, rather than the cause of lower respiratory infection; for example, one-quarter of asymptomatic children had a positive test.[51,52] Newly available PCR assays that include bacterial and viral targets utilize sputum or bronchial samples. However, as previously mentioned, obtaining high-quality sputum samples in the ED is challenging and will impact the diagnostic yield of such assays.[20] Bronchiolar lavage likely provides better accuracy, but it is not feasible for routine use in the ED.

However, counter-arguments emerging in the literature should be considered. A recent study demonstrated high agreement of PCR testing between oropharyngeal samples and lower respiratory tract samples in ED patients with CAP.[53] Therefore, the authors recommend determining the potential utility in your own practice based on (1) quality of procedures for sputum collection in your ED and (2) which pathogens are included on your hospital's panel.

Methicillin-resistant Staphylococcus aureus Polymerase Chain Reaction

Nasal MRSA PCR swabs are primarily used for de-escalation, stopping anti-MRSA therapy in patients who were initially covered for MRSA empirically. While unable to distinguish infection from colonization, the negative predictive value for MRSA pneumonia using the nasal swab ranges from 75% to 99%.[4,54,55]

Host-response Biomarkers

No available biomarker, in isolation, can reliably identify the presence of pneumonia or differentiate viral from bacterial pneumonia. Neither ACEP nor IDSA/ATS currently recommend their routine use.[5] However, this is an ongoing area of research and it is unclear how these assays may perform in combination (eg, viral PCR plus biomarkers) and in conjunction with estimates of pretest probability.

Procalcitonin

Procalcitonin as a laboratory marker of bacterial pneumonia deserves specific discussion, as research is ongoing and rapidly expanding. The traditional critique of procalcitonin is that a single value cannot be used to determine decision making. However, a recent study compared the outcomes of patients with suspected viral lower respiratory infection and low procalcitonin randomized to azithromycin or placebo and demonstrated noninferiority.[56] Experts debating the strengths and limitations of this study conclude that using procalcitonin in this manner, which could be directly applied to EDs, be considered.[57] However, the largest ED-based US trial, ProACT Trial, demonstrated minimal differences in antibiotic prescribing and no difference in short- or long-term mortality between those treated on a procalcitonin-guided pathway or not.[58–60] The lack of effect on antibiotic prescribing was in part driven by providers not following the procalcitonin guidance, suggesting lack of confidence in the test may be a barrier to adoption. Additionally, emergency providers may be asked to obtain procalcitonin because serial procalcitonin measurements may have utility in de-escalating inpatient antibiotic therapy[61,62]

MeMed BV

Since the publication of existing guidelines, MeMed BV (MeMed Diagnostics, Ltd) was Food and Drug Administration (FDA)-approved as a test to differentiate bacterial and viral respiratory infections. A recent study in the US ED demonstrated that while the test is clinically feasible, less than half of the MeMed BV results were viewed prior to administration of antibiotics.[63] Thus, while the data on MeMed BV are promising, further study on both implementation and outcomes are necessary before a definitive recommendation can be made.

RISK STRATIFICATION

There are many risk stratification tools available for CAP to aid the clinician in deciding appropriate patient disposition (eg, discharge, hospital admission, or ICU admission). Validated clinical decision rules include the Pneumonia Severity Index (PSI),[64] CURB-65,[65] and A-DROP.[66] For ED use, the ACEP guidelines recommend PSI and CURB-65 to support clinical judgment to assess which patients may be appropriate for discharge. The IDSA/ATS favor PSI over CURB-65.[4] A recent study showed similar performance between CURB-65 and A-DROP in ED patients.[67] The ACEP guidelines recommend using the IDSA/ATS minor criteria (see **Table 1**) to assess need for ICU admission.[5] However, the results of recent literature have been mixed regarding clinical utility of such tools in the ED[68,69] supporting the ACEP guideline assertion that these should only be one part of clinician decision-making.

SPECIAL POPULATIONS
Pediatrics

The 2011 Pediatric Infectious Diseases Society and IDSA CAP pediatric guidelines are the current standard.[6] The most common cause of pneumonia in pediatric patients is viruses. The advent of widespread vaccine use has decreased the incidence of CAP caused by *Haemophilus influenzae* type B and *Pneumococcal pneumoniae*.[51,70]

Pediatric symptoms of pneumonia are hard to distinguish from other causes of respiratory illness.[51] Treatment with antibiotics was previously guided by the World Health Organization respiratory rate criteria[70]; the goal of this criterion was to identify children at risk of death. A more recent systematic review did not find tachypnea associated with pneumonia. Instead, hypoxemia and work of breathing were associated with pneumonia diagnosis.[70,71]

Importantly, the guidelines recommend avoiding routine use of chest radiography in patients well enough to be treated as an outpatient (discharged from the ED).[6] Emergency physicians should be aware of these guidelines as a recent paper suggests overuse of chest radiograph.[72] Further, the use of diagnostic modalities for pediatric patients with fever differs between general and pediatric EDs.[73] Thus, emergency physicians should aim to follow the guidelines and only obtain chest radiograph in pediatric patients when admission is required.

Geriatrics

Pneumonia incidence[74]-related hospitalizations[15] and in-hospital mortality[75] all increase with age. Because 3 out of 4 adults $\geq$65 years of age who are hospitalized with pneumonia are initially treated in the ED,[76] emergency providers must know how to maximize diagnostic accuracy in this population. Unfortunately, CAP in older adults poses a diagnostic challenge to emergency physicians and our inpatient colleagues.[77,78] Geriatric-specific factors that contribute to this challenge include atypical presentations[17,18,79–84]; having fewer specific symptoms (ie, shortness of breath, fever) than young patients; reduced accuracy of chest radiographs[85]; and presence of comorbidities that can mimic CAP.[86,87] The utility of the current clinical definition of pneumonia is unknown in this population, and geriatric-specific pneumonia diagnostic criteria have been developed in non-ED health care settings.[88,89] While older adults residing in long-term care facilities are also at risk for drug-resistant organisms,[90] the current guidelines do not recommend any changes to standard risk factor-based empiric therapy in older adults with nonsevere CAP, regardless of living situation.[4]

Recent Foreign Travel

Depending on the site of recent travel, pulmonary symptoms in a returning traveler may have an atypical cause based on location; for example, in travelers to South and Central Asia, diphtheria, tuberculosis, and avian flu are common but rare causes such as Nipah virus may need to be considered.[91,92] Clinicians should consider testing and treatment for atypical causes based on endemic and potential novel pulmonary diseases found in the areas of recent travel. The Centers for Disease Control and Prevention (CDC) maintains online resources for clinicians including but not limited to regions of common exposure, presentation, incubation periods, and treatment.[93] An infectious disease specialist should also be consulted, when there is suspicion of pneumonia due to an unusual or novel pathogen acquired while traveling. For example, at the time of this writing, the CDC includes COVID-19, avian influenza, Middle East respiratory syndrome, among others for consideration.[93]

Immunocompromised

Immunocompromised patients are at higher risk for atypical causes of pneumonia across the age span,[51,94] but there is no consensus on how this should affect the empiric antibiotic treatment.[94] Immunocompromised patients are excluded from the CAP guidelines. Clinicians should consider early infectious disease consultation in these patients.

Patients at Risk for Aspiration

Aspiration pneumonia has been proposed as a common cause of pneumonia, particularly in older adults.[95–97] Whether or not anaerobic coverage is necessary in suspected aspiration, pneumonia is not clear according to a recent systematic review and meta-analysis.[98] The IDSA/ATS guidelines suggest only adding anaerobic coverage if lung abscess or empyema is suspected.[4]

TREATMENT RECOMMENDATIONS

The IDSA/ATS guidelines state, and the ACEP agrees, "there is no current diagnostic test accurate enough or fast enough to determine that CAP is solely due to a virus at presentation, our recommendations are to initially treat empirically for possible bacterial infection or coinfection."[4] Thus, empiric treatment with antibiotics is the current recommendation. The COVID-19 pneumonia may represent an exception to this recommendation. Empiric therapy recommendations in this section focus on the adult population. For outpatients with no comorbidities, treatment primarily focuses on coverage of S pneumoniae with either amoxicillin or doxycycline (**Table 1**). Doxycycline has the advantage that it covers atypical organisms and may provide H influenza and S aureus coverage. While azithromycin monotherapy historically has been used for outpatient pneumonia, macrolide resistance has increased and azithromycin should only be used if a local antibiogram shows macrolide resistance of less than 25%. Many patients presenting to the ED with pneumonia will have additional comorbidities placing them at risk for resistant pathogens and poor outcomes if initial empiric therapy is inadequate. Thus, in addition to S pneumoniae coverage, outpatients with significant comorbidities should receive a regimen that covers H influenzae and Moraxella catarrhalis, S aureus, some gram-negative bacteria, and atypical pathogens. This can be accomplished with either combination therapy consisting of a beta-lactam and a beta-lactamase inhibitor (amoxicillin-clavulanate) plus doxycycline or a macrolide or monotherapy with a respiratory fluoroquinolone (levofloxacin or moxifloxacin). However, providers should consider the potential for collateral damage with fluoroquinolones, including tendinitis, tendon rupture, and peripheral and central nervous system effects. Additionally, a new fluoroquinolone black box warning was issued in 2018 regarding risk for aortic aneurysm or dissection and potential mental health side effects.[99] These black box warnings pertain to older adult patients disproportionately.

For patients being admitted to the hospital, a beta-lactam plus a macrolide or doxycycline are the favored combination,[4,7] but local resistance patterns as well as patient-specific risk factors will strongly impact the recommended empiric therapy (see **Table 1**). The IDSA/ATS guidelines focus on previous growth of MRSA or P aeruginosa from respiratory cultures, hospitalization with parenteral antibiotics in the past 90 days as risk factors that should prompt broad-spectrum empiric therapy. The guidelines also encourage the development of locally validated risk factors for MRSA or P aeruginosa when selecting empiric regimens; the feasibility of this recommendation and the potential impact on ED empiric therapy selection have just begun to be studied.[100] In patients receiving empiric therapy for MRSA and P aeruginosa, it is important to obtain sputum cultures and nasal MRSA PCR screening, which if negative may allow de-escalation and less exposure to broad-spectrum antibiotics.

There are recent data confirming that patients meeting the IDSA/ATS criteria for severe CAP[4] have higher rates of positive blood cultures and higher organ failure scores and mortality. While a resistant organism was isolated in about 10% of these cases, which supports maintaining a low threshold for broad empiric coverage in severe

Table 1
Antimicrobial treatment considerations

Setting and Severity	Patient Characteristics	Antimicrobial Recommendations
Outpatient	No comorbidities or risk factors for MRSA or P aeruginosa	Amoxicillin (high dose) OR Doxycycline OR Macrolide[a] (only if local pneumococcal resistance is <25%)
	Comorbidities, including chronic heart, lung, liver or renal disease, diabetes mellitus, alcoholism, malignancy, or asplenia	Combination therapy • Amoxicillin/clavulanate OR cephalosporin[b] • Atypical coverage (doxycycline OR macrolide)[a] OR Respiratory fluoroquinolone monotherapy[c,d]
Inpatient, nonsevere pneumonia	No prior respiratory cultures with MRSA or P aeruginosa	Beta-lactam[e] PLUS atypical coverage[a] OR Respiratory fluoroquinolone monotherapy[c,d]
	Prior respiratory isolate with MRSA or local validated risk factors for MRSA [f]	Add vancomycin or linezolid
	Prior respiratory isolate with P aeruginosa within 1 y, local validated risk factors or advanced structural lung disease[f]	Antipseudomonal beta-lactam[h] PLUS atypical coverage[a] OR respiratory fluoroquinolone
	Recent hospitalization with parenteral antibiotics[f,h]	Beta-lactam[e] PLUS macrolide[a] OR Respiratory fluoroquinolone monotherapy[c,d]

(continued on next page)

Table 1
(continued)

Setting and Severity	Patient Characteristics	Antimicrobial Recommendations
Inpatient, severe pneumonia	No prior respiratory cultures with MRSA or *P aeruginosa*	Beta-lactam[e] PLUS macrolide[a] OR Respiratory fluoroquinolone monotherapy[c,d]
	Prior respiratory isolate with *MRSA*[f] or recent hospitalization with parenteral antibiotics and locally validated risk factors for MRSA[f]	Beta-lactam[f] PLUS macrolide[a] OR Respiratory fluoroquinolone[c,d] PLUS vancomycin or linezolid
	Prior respiratory isolate with *P aeruginosa*[g] or recent hospitalization with parenteral antibiotics and locally validated risk factors for *P aeruginosa*[g]	Antipseudomonal beta-lactam[h] PLUS macrolide[a]

[a] Azithromycin, clarithromycin, or doxycycline.
[b] Cefpodoxime, cefuroxime.
[c] Levofloxacin, moxifloxacin, gemifloxacin
[d] Fluoroquinolones should be reserved only if other agents are not clinically appropriate given the potential risks (hypoglycemia, mental status changes, effects on tendons, joint, muscles and nerves, and aortic aneurysm/dissection)[105].
[e] Ampicillin/sulbactam, cefotaxime, ceftriaxone.
[f] Obtain cultures and/or nasal MRSA PCR.
[g] Should be driven by local antibiogram but may include piperacillin/tazobactam, cefepime, ceftazidime, imipenem, meropenem, or aztreonam.
[h] Only initiate coverage for MRSA if results positive.

CAP, a much higher proportion received vancomycin and/or piperacillin–tazobactam.[101] These findings underscore the recommendation above to obtain all appropriate diagnostic studies, which might allow later de-escalation of broad-spectrum therapy.

A common clinical practice in EDs is to give 1 dose of intravenous antibiotics followed by initiation of an oral regimen, based on factors such as antimicrobial bioavailability, intestinal absorption, and ability to tolerate oral medications. The ACEP found a lack of evidence to support or refute this practice.[5] In the absence of clear clinical benefit, increased cost and potential increased length of ED stay, we do not advise this practice.

A routine addition of corticosteroids to antibiotics in CAP is not recommended.[4] Recently published studies evaluating the use of hydrocortisone and methylprednisolone in patients with severe CAP have shown mixed results, though the expert consensus seems favor giving steroids in this setting.[102,103] Additionally, corticosteroids may have a role in patients with shock, acute respiratory distress syndrome and COVID-19 pneumonia.[4,7]

The recommended duration of antimicrobial therapy for CAP is a minimum of 5 days, depending on the antibiotic and measures of clinical stability and improvement.[4] For patients being discharged from the ED, a prescription for 5 days of therapy is often appropriate. Clear discharge instructions should be provided regarding expected recovery and return precautions. A recent randomized controlled trial comparing antibiotic duration in pediatric CAP found that a 5 day course was superior to 10 days.[104]

SUMMARY

The core principles of pneumonia diagnosis have not changed since 2018. However, the literature regarding diagnostic modalities and treatment strategies is rapidly changing. Keeping abreast of guidelines on CAP diagnosis and treatment is therefore critical for high-quality clinical care. Clinicians should consider specific challenges in certain populations (eg, pediatrics, geriatrics, and international travelers) as well as patient-specific risk factors when selecting empiric antimicrobial therapy.

DISCLOSURE

Dr K.M. Hunold is funded by the NIH under award K76AG074941 and R01AG071018. Dr N. Brummel is supported by the NIH under awards R01HD107103 and R01AG077644.

REFERENCES

1. Branch TAaHCS. National hospital Ambulatory medical care Survey: 2020 emergency department summary Tables. Centers for Disease Control; 2020.
2. Lim WS, Baudouin SV, George RC, et al. BTS guidelines for the management of community acquired pneumonia in adults: update 2009. Thorax 2009;64(Suppl 3). iii1-55.
3. Ramirez JA, Wiemken TL, Peyrani P, et al. Adults Hospitalized With Pneumonia in the United States: Incidence, Epidemiology, and Mortality. Clin Infect Dis 2017;65:1806–12.
4. Metlay JP, Waterer GW, Long AC, et al. Diagnosis and Treatment of Adults with Community-acquired Pneumonia. An Official Clinical Practice Guideline of the American Thoracic Society and Infectious Diseases Society of America. Am J Respir Crit Care Med 2019;200:e45–67.

5. Pneumonia ACoEPCPSWCoC-A. Critical Issues in the Management of Adult Patients Presenting to the Emergency Department With Community-Acquired Pneumonia. Ann Emerg Med 2020;77(1):e1–57.

6. Bradley JS, Byington CL, Shah SS, et al. The management of community-acquired pneumonia in infants and children older than 3 months of age: clinical practice guidelines by the Pediatric Infectious Diseases Society and the Infectious Diseases Society of America. Clin Infect Dis 2011;53:e25–76.

7. Martin-Loeches I, Torres A, Nagavci B, et al. Correction: ERS/ESICM/ESCMID/ALAT guidelines for the management of severe community-acquired pneumonia. Intensive Care Med 2023;49(8):1040–1.

8. Mandell LA, Niederman MS. Aspiration Pneumonia. N Engl J Med 2019;380:651–63.

9. Gleeson K, Eggli DF, Maxwell SL. Quantitative aspiration during sleep in normal subjects. Chest 1997;111:1266–72.

10. Burk M, El-Kersh K, Saad M, et al. Viral infection in community-acquired pneumonia: a systematic review and meta-analysis. Eur Respir Rev 2016;25:178–88.

11. Shoar S, Musher DM. Etiology of community-acquired pneumonia in adults: a systematic review. Pneumonia (Nathan) 2020;12:11.

12. Musher DM, Jesudasen SS, Barwatt JW, et al. Normal Respiratory Flora as a Cause of Community-Acquired Pneumonia. Open Forum Infect Dis 2020;7:ofaa307.

13. Gadsby NJ, Russell CD, McHugh MP, et al. Comprehensive Molecular Testing for Respiratory Pathogens in Community-Acquired Pneumonia. Clin Infect Dis 2016;62:817–23.

14. Jain S, Williams DJ, Arnold SR, et al. Community-acquired pneumonia requiring hospitalization among U.S. children. N Engl J Med 2015;372:835–45.

15. Jain S, Self WH, Wunderink RG, et al. Community-Acquired Pneumonia Requiring Hospitalization among U.S. Adults. N Engl J Med 2015;373:415–27.

16. Yang S, Lin S, Khalil A, et al. Quantitative PCR assay using sputum samples for rapid diagnosis of pneumococcal pneumonia in adult emergency department patients. J Clin Microbiol 2005;43:3221–6.

17. Bartlett JG, Mundy LM. Community-acquired pneumonia. N Engl J Med 1995;333:1618–24.

18. Marrie TJ. Community-acquired pneumonia. Clin Infect Dis 1994;18:501–13 [quiz 14-5].

19. Gelfer G, Leggett J, Myers J, et al. The clinical impact of the detection of potential etiologic pathogens of community-acquired pneumonia. Diagn Microbiol Infect Dis 2015;83:400–6.

20. Markussen DL, Ebbesen M, Serigstad S, et al. The diagnostic utility of microscopic quality assessment of sputum samples in the era of rapid syndromic PCR testing. Microbiol Spectr 2023;11:e0300223.

21. Ahmad FBCJ, Xu J, Anderson RN. COVID-19 Mortality Update — United States, 2022. MMWR Morb Mortal Wkly Rep 2023;493–6.

22. Rodriguez A, Moreno G, Gomez J, et al. Severe infection due to the SARS-CoV-2 coronavirus: Experience of a tertiary hospital with COVID-19 patients during the 2020 pandemic. Med Intensiva 2020;44(9):525–33.

23. Langford BJ, So M, Raybardhan S, et al. Bacterial co-infection and secondary infection in patients with COVID-19: a living rapid review and meta-analysis. Clin Microbiol Infect 2020;26:1622–9.

24. Russell CD, Fairfield CJ, Drake TM, et al. Co-infections, secondary infections, and antimicrobial use in patients hospitalised with COVID-19 during the first

pandemic wave from the ISARIC WHO CCP-UK study: a multicentre, prospective cohort study. Lancet Microbe 2021;2:e354–65.

25. Patton MJ, Orihuela CJ, Harrod KS, et al. COVID-19 bacteremic co-infection is a major risk factor for mortality, ICU admission, and mechanical ventilation. Crit Care 2023;27:34.

26. Brueggemann AB, Jansen van Rensburg MJ, Shaw D, et al. Changes in the incidence of invasive disease due to Streptococcus pneumoniae, Haemophilus influenzae, and Neisseria meningitidis during the COVID-19 pandemic in 26 countries and territories in the Invasive Respiratory Infection Surveillance Initiative: a prospective analysis of surveillance data. Lancet Digit Health 2021;3: e360–70.

27. Kalil AC, Thomas PG. Influenza virus-related critical illness: pathophysiology and epidemiology. Crit Care 2019;23:258.

28. Chadha M, Hirve S, Bancej C, et al. Human respiratory syncytial virus and influenza seasonality patterns-Early findings from the WHO global respiratory syncytial virus surveillance. Influenza Other Respir Viruses 2020;14:638–46.

29. Chung JR, Rolfes MA, Flannery B, et al. Effects of Influenza Vaccination in the United States During the 2018-2019 Influenza Season. Clin Infect Dis 2020;71: e368–76.

30. Leuchter RK, Jackson NJ, Mafi JN, et al. Association between Covid-19 Vaccination and Influenza Vaccination Rates. N Engl J Med 2022;386:2531–2.

31. Gentilotti E, De Nardo P, Cremonini E, et al. Diagnostic accuracy of point-of-care tests in acute community-acquired lower respiratory tract infections. A systematic review and meta-analysis. Clin Microbiol Infect 2022;28:13–22.

32. Wootton D, Feldman C. The diagnosis of pneumonia requires a chest radiograph (x-ray)-yes, no or sometimes? Pneumonia (Nathan) 2014;5:1–7.

33. Gezer NS, Balci P, Tuna KC, et al. Utility of chest CT after a chest X-ray in patients presenting to the ED with non-traumatic thoracic emergencies. Am J Emerg Med 2017;35:623–7.

34. Claessens YE, Debray MP, Tubach F, et al. Early Chest Computed Tomography Scan to Assist Diagnosis and Guide Treatment Decision for Suspected Community-acquired Pneumonia. Am J Respir Crit Care Med 2015;192:974–82.

35. Kroft LJM, van der Velden L, Giron IH, et al. Added Value of Ultra-low-dose Computed Tomography, Dose Equivalent to Chest X-Ray Radiography, for Diagnosing Chest Pathology. J Thorac Imaging 2019;34:179–86.

36. van den Berk IAH, Kanglie M, van Engelen TSR, et al. Ultra-low-dose CT versus chest X-ray for patients suspected of pulmonary disease at the emergency department: a multicentre randomised clinical trial. Thorax 2023;78:515–22.

37. Bouam M, Binquet C, Moretto F, et al. Delayed diagnosis of pneumonia in the emergency department: factors associated and prognosis. Front Med 2023; 10:1042704.

38. Claessens YE, Berthier F, Baque-Juston M, et al. Early chest CT-scan in emergency patients affected by community-acquired pneumonia is associated with improved diagnosis consistency. Eur J Emerg Med 2022;29:417–20.

39. Seo H, Cha SI, Shin KM, et al. Community-Acquired Pneumonia with Negative Chest Radiography Findings: Clinical and Radiological Features. Respiration 2019;97:508–17.

40. Buhumaid RE, St-Cyr Bourque J, Shokoohi H, et al. Integrating point-of-care ultrasound in the ED evaluation of patients presenting with chest pain and shortness of breath. Am J Emerg Med 2019;37:298–303.

41. Pagano A, Numis FG, Visone G, et al. Lung ultrasound for diagnosis of pneumonia in emergency department. Intern Emerg Med 2015;10:851–4.

42. Murali A, Prakash A, Dixit R, et al. Lung Ultrasound: A Complementary Imaging Tool for Chest X-Ray in the Evaluation of Dyspnea. Indian J Radiol Imaging 2023; 33:162–72.

43. Zhang D, Yang D, Makam AN. Utility of Blood Cultures in Pneumonia. Am J Med 2019;132:1233–8.

44. Joint Commission. Specifications manual for national hospital inpatient quality measures. 2024. Available at: https://www.jointcommission.org/measurement/specification-manuals/chart-abstracted-measures/.). [Accessed 31 January 2024].

45. Cartuliares MB, Rosenvinge FS, Mogensen CB, et al. Expiratory Technique versus Tracheal Suction to Obtain Good-Quality Sputum from Patients with Suspected Lower Respiratory Tract Infection: A Randomized Controlled Trial. Diagnostics 2022;12.

46. Cartuliares MB, Sundal LM, Gustavsson S, et al. Limited value of sputum culture to guide antibiotic treatment in a Danish emergency department. Dan Med J 2020;67.

47. Kim P, Deshpande A, Rothberg MB. Urinary Antigen Testing for Respiratory Infections: Current Perspectives on Utility and Limitations. Infect Drug Resist 2022;15:2219–28.

48. van der Eerden MM, Vlaspolder F, de Graaff CS, et al. Comparison between pathogen directed antibiotic treatment and empirical broad spectrum antibiotic treatment in patients with community acquired pneumonia: a prospective randomised study. Thorax 2005;60:672–8.

49. Piso RJ, Iven-Koller D, Koller MT, et al. The routine use of urinary pneumococcal antigen test in hospitalised patients with community acquired pneumonia has limited impact for adjustment of antibiotic treatment. Swiss Med Wkly 2012; 142:w13679.

50. Wheat LJ, Knox KS, Hage CA. Approach to the diagnosis of histoplasmosis, blastomycosis and coccidioidomycosis. Curr Treat Options Infect Dis 2014;6: 337–51.

51. Katz SE, Williams DJ. Pediatric community-acquired pneumonia in the united states: changing epidemiology, diagnostic and therapeutic challenges, and areas for future research. Infect Dis Clin North Am 2018;32:47–63.

52. Self WH, Williams DJ, Zhu Y, et al. Respiratory viral detection in children and adults: comparing asymptomatic controls and patients with community-acquired pneumonia. J Infect Dis 2016;213:584–91.

53. Serigstad S, Knoop ST, Markussen DL, et al. Diagnostic utility of oropharyngeal swabs as an alternative to lower respiratory tract samples for PCR-based syndromic testing in patients with community-acquired pneumonia. J Clin Microbiol 2023;61:e0050523.

54. Mergenhagen KA, Starr KE, Wattengel BA, et al. Determining the utility of methicillin-Resistant Staphylococcus aureus nares screening in antimicrobial stewardship. Clin Infect Dis 2020;71:1142–8.

55. Smith MN, Brotherton AL, Lusardi K, et al. Systematic review of the clinical utility of methicillin-resistant Staphylococcus aureus (MRSA) nasal screening for MRSA Pneumonia. Ann Pharmacother 2019;53:627–38.

56. Tsalik EL, Rouphael NG, Sadikot RT, et al. Efficacy and safety of azithromycin versus placebo to treat lower respiratory tract infections associated with low

procalcitonin: a randomised, placebo-controlled, double-blind, non-inferiority trial. Lancet Infect Dis 2023;23:484–95.

57. Sivapalan P, Jensen JS. Procalcitonin to reduce antimicrobial overuse in patients with lower respiratory tract infection: time for re-evaluation of our prescription culture? Lancet Infect Dis 2023;23:390–1.

58. Huang DT, Yealy DM, Angus DC, et al. Longer-Term Outcomes of the ProACT Trial. N Engl J Med 2020;382:485–6.

59. Huang DT, Yealy DM, Filbin MR, et al. Procalcitonin-Guided Use of Antibiotics for Lower Respiratory Tract Infection. N Engl J Med 2018;379:236–49.

60. Pulia MS, Schulz LT, Fox BC. Procalcitonin-Guided Antibiotic Use. N Engl J Med 2018;379:1971–2.

61. Pepper DJ, Sun J, Rhee C, et al. Procalcitonin-Guided Antibiotic Discontinuation and Mortality in Critically Ill Adults: A Systematic Review and Meta-analysis. Chest 2019;155:1109–18.

62. Schuetz P, Wirz Y, Sager R, et al. Procalcitonin to initiate or discontinue antibiotics in acute respiratory tract infections. Cochrane Database Syst Rev 2017; 10:CD007498.

63. Novak D, Masoudi A, Shaukat B, et al. MeMed BV testing in emergency department patients presenting with febrile illness concerning for respiratory tract infection. Am J Emerg Med 2023;65:195–9.

64. Fine MJ, Auble TE, Yealy DM, et al. A prediction rule to identify low-risk patients with community-acquired pneumonia. N Engl J Med 1997;336:243–50.

65. Lim WS, van der Eerden MM, Laing R, et al. Defining community acquired pneumonia severity on presentation to hospital: an international derivation and validation study. Thorax 2003;58:377–82.

66. Miyashita N, Matsushima T, Oka M, et al. The JRS guidelines for the management of community-acquired pneumonia in adults: an update and new recommendations. Intern Med 2006;45:419–28.

67. Limapichat T, Supavajana S. Comparison between the Severity Scoring Systems A-DROP and CURB-65 for Predicting Safe Discharge from the Emergency Department in Patients with Community-Acquired Pneumonia. Emerg Med Int 2022;2022:6391141.

68. Ferrari R, Viale P, Muratori P, et al. Rebounds after discharge from the emergency department for community-acquired pneumonia: focus on the usefulness of severity scoring systems. Acta Biomed 2018;88:519–28.

69. Sharp AL, Jones JP, Wu I, et al. CURB-65 Performance Among Admitted and Discharged Emergency Department Patients With Community-acquired Pneumonia. Acad Emerg Med 2016;23:400–5.

70. Nascimento-Carvalho CM. Community-acquired pneumonia among children: the latest evidence for an updated management. J Pediatr 2020;96(Suppl 1): 29–38.

71. Shah SN, Bachur RG, Simel DL, et al. Does This Child Have Pneumonia?: The Rational Clinical Examination Systematic Review. JAMA 2017;318:462–71.

72. McLaren SH, Mistry RD, Neuman MI, et al. Guideline Adherence in Diagnostic Testing and Treatment of Community-Acquired Pneumonia in Children. Pediatr Emerg Care 2021;37:485–93.

73. Ramgopal S, Aronson PL, Marin JR. United States' Emergency Department Visits for Fever by Young Children 2007-2017. West J Emerg Med 2020;21: 146–51.

74. Morimoto K, Suzuki M, Ishifuji T, et al. The burden and etiology of community-onset pneumonia in the aging Japanese population: a multicenter prospective study. PLoS One 2015;10:e0122247.

75. Olasupo O, Xiao H, Brown JD. Relative Clinical and Cost Burden of Community-Acquired Pneumonia Hospitalizations in Older Adults in the United States-A Cross-Sectional Analysis. Vaccines (Basel) 2018;6.

76. Yealy DM, Auble TE, Stone RA, et al. The emergency department community-acquired pneumonia trial: Methodology of a quality improvement intervention. Ann Emerg Med 2004;43:770–82.

77. Chandra A, Nicks B, Maniago E, et al. A multicenter analysis of the ED diagnosis of pneumonia. Am J Emerg Med 2010;28:862–5.

78. Hunold KM, Schwaderer AL, Exline M, et al. Diagnosing Dyspneic Older Adult Emergency Department Patients: A Pilot Study. Acad Emerg Med 2020;28(6): 675–8.

79. Metlay JP, Schulz R, Li YH, et al. Influence of age on symptoms at presentation in patients with community-acquired pneumonia. Arch Intern Med 1997;157: 1453–9.

80. Grosmaitre P, Le Vavasseur O, Yachouh E, et al. Significance of atypical symptoms for the diagnosis and management of myocardial infarction in elderly patients admitted to emergency departments. Arch Cardiovasc Dis 2013;106: 586–92.

81. Thompson L, Wood C, Wallhagen M. Geriatric acute myocardial infarction: a challenge to recognition, prompt diagnosis, and appropriate care. Crit Care Nurs Clin North Am 1992;4:291–9.

82. Woon VC, Lim KH. Acute myocardial infarction in the elderly–the differences compared with the young. Singapore Med J 2003;44:414–8.

83. Limpawattana P, Phungoen P, Mitsungnern T, et al. Atypical presentations of older adults at the emergency department and associated factors. Arch Gerontol Geriatr 2016;62:97–102.

84. Peters M. The older adult in the emergency department: aging and atypical illness presentation. J Emerg Nurs 2010;36:29–34.

85. Bourcier JE, Paquet J, Seinger M, et al. Performance comparison of lung ultrasound and chest x-ray for the diagnosis of pneumonia in the ED. Am J Emerg Med 2014;32:115–8.

86. Banerjee S. Multimorbidity–older adults need health care that can count past one. Lancet 2015;385:587–9.

87. Dharmarajan K, Strait KM, Tinetti ME, et al. Treatment for Multiple Acute Cardiopulmonary Conditions in Older Adults Hospitalized with Pneumonia, Chronic Obstructive Pulmonary Disease, or Heart Failure. J Am Geriatr Soc 2016;64: 1574–82.

88. Loeb M, Bentley DW, Bradley S, et al. Development of minimum criteria for the initiation of antibiotics in residents of long-term-care facilities: results of a consensus conference. Infect Control Hosp Epidemiol 2001;22:120–4.

89. Stone ND, Ashraf MS, Calder J, et al. Surveillance definitions of infections in long-term care facilities: revisiting the McGeer criteria. Infect Control Hosp Epidemiol 2012;33:965–77.

90. Henig O, Kaye KS. Bacterial Pneumonia in Older Adults. Infect Dis Clin North Am 2017;31:689–713.

91. Duong TN, Waldman SE. Importance of a Travel History in Evaluation of Respiratory Infections. Curr Emerg Hosp Med Rep 2016;4:141–52.

92. Trimble A, Moffat V, Collins AM. Pulmonary infections in the returned traveller. Pneumonia (Nathan) 2017;9:1.
93. General Approach to the Returned Traveler. 2023. (Accessed October 2023, Available at: https://wwwnc.cdc.gov/travel/yellowbook/2024/posttravel-evaluation/general-approach-to-the-returned-traveler.)
94. Ramirez JA, Musher DM, Evans SE, et al. Treatment of Community-Acquired Pneumonia in Immunocompromised Adults: A Consensus Statement Regarding Initial Strategies. Chest 2020;158:1896–911.
95. Manabe T, Teramoto S, Tamiya N, et al. Risk Factors for Aspiration Pneumonia in Older Adults. PLoS One 2015;10:e0140060.
96. Marrie TJ. Epidemiology of community-acquired pneumonia in the elderly. Semin Respir Infect 1990;5:260–8.
97. Makhnevich A, Feldhamer KH, Kast CL, et al. Aspiration Pneumonia in Older Adults. J Hosp Med 2019;14:429–35.
98. Yoshimatsu Y, Aga M, Komiya K, et al. The Clinical Significance of Anaerobic Coverage in the Antibiotic Treatment of Aspiration Pneumonia: A Systematic Review and Meta-Analysis. J Clin Med 2023;12.
99. FDA In Brief. FDA warns that fluoroquinolone antibiotics can cause aortic aneurysm in certain patients. U.S. Food & Drug Administration, 2018. 2023. Available at: https://www.fda.gov/news-events/fda-brief/fda-brief-fda-warns-fluoroquinolone-antibiotics-can-cause-aortic-aneurysm-certain-patients.). [Accessed 20 October 2023].
100. Frazee BW, Singh A, Labreche M, et al. Methicillin-resistant Staphylococcus aureus and Pseudomonas aeruginosa community acquired pneumonia: Prevalence and locally derived risk factors in a single hospital system. J Am Coll Emerg Physicians Open 2023;4:e13061.
101. Haessler S, Guo N, Deshpande A, et al. Etiology, Treatments, and Outcomes of Patients With Severe Community-Acquired Pneumonia in a Large U.S. Sample. Crit Care Med 2022;50:1063–71.
102. Dequin PF, Meziani F, Quenot JP, et al. Hydrocortisone in Severe Community-Acquired Pneumonia. N Engl J Med 2023;388:1931–41.
103. GU Meduri, Shih MC, Bridges L, et al. Low-dose methylprednisolone treatment in critically ill patients with severe community-acquired pneumonia. Intensive Care Med 2022;48:1009–23.
104. Williams DJ, Creech CB, Walter EB, et al. Short- vs Standard-Course Outpatient Antibiotic Therapy for Community-Acquired Pneumonia in Children: The SCOUT-CAP Randomized Clinical Trial. JAMA Pediatr 2022;176:253–61.
105. Fluoroquinolone Antimicrobial Drugs Information. U.S. Food & Drug Adminisration 2018. 2023. Available at: https://www.fda.gov/drugs/information-drug-class/fluoroquinolone-antimicrobial-drugs-information.). [Accessed 29 June 2023].

Orthopedic Articular and Periarticular Joint Infections

Pim Jetanalin, MD[a],*, Yanint Raksadawan, MD[b],
Pholaphat Charles Inboriboon, MD, MPH[c]

KEYWORDS

- Septic arthritis • Septic bursitis • Prosthetic joint infection • Monoarticular arthritis

KEY POINTS

- Septic arthritis is a "cannot miss" diagnosis of acute nontraumatic joint pain.
- Synovial fluid analysis must be interpreted in the context of a patient's risk factors.
- Diagnosing prosthetic joint infections requires a high index of suspicion given its varied presentation.
- All patients with suspected septic arthritis or prosthetic joint infections should be admitted and orthopedics surgery should be consulted.

INTRODUCTION

Acute joint pain is commonly seen in the emergency department. The emergency physician must be adept in recognizing and treating the various causes of acute joint pain (**Box 1** differential diagnosis). Septic arthritis is an orthopedic emergency. If not promptly treated, it can result in serious complications including joint destruction and systemic infection that can lead to death.

The prevalence of septic arthritis is 2 to 10 in 100,000 in the general population.[1–4] Those in the extremes of ages: the first decade of life and the sixth decade of life are at the highest risk.[5–7] Patient-specific risk factors include injection drug use (IDU),[8] hemodialysis (HD),[8] immunocompromised states,[8] using immmunomodulators,[8] diabetes mellitus (DM),[5] and rheumatoid arthritis (RA; **Table 1** risk factors).[1,6] Joint-specific risk factors include pre-existing joint disease,[8] recent trauma,[5,6] previous articular procedures,[8] and periarticular soft tissue infection.[8] The most frequently identified pathogens are *Staphylococcus aureus* (54%–55%)[5,6,9] and *Streptococcus*

[a] Department Medicine, Division of Rheumatology, University of Illinois at College of Medicine, 818 South Wolcott Avenue, 6th Floor, MC 733, Chicago, IL 60612, USA; [b] Department of Medicine, Weiss Memorial Hospital, Medical Education, 4646 N. Marine Drive, Chicago, IL 60640, USA; [c] Department of Emergency Medicine, University of Illinois at College of Medicine, 808 South Wood Street MC 724, Chicago, IL, USA
* Corresponding author.
E-mail address: pimlin@uic.edu

Emerg Med Clin N Am 42 (2024) 249–265
https://doi.org/10.1016/j.emc.2024.01.002
0733-8627/24/Published by Elsevier Inc.

emed.theclinics.com

Box 1
Differential diagnosis of acute joint pain

Differential diagnosis for acute joint pain
  Trauma
    Fracture
    Hemarthrosis
    Periarticular injury/internal derangement
  Infectious
    Septic arthritis
    Disseminated gonoccocal infection
    Septic bursitis
    Transient synovitis
    Lyme arthritis
  Crystalline diseases
    Gout
    Calcium pyrophosphate dihydrate deposition disease
    Basic calcium phosphate
    Hydroxyapatite deposition disease
    Calcium oxalate deposition disease
  Inflammatory arthritis
    Atypical presentation/early presentation of polyarticular arthritis
    Spondyloarthropathy
    Juvenile idiopathic arthritis
    Palindromic rheumatism
  Other
    Pigmented villonodular synovitis
    Lipoma arborescens
    Synovial osteochondromatosis
    Synovioma/sarcoma/metastatic disease
    Neuropathic (Charcot joint)

---

spp (7.5%).[5,6] Methicillin-resistant *S aureus* (MRSA) accounts for 23% to 50% of isolates in contemporary case series.(Frazee 5)[90] Septic arthritis most commonly from hematogenous seeding but can also occur through local inoculation. Hence, a focused yet comprehensive history and physical examination are essential to diagnosing septic arthritis and the potential pathogen.

CLINICAL PRESENTATION

Patients typically present with acute onset joint pain, swelling, and limited range of motion. Joint pain (85%) and swelling (78%) are the most sensitive symptoms.[10] Patients

---

Table 1
Risk factors for septic arthritis

Patient-Specific Risk Factors	Local Risk Factors
• Immunocompromised states	• Pre-existing joint disease
• Using immunomodulators	• Previous articular procedures
• IDU	• Recent trauma
• HD	• Adjacent soft tissue infection
• DM	• Cutaneous ulcer
• RA	
• Extreme ages	
• Occupational risk factors	

may experience constitutional symptoms such as fever, sweats, and rigor. However, lack of these symptoms does not rule out septic arthritis as only 40% to 75% of patients have fever,[6,9–11] and 27% and 19% have sweats and rigor, respectively.[10]

The majority of patients with septic arthritis present with monoarticular arthritis. However, up to 22% have more than one joint involvement.[12] Therefore, septic arthritis cannot be excluded based on the number of joints affected.[12] Large joints are the most commonly affected, with knees representing more than 50% of cases.[5,6,8] Other commonly affected joints include the hip and shoulder. A history of IDU is a risk factor for septic arthritis involving fibrocartilaginous joints, such as the sacroiliac joint, sternoclavicular joint, or intervertebral disk.[13]

Risk factors for septic arthritis should be sought. In addition to IDU, these include pre-existing inflammatory joint diseases, such as RA and gout, a recent joint procedure and an immunosuppressed state, including use of immunosuppressive therapy and underlying systemic disease, including diabetes milletus, including diabetes. In patients with underlying inflammatory joint conditions, particularly RA, strongly consider septic arthritis if the patient develops new onset of acute arthritis in the setting of well-controlled disease, has a change in their typical flare pattern, or presents with constitutional symptoms. Maintain a high index of suspicion in patients who are immunocompromised, have prosthetic joints, or are infected with atypical organisms because they may present with a more insidious course.

Special Populations

Immunocompromised hosts

Immunocompromised hosts, such as patients with acquired immunodeficiency syndrome and patients who require immunosuppressive medications may present atypically with septic arthritis. Patients may have a chronic indolent course with pain for months rather than an acute onset.[14,15] Some may present without the typical physical examination findings such as joint swelling and only present with pain and range of motion (ROM) limitation.[16] Some may present with an infection due to more than one pathogen.[17]

These patients are also prone to infections due to rare pathogens. Septic arthritis may be the first manifestation of a disseminated infection with a rare pathogen, such as Listeria monocytogenes,[1] Mycobacterium avium complex,[18] Histoplasma capsulatum,[19] Aspergillus fumigatus,[20] Brucella spp,[21] Salmonella enteritidis,[22] Mycoplasma pneumoniae,[23] or Blastomyces dermatitidis[14] (Fig. 1). This wide variety of potential pathogens underscores the importance of obtaining synovial fluid cultures.

Underlying rheumatologic disease

Patients with certain underlying rheumatologic conditions also have an increased risk for septic arthritis, both because of immunosuppressive medications and pre-existing joint pathology. Other risk factors that increase risk in this patient population include older age, male sex, HTN, DM, and seropositive RA diagnosis.[24] Tumor necrosis factor inhibitors, which are one of the most widely used biologics in RA and spondyloarthropathies, have been shown to increase the risk of septic arthritis.[24,25] In contrast to the general population, a retrospective study found that the most common pathogen for septic arthritis in patients with SLE was Salmonella, followed by Mycobacterium, and then S aureus.[26] High-dose steroids in patients with systemic lupus erythematosus were found to be a predisposing factor for salmonella infection.[27]

Physical examination

The affected joint should be exposed and assessed. Generalized tenderness, erythema, warmth, and pain with both passive and active range of motion should increase

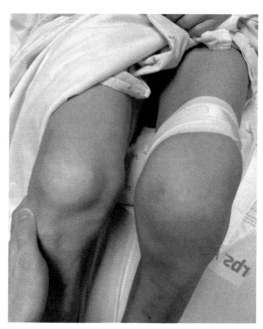

Fig. 1. A 64 year old man with a history liver transplant on immunosuppressive therapy presented with subacute onset of left knee pain, swelling, and decreased ROM. Patient was found to have disseminated blastomycosis.

your suspicion for septic arthritis. On the contrary, in periarticular pathology (ie, tendinitis, bursitis, and periarticular gout), range of motion is relatively preserved and pain only occurs during active ROM. Swelling, point of tenderness, and erythema are typically more localized.[28]

In addition to a focused joint examination, a focused physical examination including a skin examination looking for lesions, pustules, wounds, cellulitis, and other skin or soft tissue infections should be performed. In patients with fibrocartilaginous joint infections, patients should be examined for other sources of infection, such as skin abscess and infectious endocarditis.

Diagnostic tests

Diagnosis can be challenging due to lack of both reliable and specific laboratory and imaging findings. Patients may have leukocytosis or elevated acute phase reactants. C-reactive protein (CRP) is of particular diagnostic value because it is more sensitive than the white blood cell (WBC) count or erythrocyte sedimentation rate (ESR).[6,9] Only two-thirds of patients with septic arthritis have a leukocytosis greater than 11,000 cells/mm^3.[6,11] It is important to note that these laboratory values are nonspecific and can be seen in other types of inflammatory arthritis as well as in nonjoint infections such as osteomyelitis and bursitis.

In early septic arthritis, plain radiographs may be normal or it may reveal periarticular osteopenia, soft tissue swelling, and effusions.[29,30] In advanced disease, there can be joint space narrowing, nonspecific erosion, and destruction.[29,31] CT and MRI are more sensitive in detecting soft tissue changes[30] and can help identify which anatomic compartment is affected.[32] MRI is the most sensitive modality for detecting inflammatory arthritis, including septic arthritis. Early in the disease process, joint effusion and synovial inflammation is seen. This is followed by early marrow signal abnormality and subsequent cartilage loss and subchondral bone erosion.[33] Ultrasound can help detect joint effusions that may be missed by plain radiographs.[34] In the case of hip ultrasounds, the lack of an effusion has a high negative predictive value for septic arthritis.[35] Additionally, it can be used as a point-of-care tool to guide joint aspiration.[36,37]

ARTHROCENTESIS AND SYNOVIAL FLUID ANALYSIS

Arthrocentesis should be performed in all patients with suspected septic arthritis. It can be performed using anatomic landmarks or with the assistance of imaging modalities such as ultrasound and fluoroscopy. Needle aspiration through overlying cellulitis is generally contraindicated; however, some advocate going through infected skin when it cannot be avoided given the risk of delayed diagnosis and treatment.[10] In cases in which arthrocentesis does not yield an adequate amount of fluid, sterile saline can be used to irrigate the joint to obtain fluid for gram stain and culture analysis.[38]

Synovial fluid analysis is an essential diagnostic test in the evaluation of possible septic arthritis. Synovial fluid should be sent for cell count with differential, gram stain, culture, and crystal analysis. Gram stain is positive in about half of patients with septic arthritis. Cultures are considered the gold standard but are only positive in 71% of patients with native joints infections and in 82% of patients with prosthetic joints infections.[11] Given the relatively low yield of gram stains and that culture results are not immediately available, synovial cell count is essential for determining the likelihood of septic arthritis. The likelihood ratio of having septic arthritis increases with an increasing synovial fluid WBC count[10] (**Tables 2** and **3**). Patients with synovial WBC count greater than 50,000 cells/mm^3 should be treated empirically for septic arthritis. Immunocompromised patients may have a lower than expected synovial WBC count.[39] It is important to note that crystalline disease (gout and calcium pyrophosphate disease) with or without acute flare can coexist with septic arthritis. Therefore, the presence of crystals does not rule out septic arthritis.[40]

Treatment

Patients with suspected septic arthritis should be admitted and orthopedics should be consulted. Immediate orthopedic consult is particularly crucial in suspected prosthetic joint infection (PJI). In clinically uncertain cases, patients should be admitted for close monitoring and further evaluation while awaiting culture results.

Treatment of septic arthritis includes both antibiotics and removal of infected synovial fluid. Empiric antibiotic selection is guided by the results of gram stain, patient risk

Table 2	
Synovial cell count and likelihood of septic arthritis	
Synovial Fluid WBC Count	**Likelihood Ratio**
WBC <25,000	0.32
WBC >25,000	2.9
WBC >50,000	7.7
WBC >100,000	28
Synovial PMN >90%	3.4
Synovial PMN <90%	0.34

Table 3
Diagnostic characteristics of synovial fluid

Characteristics of Synovial Fluid	Normal	Noninflammatory	Bacterial Septic Arthritis	Disseminated Gonococcal Infection	PJI
Appearance	Transparent	Transparent	Cloudy	Cloudy	—
Viscosity	High	High	Variable	Variable	—
WBC count (cells/mm^3)	<200	200–2000	2000–>50,000	13,000–100,000	>10,000 in early onset >3000 in late onset
Neutrophils (%)	<10	<10	>90	90	>90 in acute >80 in chronic
Gram stain	Negative	Negative	Positive	<50% showing intracellular and extracellular gram-negative diplococci	Positive
Culture	Negative	Negative	Positive	<50% of cases	Positive

factors, and the list of common causative pathogens (**Table 4**). For patients in communities with high MRSA prevalence, known MRSA colonization, or other risk factors for MRSA infection, vancomycin is recommended.[39,41] Cefazolin is recommended for patients at low risk for MRSA.[39] Immunocompromised, elderly, or IDU populations are at risk for gram-negative infections, particularly *Pseudomonas aeruginosa*, and addition of an antipseudomonal beta-lactam such as cefepime or piperacillin-tazobactam should be considered.[39,41] There is no consensus on the duration of antibiotic therapy, with recommendations ranging from 2 to 6 weeks, including step-down oral antibiotics.[39] Clinical improvement and acute phase reactants can be used to assess response to treatment and duration of therapy.[42]

In addition to establishing the diagnosis of septic arthritis, arthrocentesis aids in treatment, decreasing the organism load, inflammatory mediators,[43] and intra-articular pressures that can lead to localized joint destruction. Patients can be treated medically with serial arthrocentesis or surgically with arthroscopy or open arthrotomy. Though there is a higher rate of treatment failure in patients treated with serial arthrocentesis, patients that undergo surgery tend to have longer hospital stays, are less likely to achieve full recovery, and are more likely to have residual joint deformities.[44,45] Patients with underlying joint disease, abscess formation, positive synovial culture, hip joint involvement, or osteomyelitis are more likely to require surgical treatment.[46]

Prosthetic Joint Infection

PJI is a feared complication of joint replacement that causes significant morbidity and mortality and is the most common cause of total knee arthroplasty failure.[47] PJI has an incident rate of 1.4% to 1.7%.[48,49] The prevalence of PJI has increased 2.5-fold from 2005 to 2013 in primary knee replacements, and 7.5-fold in revision knee replacements.[50] Risk factors for developing PJI include male sex,[48] young age,[48] type 2 DM,[48] posttraumatic arthritis,[48] patellar resurfacing,[48] discharge to a convalescent home,[48] malnutrition,[51] morbid obesity,[51] immunocompromised state,[51] preoperative anemia,[52] and *S aureus* colonization.[51]

Table 4
Empiric antibiotic regimens for patients with suspected septic arthritis

Synovial Fluid Gram Stain	Antibiotic Coverage	Dose
Gram-positive cocci in clusters (presumed *Staphylococcus*)	Cefazolin	2 g IV every 8 h
Gram-positive cocci in clusters (presumed MRSA in high-prevalence area)	Vancomycin	1 g IV every 12 h
Gram-positive cocci in chains (presumed *Streptococcus*)	Cefazolin	2 g IV every 8 h
Gram-negative diplococci (presumed gonococcus) or clinical presentation suggestive of disseminated gonoccal infection	Ceftriaxone +Azithromycin	1 g IV every 24 h 1 g PO (single dose)
Gram-negative bacilli	Cefepime or Piperacillin-tazobactam	2 g IV every 8 h or 4.5 g IV every 6 h

In the absence of an organism on gram stain, consider vancomycin 1 g IV every 12 h (cefazolin may be used in patients at low risk for MRSA in a low prevalence area). An antipseudomonal beta-lactam, such as cefepime or piperacillin-tazobactam, should be added in the elderly, immunocompromised, critically ill, or intravenous drug users.

John J Ross. Septic Arthritis of Native Joints. Infect Dis Clin North Am. 2017 Jun;31(2):203-218.[39]

The most common pathogens are *S aureus* and coagulase-negative *Staphylococcus*.[52–54] *Candida* infection has been reported in patients with systemic autoimmune diseases and in those who are immunocompromised or have chronic diseases such as renal disease.[55]

PJI can be divided into 3 categories, by time of onset: early (<3 months), delayed (3–12 months), and late (>12 months; **Table 5**). Early infection is typically caused by relatively virulent pathogens introduced during surgery, including *S aureus* and gram-negative bacteria. Delayed infection is usually caused by less virulent pathogens introduced during surgery. Late PJI often occurs through hematogenous seeding of the prosthetic joint from a remote source of infection.[53]

In addition to the classic symptoms of septic arthritis, features that are highly suspicious for PJI include persistent drainage from operative wound, the presence of a sinus tract, acute onset of pain over a prosthetic joint that was previously asymptomatic, and persistent pain after joint replacement without a pain-free period.[56] An orthopedic specialist should be consulted immediately in patients with suspected PJI.

Plain x-rays of the prosthetic joint may be of limited diagnostic utility in suspected PJI because radiographic findings may lag by 1 to 2 weeks from the onset of clinical findings. MRI is a more sensitive imaging modality, but it may be limited by metal artifact from the prosthetic joint.[57]

Synovial WBC elevation is not able to differentiate between infectious and other inflammatory arthropathies.[57,58] Preoperative synovial aspiration culture (bedside arthrocentesis of the infected joint) is positive in only 45.2% of knee PJI and 44.4% of hip PJI.[59] It cannot be used alone to rule out PJI because the false-negative rate is as high as 20.7% in knee PJI and 15% in hip PJI.[59]

The 2018 definition of periprosthetic hip and knee infection criteria has a sensitivity and specificity of 97.7% and 99.5% (**Fig. 2**: PJI Diagnostic Criteria).[60] PJI is diagnosed

Table 5
Characteristic of prosthetic joint infection based upon onset

Time to Infection After Implantation	Early Onset	Delayed Onset (3–12 mo)	Late Onset
Synovial fluid			
WBC (cells/µL)	>10,000	>3000	>3000
Neutrophils (%)	>90	>80	>80
Clinical symptoms	Wound drainage, erythema, joint pain, fever	Possible sinus tract formation, subacute joint pain	Systemic symptoms with bacteremia, pain
Serum ESR (mm/h)	Not useful	>30	>30
Serum CRP (mg/L)	>100	>10	>10
Common pathogens	Virulent organisms: S aureus Aerobic gram-negative bacilli Polymicrobial Anaerobic	Low virulence organisms: Coagulase-negative staphylococci Enterococcus, Cutibacterium	S aureus β-Hemolytic streptococci Gram-negative bacilli

Modified from Beam E, Osmon D. Prosthetic Joint Infection Update. Infect Dis Clin North Am. 2018;32(4):843-859. https://doi.org/10.1016/j.idc.2018.06.005.[53]

when 1 of 2 major criteria is present, or scoring 6 or more based on minor criteria. Major criteria are 2 positive cultures growing the same organism and the presence of a sinus tract with evidence of communication to the joint, including visualization of the prosthesis. Minor criteria are based on serum and synovial fluid testing. Serum ESR, CRP, and d-dimer should be ordered and synovial cell count with differential and synovial CRP and alpha-defensin should be obtained. Synovial fluid alpha-defensin has high sensitivity and specificity for PJI.[60,61]

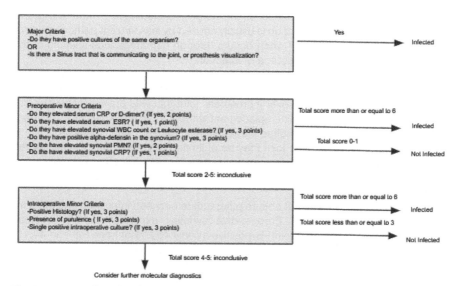

Fig. 2. A scoring-based definition for periprosthetic joint infection (PJI).

When patients are clinically stable, the The Infectious Diseases Society of America (IDSA) recommends withholding antimicrobial therapy for at least 2 weeks to increase the likelihood of positive culture.[62] Definitive PJI treatment requires antibiotic therapy plus surgical debridement or joint replacement. A 12 week course of oral antibiotic therapy decreases the risk of treatment failure.[63,64]

Gonococcal Arthritis (Disseminated Gonococcal Infection)

Gonococcal arthritis is seen predominantly in sexually active young adults with a 3:1 female predominance.[65] It is postulated that localized infections in female individuals are typically asymptomatic, which leads to delayed diagnosis and progression to disseminated infection.[66] Gonococcal arthritis classically presents as a triad of migratory polyarthritis, tenosynovitis, and skin lesions. However, only about a quarter of patients present with all of these symptoms.[67] Patients may present with migratory polyarthralgias or polyarthritis. True arthritis is only present in 50% of patients, and commonly affected joints include the knee, ankle, elbow, and wrist. Tenosynovitis is typically noted in the wrist, ankles, finger, or toe joints. Dermatitis is present in about 75% of patients and is often present on the extremities as nonpainful nonpruritic macules, papules, pustules, or vesicles (**Fig. 3**). Lesions are rarely noted on the face.[65,66,68]

Synovial fluid WBC count is typically lower than in classic septic arthritis, ranging from 13,000 to 100,000 with neutrophil predominance.[67] *Neisseria gonorrhoeae* is identified by gram stain in about half of confirmed cases of gonococcal arthritis, and synovial cultures are positive in less than half of cases.[65] Synovial nucleic acid amplification tests (NAAT) can detect infection in synovial fluid, although this test is neither widely available nor standardized.[65] In addition to the traditional septic arthritis evaluation, a comprehensive sexual history should be obtained in patients with suspected gonoccocal arthritis, with cultures or NAAT of multiple mucosal sites (oropharyngeal, cervical, urethral, and anorectal) recommended. Upward of 80% of patients with gonococcal arthritis are diagnosed based on clinical presentation and nonsynovial, mucosal NAAT, or cultures.[66] Blood cultures are positive in less than 50%, and cultures of skin lesions have a very low yield.

With early recognition and prompt treatment, 95% of patients will have a full recovery.[69] The Centers for Disease Control and Prevention recommends hospitalization and infectious disease consultation for the treatment of gonoccocal arthritis. The initial recommended treatment is ceftriaxone 1 g intravenously (IV) or intramuscularly every 24 hours. An

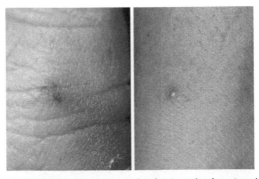

Fig. 3. Skin lesions in disseminated gonococcal infection. (Joshua Landy, Dennis Djogovic, Wendy Sligl, Gonococcal septic shock, acute respiratory distress syndrome, and multisystem organ failure: a case report, International Journal of Infectious Diseases, 14, Suppl 3, 2010, e239-e241, https://doi.org/10.1016/j.ijid.2009.08.021.)

alternative option is either cefotaxime 1 g IV every 8 hours or ceftizoxime 1 g every 8 hours. Patients generally should be tested and empirically treated for chlamydial infection also, and should undergo testing for other sexually transmitted infections.[70]

Septic Bursitis

Septic bursitis is frequently due to direct trauma rather than hematogenous infection. The olecranon and prepatellar bursa are the most commonly affected sites because of their location and frequency of adjacent trauma.[71] Deep septic bursitis is uncommon and diagnosis is often delayed.[72] The annual incidence of acute olecranon and prepatellar bursitis is 10 in 100,000, with one-third of the cases being septic.[73] Cases are predominantly male individuals (80%–89%),[74–77] with a mean age of onset reported at 49.7 to 57 years of age.[74–78]

The most prominent risk factor for septic bursitis is repetitive motion and trauma,[71,77,78] which is present in 47% to 77% of cases.[79] There is a well-known association between occupation and certain types of bursitis. For example, occupations that involve constant kneeling are associated with prepatellar bursitis, sometime referred to as "housemaid's knee." This condition is also seen in Carpet layers. Janitors and laborers are more likely to experience olecranon bursitis, while automobile mechanics and carpenters have an increased risk of developing both olecranon and prepatellar bursitis.[71] Other risk factors for septic bursitis include underlying comorbid conditions such as HD,[71] chronic obstructive pulmonary disease (COPD),[71] DM,[71] chronic alcohol use,[71,77] previous traumatic bursitis,[71] RA,[71] gout,[71] and steroid use.[71]

S aureus, including MRSA, is the predominant pathogen[74,78,80–82] accounting for 87.5% to 94.4%[77,82] of cases. Less common potential pathogens include skin flora such as *S epidermidis* and streptococcal species.[83] Septic bursitis due to exotic pathogens has been described in immunocompromised individuals, including *Mycobacterium kansasii*,[84] *Candida* spp,[81,85] *Salmonella*,[86] and *Cryptococcus neoformans*.[81]

Clinical presentation

Patients typically present with localized tenderness, erythema, and warmth over the bursa area (**Fig. 4**). In contrast to septic arthritis, the joint motion is usually preserved.[71] It may be difficult to determine whether bursitis is septic or aseptic. In comparison to aseptic bursitis, septic bursitis has an increased frequency of tenderness (88 vs 36%), erythema (83 vs 27%), warmth (84 vs 56%), trauma (50 vs 25%), and fever (38 vs 0%; **Table 6**).[79]

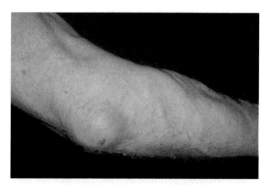

Fig. 4. Septic olecranon bursitis note the localized erythema and swelling over the olecranon bursa. (Danielle Reilly, Srinath Kamineni, Olecranon bursitis, Journal of Shoulder and Elbow Surgery, 25 (1), 2016, 158-167, https://doi.org/10.1016/j.jse.2015.08.032.)

Table 6
Frequency of symptoms associated with septic and aseptic bursitis

	Septic Bursitis	Aseptic Bursitis
Tenderness (%)	88	36
Erythema (%)	83	27
Warmth (%)	84	56
Trauma (%)	50	25
Fever (%)	38	0

Diagnostic tests

Leukocytosis and elevated CRP are more indicative of septic rather than aseptic bursitis.[87] Imaging studies such as CT and MRI, though rarely necessary, are sensitive and may be helpful in identifying which anatomic compartment the infection is located in and can rule out other conditions such as cellulitis, myositis, and so forth.[32] Ultrasound can be used to detect bursal distension and guide bursa aspiration.[88]

While symptoms can help differentiate septic from aseptic bursitis, bursal fluid analysis is required to confirm the etiology. Purulent aspirate favors an infectious etiology.[87] In septic bursitis, fluid WBC count is typically highly elevated (>200,000 cells/mm^3), with neutrophil predominance. Conversely, the WBC count in aseptic bursitis is usually less than 1500 cells/mm^3 with lymphocyte predominance. Crystal-induced (gouty) bursitis usually shows a fluid WBC in the intermediate range of 1000 to 6000 cells/mm^3.[83] Although not commonly performed in practice, bursal glucose less than 31 mg/dL or less than 50% the serum glucose level also suggests septic bursitis. Gram stains can be negative in 30% of cases.[83] When possible, bursal fluid should be sent for cultures to identify the pathogen.

Treatment

Since the predominant pathogens are *Staphylococcus* and *Streptococcus* species, the antibiotic of choice should cover this pathogen, such as a first-generation cephalosporin or penicillinase-resistant penicillin.[83,87] In severe infections, and patients at increased risk, MRSA coverage should be provided while awaiting culture results. There is differing opinion on the need for bursal fluid aspiration prior to the start of antibiotics. Up to 88% of patients with suspected uncomplicated septic bursitis treated empirically with antibiotics without bursal aspiration had resolution of symptoms.[76] This approach may lead to decreased complications from bursal aspiration.

Patients with mild-to-moderate septic bursitis can be managed with a 2 week course of oral antibiotics.[74] Failure to reach resolution within 10 days is considered failure of antibiotic treatment.[89] Patients with severe bursitis (extensive localized infection or systemic symptoms) or immunosuppression should be admitted for intravenous antibiotics followed by oral antibiotics for a total of 2 weeks.[74] Patients with complicated septic bursitis may ultimately need bursectomy for definitive treatment.

SUMMARY

Acute joint pain has a broad differential that includes both articular and periarticular causes of pain. Obtain a focused history that assesses for risk factors including the presence of an immunocompromise or immunosuppression, or the presence of orthopedic hardware, where the presentation can be indolent, the diagnosis more difficult and treatment course more complicated. A detailed joint examination can help distinguish between articular and periarticular causes. Localized swelling and tenderness is suggestive of extra-articular causes such as bursitis and tendinitis, whereas generalized joint tenderness and very painful range of motion is suggestive of intra-articular pathology. If there is clinical concern for septic arthritis, obtain synovial fluid for analysis. Interpret the results in the setting of the patient's clinical picture and associated risk factors. For suspected PJI, consult an orthopedic specialist immediately. In cases when the diagnosis is unclear, err on the side of caution and admit patients for close monitoring and further evaluation.

CLINICS CARE POINTS

- Septic arthritis typically presents with acute monoarticular arthritis but 1 in 5 patients have more than 1 joint involved.
- The lack of systemic symptoms or laboratory findings such as fever or leukocytosis does not rule out septic arthritis.
- Patients with prosthetic joints or those who are immunocompromised may have an insidious presentation.
- *Salmonella* is the most common pathogen in patients with SLE, particularly with high-dose steroid use.
- Crystalline disease can coexist with septic arthritis. Therefore, the presence of crystals does not exclude septic arthritis.
- When there is concern for septic arthritis, arthrocentesis must be performed unless there is a strong contraindication.
- The classic triad of disseminated gonococcal infection includes migratory polyarthritis, tenosynovitis, and skin lesions. When there is a suspicion of disseminated gonococcal infection with arthritis, in addition to synovial fluid cultures, which have low yield, NAAT and culture of other mucosal sites should be obtained, along with blood cultures.
- Patients with septic bursitis typically present with localized pain, tenderness, warmth, and swelling but joint ROM is preserved.

DISCLOSURE

The authors have nothing to disclose.

REFERENCES

1. Favero M, Schiavon F, Riato L, et al. Rheumatoid arthritis is the major risk factor for septic arthritis in rheumatological settings. Autoimmun Rev 2008;8(1):59–61.
2. McBride S, Mowbray J, Caughey W, et al. Epidemiology, Management, and Outcomes of Large and Small Native Joint Septic Arthritis in Adults. Clin Infect Dis 2020;70(2):271–9.
3. Lim SY, Lu N, Choi HK. Septic arthritis in gout patients: a population-based cohort study. Rheumatology 2015;54(11):2095–9.
4. Mathews CJ, Weston VC, Jones A, et al. Bacterial septic arthritis in adults. Lancet 2010;375(9717):846–55.
5. Lim SY, Pannikath D, Nugent K. A retrospective study of septic arthritis in a tertiary hospital in West Texas with high rates of methicillin-resistant Staphylococcus aureus infection. Rheumatol Int 2015;35(7):1251–6.
6. Weston VC, Jones AC, Bradbury N, et al. Clinical features and outcome of septic arthritis in a single UK Health District 1982-1991. Ann Rheum Dis 1999;58(4):214–9.

7. Frazee BF, Fee C, Lambert L. How Common is MRSA in Adult Septic Arthritis. Ann Emerg Med 2009;54(5):695–700.
8. Rego de Figueiredo I, Vieira Alves R, Guerreiro Castro S, et al. Septic arthritis incidence and risk factors: a 5-year cross-sectional study. Infect Dis Lond Engl 2019; 51(8):635–7.
9. George J, Chandy VJ, Premnath J, et al. Microbiological profile of septic arthritis in adults: Lessons learnt and treatment strategies. Indian J Med Microbiol 2019; 37(1):29–33.
10. Margaretten ME, Kohlwes J, Moore D, et al. Does This Adult Patient Have Septic Arthritis? JAMA 2007;297(13):1478–88.
11. Vassallo C, Borg AA, Farrugia D, et al. The Epidemiology and Outcomes of Septic Arthritis in the Maltese Islands: A Hospital-Based Retrospective Cohort Study. Mediterr J Rheumatol 2020;31(2):195–205.
12. Mathews CJ, Kingsley G, Field M, et al. Management of septic arthritis: a systematic review. Ann Rheum Dis 2007;66(4):440–5.
13. Peng EWK, McKillop G, Prasad S, et al. Septic Arthritis of the Manubriosternal Joint. Ann Thorac Surg 2007;83(3):1190–4.
14. Ploom S, Cooley M, Nagpal A, et al. Blastomyces dermatitidis Septic Arthritis in a Renal Transplant Patient. J Investig Med High Impact Case Rep 2023;11. https:// doi.org/10.1177/23247096231166674. 23247096231166670.
15. Miller JB, McCARTHY EF, Gelber AC. Graft-versus-host Disease Complicated by Sequential Septic Arthritis and Osteomyelitis. J Rheumatol 2020;47(3):477–8.
16. Lam V, Theyyunni N. Septic arthritis due to non-tuberculous mycobacterium without effusion. Am J Emerg Med 2021;43:287–287.e7.
17. Chang JW, Tsai HL, Yang LY. Successful treatment of refractory septic arthritis caused by salmonella and staphylococcus aureus with preservation of graft function in a long-term renal transplant recipient by total withdrawal of immunosuppressants. Clin Nephrol 2010;73(1):72–5.
18. Chalhoub N, Georgescu C, Altorok N. Mycobacterium Avium Complex Septic Arthritis in a Patient Treated by Infliximab. Am J Therapeut 2016;23(5):e1222–5.
19. Sen D, Birns J, Rahman A. Articular presentation of disseminated histoplasmosis. Clin Rheumatol 2007;26(5):823–4.
20. Lodge BA, Ashley ED, Steele MP, et al. Aspergillus fumigatus empyema, arthritis, and calcaneal osteomyelitis in a lung transplant patient successfully treated with posaconazole. J Clin Microbiol 2004;42(3):1376–8.
21. Einollahi B, Hamedanizadeh AK, Alavian SM. Brucellosis arthritis–a rare complication of renal transplantation: a case report. Transplant Proc 2003;35(7):2698.
22. Katsarolis I, Tsiodras S, Panagopoulos P, et al. Septic arthritis due to Salmonella enteritidis associated with infliximab use. Scand J Infect Dis 2005;37(4):304–5.
23. O'Sullivan MVN, Isbel NM, Johnson DW, et al. Disseminated pyogenic Mycoplasma pneumoniae infection in a renal transplant recipient, detected by broad-range polymerase chain reaction. Clin Infect Dis 2004;39(9):e98–9.
24. Kim HW, Han M, Jung I, et al. Incidence of septic arthritis in patients with ankylosing spondylitis and seropositive rheumatoid arthritis following TNF-inhibitor therapy. Rheumatol Oxf Engl 2022. https://doi.org/10.1093/rheumatology/keac721. keac721.
25. Galloway JB, Hyrich KL, Mercer LK, et al. Risk of septic arthritis in patients with rheumatoid arthritis and the effect of anti-TNF therapy: results from the British Society for Rheumatology Biologics Register. Ann Rheum Dis 2011;70(10):1810–4.
26. Qiao L, Xu D, Zhao Y, et al. A retrospective study of joint infections in patients with systemic lupus erythematosus. Clin Rheumatol 2017;36(9):2011–7.

27. Gerona JG, Navarra SV. Salmonella infections in patients with systemic lupus erythematosus: a case series. Int J Rheum Dis 2009;12(4):319–23.

28. Horowitz DL, Katzap E, Horowitz S, et al. Approach to septic arthritis. Am Fam Physician 2011;84(6):653–60.

29. Chan BY, Crawford AM, Kobes PH, et al. Septic Arthritis: An Evidence-Based Review of Diagnosis and Image-Guided Aspiration. AJR Am J Roentgenol 2020; 215(3):568–81.

30. Learch TJ. Imaging of infectious arthritis. Semin Muscoskel Radiol 2003;7(2): 137–42.

31. Ellanti P, Moriarity A, Barry S, et al. Radiographic progression of septic arthritis of the hip. BMJ Case Rep 2015;2015. https://doi.org/10.1136/bcr-2015-212079. bcr2015212079.

32. Fayad LM, Carrino JA, Fishman EK. Musculoskeletal infection: role of CT in the emergency department. Radiogr Rev Publ Radiol Soc N Am Inc 2007;27(6): 1723–36.

33. Learch TJ, Farooki S. Magnetic resonance imaging of septic arthritis. Clin Imag 2000;24(4):236–42.

34. Boniface K, Pyle M, Jaleesah N, et al. Point-of-Care Ultrasound for the Detection of Hip Effusion and Septic Arthritis in Adult Patients With Hip Pain and Negative Initial Imaging. J Emerg Med 2020;58(4):627–31.

35. Chin TY, Peh WC. Imaging update on musculoskeletal infections. J Clin Orthop Trauma 2021;22:101600.

36. Iagnocco A, Vavala C, Scirocco C, et al. Unilateral painful, swollen and erythematosus knee. Case report. Med Ultrason 2012;14(3):251–3.

37. Thom C, Pozner J, Kongkatong M, et al. Ultrasound-Guided Talonavicular Arthrocentesis. J Emerg Med 2021;60(5):633–6.

38. EL-Gabalawy H, Tanner S. Chapter 56: Synovial fluid analyses, synovial biopsy and synovial pathology. In: Firestein GS, Budd RC, Gabriel SE, et al, editors. *Firestein & kelley's textbook of rheumatology-E-book*. Elsevier Health Sciences; 2020. p. 841–58.

39. Ross JJ. Septic Arthritis of Native Joints. Infect Dis Clin North Am 2017;31(2): 203–18.

40. Yu KH, Luo SF, Liou LB, et al. Concomitant septic and gouty arthritis–an analysis of 30 cases. Rheumatol Oxf Engl 2003;42(9):1062–6.

41. Hassan AS, Rao A, Manadan AM, et al. Peripheral Bacterial Septic Arthritis: Review of Diagnosis and Management. J Clin Rheumatol Pract Rep Rheum Musculoskelet Dis 2017;23(8):435–42.

42. Weston V, Coakley G, British Society for Rheumatology BSR Standards, Guidelines and Audit Working Group, et al. British Society for Rheumatology (BSR) Standards, Guidelines and Audit Working Group, et al. Guideline for the management of the hot swollen joint in adults with a particular focus on septic arthritis. J Antimicrob Chemother 2006;58(3):492–3.

43. Mathews CJ, Coakley G. Septic arthritis: current diagnostic and therapeutic algorithm. Curr Opin Rheumatol 2008;20(4):457–62.

44. Lieber SB, Alpert N, Fowler ML, et al. Clinical characteristics and outcomes of patients with septic arthritis treated without surgery. Eur J Clin Microbiol Infect Dis 2020;39(5):897–901.

45. Mabille C, El Samad Y, Joseph C, et al. Medical versus surgical treatment in native hip and knee septic arthritis. Infect Dis Now 2021;51(2):164–9.

46. Ruangpin C, Rodchuae M, Katchamart W. Factors Related to Surgical Treatment and Outcomes of Thai Patients With Septic Arthritis. JCR J Clin Rheumatol 2019; 25(4):176.
47. Zardi EM, Franceschi F. Prosthetic joint infection. A relevant public health issue. J Infect Public Health 2020;13(12):1888–91.
48. McMaster Arthroplasty Collaborative (MAC). Incidence and Predictors of Prosthetic Joint Infection Following Primary Total Knee Arthroplasty: A 15-Year Population-Based Cohort Study. J Arthroplasty 2022;37(2):367–72.e1.
49. Marang-van de Mheen PJ, Bragan Turner E, Liew S, et al. Variation in Prosthetic Joint Infection and treatment strategies during 4.5 years of follow-up after primary joint arthroplasty using administrative data of 41397 patients across Australian, European and United States hospitals. BMC Musculoskelet Disord 2017; 18(1):207.
50. Lenguerrand E, Whitehouse MR, Beswick AD, et al. Description of the rates, trends and surgical burden associated with revision for prosthetic joint infection following primary and revision knee replacements in England and Wales: an analysis of the National Joint Registry for England, Wales, Northern Ireland and the Isle of Man. BMJ Open 2017;7(7):e014056.
51. Kapadia BH, Berg RA, Daley JA, et al. Periprosthetic joint infection. Lancet 2016; 387(10016):386–94.
52. Cochrane NH, Wellman SS, Lachiewicz PF. Early Infection After Aseptic Revision Knee Arthroplasty: Prevalence and Predisposing Risk Factors. J Arthroplasty 2022;37(6S):S281–5.
53. Beam E, Osmon D. Prosthetic Joint Infection Update. Infect Dis Clin North Am 2018;32(4):843–59.
54. Tsai Y, Chang CH, Lin YC, et al. Different microbiological profiles between hip and knee prosthetic joint infections. J Orthop Surg Hong Kong 2019;27(2). https://doi.org/10.1177/2309499019847768. 2309499019847768.
55. Cobo F, Rodríguez-Granger J, López EM, et al. Candida-induced prosthetic joint infection. A literature review including 72 cases and a case report. Infect Dis Lond Engl 2017;49(2):81–94.
56. Arvieux C, Common H. New diagnostic tools for prosthetic joint infection. Orthop Traumatol Surg Res OTSR 2019;105(1S):S23–30.
57. Nodzo SR, Bauer T, Pottinger PS, et al. Conventional Diagnostic Challenges in Periprosthetic Joint Infection. J Am Acad Orthop Surg 2015;23(suppl):S18.
58. Luo TD, Jarvis DL, Yancey HB, et al. Synovial Cell Count Poorly Predicts Septic Arthritis in the Presence of Crystalline Arthropathy. J Bone Jt Infect 2020;5(3):118–24.
59. Shanmugasundaram S, Ricciardi BF, Briggs TWR, et al. Evaluation and Management of Periprosthetic Joint Infection-an International, Multicenter Study. HSS J Musculoskelet J Hosp Spec Surg 2014;10(1):36–44.
60. Parvizi J, Tan TL, Goswami K, et al. The 2018 Definition of Periprosthetic Hip and Knee Infection: An Evidence-Based and Validated Criteria. J Arthroplasty 2018; 33(5):1309–14.e2.
61. Li B, Chen F, Liu Y, et al. Synovial Fluid α-Defensin as a Biomarker for Peri-Prosthetic Joint Infection: A Systematic Review and Meta-Analysis. Surg Infect 2017;18(6):702–10.
62. Tubb CC, Polkowksi GG, Krause B. Diagnosis and Prevention of Periprosthetic Joint Infections. J Am Acad Orthop Surg 2020;28(8):e340–8.
63. Yang J, Parvizi J, Hansen EN, et al. 2020 Mark Coventry Award: Microorganism-directed oral antibiotics reduce the rate of failure due to further infection after two-

stage revision hip or knee arthroplasty for chronic infection: a multicentre randomized controlled trial at a minimum of two years. Bone Jt J 2020;102-B-(6_Supple_A):3–9.

64. Bernard L, Arvieux C, Brunschweiler B, et al. Antibiotic Therapy for 6 or 12 Weeks for Prosthetic Joint Infection. N Engl J Med 2021;384(21):1991–2001.

65. García-De La Torre I, Nava-Zavala A. Gonococcal and nongonococcal arthritis. Rheum Dis Clin North Am 2009;35(1):63–73.

66. Bardin T. Gonococcal arthritis. Best Pract Res Clin Rheumatol 2003;17(2):201–8.

67. Moussiegt A, François C, Belmonte O, et al. Gonococcal arthritis: case series of 58 hospital cases. Clin Rheumatol 2022;41(9):2855–62.

68. Rice PA. Gonococcal arthritis (disseminated gonococcal infection). Infect Dis Clin North Am 2005;19(4):853–61.

69. Harrington L, Schneider JI. Atraumatic joint and limb pain in the elderly. Emerg Med Clin North Am 2006;24(2):389–412, vii.

70. Workowski KA, Bachmann LH, Chan PA, et al. Sexually Transmitted Infections Treatment Guidelines, 2021. MMWR Recomm Rep Morb Mortal Wkly Rep Recomm Rep 2021;70(4):1–187.

71. Zimmermann B, Mikolich DJ, Ho G. Septic bursitis. Semin Arthritis Rheum 1995; 24(6):391–410.

72. Lormeau C, Cormier G, Sigaux J, et al. Management of septic bursitis. Joint Bone Spine 2019;86(5):583–8.

73. Baumbach SF, Wyen H, Perez C, et al. Evaluation of current treatment regimens for prepatellar and olecranon bursitis in Switzerland. Eur J Trauma Emerg Surg 2013;39(1):65–72.

74. Nguyen K, Coquerelle P, Houvenagel E, et al. Characteristics and management of olecranon or prepatellar septic bursitis. Infect Dis Now 2023;53(2):104652.

75. Charret L, Bart G, Hoppe E, et al. Clinical characteristics and management of olecranon and prepatellar septic bursitis in a multicentre study. J Antimicrob Chemother 2021;76(11):3029–32.

76. Beyde A, Thomas AL, Colbenson KM, et al. Efficacy of empiric antibiotic management of septic olecranon bursitis without bursal aspiration in emergency department patients. Acad Emerg Med 2022;29(1):6–14.

77. Gómez-Rodríguez N, Méndez-García MJ, Ferreiro-Seoane JL, et al. [Infectious bursitis: study of 40 cases in the pre-patellar and olecranon regions]. Enferm Infecc Microbiol Clín 1997;15(5):237–42.

78. Sb L, Ml F, C Z, et al. Clinical characteristics and outcomes of septic bursitis. Infection 2017;45(6). https://doi.org/10.1007/s15010-017-1030-3.

79. Reilly D, Kamineni S. Olecranon bursitis. J Shoulder Elbow Surg 2016;25(1): 158–67.

80. Thompson GR, Manshady BM, Weiss JJ. Septic Bursitis. JAMA 1978;240(21): 2280–1.

81. Chartash EK, Good PK, Gould ES, et al. Septic subdeltoid bursitis. Semin Arthritis Rheum 1992;22(1):25–9.

82. Martinez-Taboada VM, Cabeza R, Cacho PM, et al. Cloxacillin-based therapy in severe septic bursitis: retrospective study of 82 cases. Joint Bone Spine 2009; 76(6):665–9.

83. McAfee JH, Smith DL. Olecranon and prepatellar bursitis. Diagnosis and treatment. West J Med 1988;149(5):607–10.

84. Mathew SD, Tully CC, Borra H, et al. Septic subacromial bursitis caused by Mycobacterium kansasii in an immunocompromised host. Mil Med 2012;177(5): 617–20.

85. Skedros JG, Keenan KE, Trachtenberg JD. Candida glabrata olecranon bursitis treated with bursectomy and intravenous caspofungin. J Surg Orthop Adv 2013;22(2):179–82.
86. Burke CC, Martel-Laferriere V, Dieterich DT. Septic bursitis, a potential complication of protease inhibitor use in hepatitis C virus. Clin Infect Dis 2013;56(10): 1507–8.
87. Baumbach SF, Lobo CM, Badyine I, et al. Prepatellar and olecranon bursitis: literature review and development of a treatment algorithm. Arch Orthop Trauma Surg 2014;134(3):359–70.
88. Costantino TG, Roemer B, Leber EH. Septic arthritis and bursitis: emergency ultrasound can facilitate diagnosis. J Emerg Med 2007;32(3):295–7.
89. Brown OS, Smith TO, Parsons T, et al. Management of septic and aseptic prepatellar bursitis: a systematic review. Arch Orthop Trauma Surg 2022;142(10): 2445–57.
90. Frazee BW, Fee C, Lambert L. How common is MRSA in adult septic arthritis? Ann Emerg Med 2009;54(5):695–700.

Diabetic Foot Infections in the Emergency Department

Bradley W. Frazee, MD*

KEYWORDS

- Diabetic foot infection • Diabetic foot ulcer • Peripheral arterial disease
- Osteomyelitis • Necrotizing soft tissue infection

KEY POINTS

- Remove bandages to examine the foot carefully.
- Routinely obtain plain x-rays.
- Consult guidelines for proper infection categorization and antimicrobial selection.
- Debridement is frequently required.
- Immediate consultation or close follow-up with a foot surgeon is mandatory.

INTRODUCTION

Among the most common diabetic complications encountered in the emergency department (ED), diabetic foot infections (DFIs) account for billions of annual health care spending in the United States and can lead to extremity amputation and near-term death. It is therefore essential that emergency providers be well acquainted with the topic of DFI, as well as the closely associated problems diabetic peripheral neuropathy, peripheral arterial disease (PAD), diabetic foot ulcer (DFU), and osteomyelitis. Providers need to be able to gauge infection severity, order and interpret initial diagnostic tests, select appropriate empiric antimicrobial therapy, decide on appropriate disposition, and recognize when emergent surgical intervention is required. Recent DFI guidelines provide detailed, evidence-based diagnostic and management recommendations. This article offers a review geared specifically for the emergency provider, including how to perform a nuanced diagnostic evaluation and provide state-of-the-art initial management.

EPIDEMIOLOGY

DFUs and DFI are among the most common diabetic complications requiring admission from the ED. Together, these diabetic foot diseases account for 2% of ED visits by

Department of Emergency Medicine, Alameda Health System, Wilma Chan Highland Hospital, 1411 East 31st Street, Oakland, CA 94602, USA
* Corresponding author.
E-mail address: bradf_98@yahoo.com

Emerg Med Clin N Am 42 (2024) 267–285
https://doi.org/10.1016/j.emc.2024.01.003
0733-8627/24/© 2024 Elsevier Inc. All rights reserved.

emed.theclinics.com

patients with diabetes, with about 80% requiring admission.[1] There exists a striking link among DFU, associated DFI, the need for amputation, and near-term mortality. The annual foot ulcer incidence among US diabetics is 6%, with roughly 50% of DFUs resulting in DFI.[2] Following a DFI, the 1 year risk of minor or major amputation is 17% to 36%.[3,4] And following DFI-related amputation, 5 year mortality is 52%, on par with many malignancies.[5] These statistics indicate that any ED patient with a DFU, DFI, or history of lower extremity amputation should be considered at very high risk. Additionally, there are significant disparities in DFI-related outcomes along socioeconomic and racial lines, with higher rates of amputation and associated mortality in Black and Latino patients and among patients with low socioeconomic status and from rural communities.[1,4] Finally, the annual US health care costs attributable just to those DFIs that are admitted through the ED sums to 8.78 billion.[1]

PATHOPHYSIOLOGY AND NATURAL HISTORY

Though DFIs—typically superficial abscesses and cellulitis—can develop in the setting of traumatic foot wounds, fungal infection, or venous stasis dermatitis, the majority of severe DFIs develop as a complication of a DFU. Hence, risk factors for, and pathophysiology of, DFUs are closely tied to those of DFI. Diabetic peripheral neuropathy is considered the essential permissive process underlying DFU and DFI: sensory neuropathy causes loss of protective sensation; motor neuropathy can lead to foot deformity and biomechanical abnormalities; autonomic neuropathy causes decreased sweating and dry, cracked skin. Repetitive vertical and shear stress leads to skin breakdown, which often goes unnoticed, and ulcer formation. Once an ulcer forms, healing is often slow and problematic, with infection supervening before skin closure can occur. Factors adversely affecting healing include PAD, large size (>1 cm^2) and location on the heal. Only about 50% of DFUs heal by 1 year, and thereafter, recurrence occurs at a rate of about 40% per year.[2,3]

The surface of chronic DFUs often become colonized with one or more pathogenic bacteria, which then can lead to clinical infection (see "Microbiology" section). New, sophisticated microscopic and molecular techniques have revealed an extensive microbiome in most DFUs, with high bioburden impairing ulcer healing. Infection is often associated with biofilms containing multiple species, which impair antibiotic penetration and are associated with antibiotic resistance.[6,7] Once clinical infection supervenes, hyperglycemia impairs neutrophil function and the avascular articular cartilage, tendons and the many compartments of the foot promote proximal spread of infection. PAD is an important risk factor for DFI development, in part, by slowing the ulcer healing process. PAD is found in 12% of patients with DFUs, but up to 49% of those presenting with DFI.[3,8]

Osteomyelitis complicates about 20% of DFIs and a much higher proportion of those serious enough to require hospitalization.[9] Ulcers and DFIs that occur on bony prominences bring their bacteriologic milieu very close to bone surface. Periosteum is largely avascular, and diabetic microvascular impairment and PAD further disrupt blood flow to the vulnerable bone. Infection and inflammation compress and obliterate vascular channels within bone. Bone devoid of blood supply can separate, forming sequestra, a safe harbor for bacteria not reached by systemic antibiotics.[10]

MICROBIOLOGY

Data on the microbiology of DFIs comes mostly from studies of nonhealing DFUs, osteomyelitis, and severe DFIs requiring hospitalization. Therefore, polymicrobial infection may be overrepresented in the literature, while nonsevere infections such as small abscesses and nonpurulent cellulitis may often be monomicrobial. Aerobic gram-positive pathogens—primarily *Staphylococcus aureus* and beta-hemolytic streptococci—are the most common class of bacterial isolates in DFI studies from the United States and Europe and are even more common in minor infections and in patients not recently treated with antibiotics.[11,12] *S aureus* is the single most frequently isolated pathogen, with methicillin-resistant *S. aureus* (MRSA) accounting for 18% to 30% of these, or about 11% of DFIs overall.[13–15] Therefore, whether or not to include MRSA coverage is a very important consideration in empiric antibiotic selection.

Polymicrobial infection and isolation of aerobic gram-negative and obligate anaerobic species occurs in 10% to 50% of infections and positively correlates with size, depth, and chronicity of the associated ulcer.[6,16–19] Additionally, recent antibiotic therapy is considered an important risk factor for resistant infections. Multidrug-resistant (MDR) gram negatives including *Pseudomonas* and extended-spectrum beta lactamase (ESBL)-producing Enterobacterales species have been common in studies conducted since 2000 in tropical and subtropical countries.[20–22] *Pseudomonas*, in particular, is considered to be more common in the following settings: recent broad-spectrum antibiotic exposure, when the ulcer is macerated or there has been chronic exposure to moisture, or when it has been isolated recently in culture.[12] Obligate anaerobes, such as *Bacteroides* species and *Peptostreptococcus*, are more commonly isolated in the setting of ischemic and necrotic wounds or a fetid odor.[23] Less pathogenic bacteria, including coagulase-negative *Staphylococcus*, Enterococci, and Corynebacteria are frequently isolated in DFIs but of unclear pathogenicity.[12,14]

CLINICAL FEATURES

Owing to underlying sensory neuropathy, patients with diabetes may be unaware that they have a foot ulcer or foot infection. Occult DFI is a notorious cause of sudden worsening of glycemic control. Therefore, careful inspection of the feet is mandatory in patients with diabetes presenting to the ED with foot pain, unexplained hyperglycemia, or systemic signs of infection. Socks and bandages must be removed. A well-lit examination should assess for the following: underlying sensory neuropathy and PAD; presence of an ulcer; signs of infection, and, if present, infection severity; and evidence of associated osteomyelitis. The physical examination alone can confirm or exclude DFI in most cases.

Neuropathy and Peripheral Arterial Disease

Examination for evidence of sensory neuropathy (loss of protective sensation) is considered a standard component of the diabetic foot examination. Assessing for loss of vibration sense on the dorsum of the great toe, with a 128 Hz tuning fork, or loss of light touch, with a 10 g monofilament, are rapid and well-established bedside tests for neuropathy. The Ipswich touch test is a simple alternative that requires no special equipment and performs well. To perform the test, the tips of digits 1, 3, and 5 on both feet are lightly touched for 1 to 2 seconds with the index finger. Failure to feel 2 or more toes being touched constitutes a positive test.[24]

Presence of PAD is another key component of the diabetic foot examination, although it is often overlooked, even in patients admitted for DFI.[25] PAD is the most significant predictor of delayed DFU healing and future amputation, and the presence of PAD indicates that revascularization may be required for successful ulcer healing and DFI treatment. Moreover, PAD, like neuropathy, is 1 of 6 elements of DFU classification (see later discussion). Clinical signs of PAD include a history of claudication and skin that is bluish, hairless, thin, and cool. Absence of pedal pulses is further evidence of PAD, with the absence of both the posterior tibial and dorsalis pedis pulses required for diagnosis. Since clinical signs and pulse palpation may not be accurate, measurement of the arterial brachial index (ABI) is recommended to confirm the impression of PAD, with an ABI of less than 0.9 considered to be confirmatory. Ischemic necrosis ("dry gangrene") due to severe PAD (**Fig. 1**), may be difficult to distinguish from infectious necrosis ("wet gangrene"), discussed further in a later section.

Diabetic Foot Ulcer

When a foot ulcer is detected on examination, the emergency provider may be asked to describe or classify the ulcer. Guidelines recommend using the Site, Ischemia, Neuropathy, Bacterial infection, Area, Depth (SINBAD) score for classification and to facilitate communication between providers[26,27] (**Table 1**). Measure and record the area, if possible uploading a photograph that includes a ruler into the medical record. An ulcer with average diameter greater than 1 cm (area >1 cm^2) is considered high risk in the SINBAD score and ulcers greater than 3 cm^2 take a median of just over 1 year to heal[28] (**Fig. 2**). Assess and record depth with the aid of bright light and an instrument to clear away exudate and devitalized tissue. Depth is graded by the tissue layers penetrated or visible at the ulcer base, as follows: involving skin and subcutaneous tissue only; reaching muscle, tendon, or joint capsule; bone visible or palpable. Ulcers that extend beyond subcutaneous tissue take a median of just over 1 year to heal.[28]

Diabetic Foot Infection and Severity Classification

Diagnosis of DFI generally requires the presence of clearly purulent secretions or 2 or more of the following: increased pain, erythema, induration, warmth, or tenderness (**Fig. 3**). Additional signs that an ulcer may be infected include the following: foul odor, friable, discolored granulation tissue, undermining of the wound edge[29] (**Fig. 4**). DFI severity should be classified according to the International Working Group on Diabetic Foot/Infectious Disease of America (IWGDF/IDSA) scheme (**Table 2**). This classification system is used to tailor empiric antibiotic selection to infection severity, as well as promote consistent communication with consultants and downstream providers.

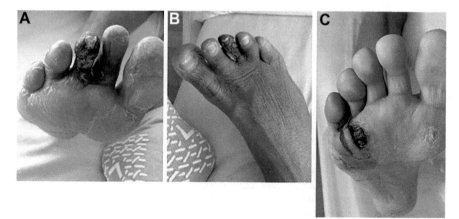

Fig. 1. Peripheral arterial disease. (*A, B*) Ischemic necrosis of the third toe showing "mummification." (*C*) Ischemic necrosis of the fifth toe associated with a nonhealing plantar ulcer. (Photos courtesy of Elly Huang, DPM.)

Table 1
SINBAD diabetic foot ulcer severity score[27]

Category	Definition	SINBAD Score
Site	Forefoot	0
	Midfoot or hindfoot	1
Ischemia	Blood flow intact (at least 1 palpable pedal pulse)	0
	Evidence of reduced blood flow (no palpable pedal pulse)	1
Neuropathy	Protective sensation intact	0
	Protective sensation lost	1
Bacterial infection	None	0
	Present	1
Area	Ulcer <1 cm^2	0
	Ulcer >1 cm^2	1
Total possible score		6

Abbreviation: Site, Ischemia, Neuropathy, Bacterial infection, Area, Depth.

A critical goal of the physical examination in DFI is to detect signs of a rapidly progressive limb-threatening necrotizing soft tissue infection (NSTI). While an NSTI can occasionally be occult or resemble a simple DFI, emergency providers must be alert to, and take seriously, any so-called hard physical examination signs of NSTI. These include necrosis, hemorrhagic bullae, crepitus, discoloration (greyish, purple, and black; **Fig. 5**). In the diabetic population, where chronic PAD is also common, it may be difficult to differentiate ischemic necrosis ("dry gangrene") from an NSTI due to infection ("wet gangrene"). We recommend that signs of necrosis be considered to be due to infection until proven otherwise.

Osteomyelitis

Physical examination signs that increase the likelihood of underlying osteomyelitis are foot ulcer area greater than 2 cm^2 and the presence of exposed bone.[30] Fever is uncommon in isolated osteomyelitis of the foot.[30] The probe to bone test is a well studied and widely accepted bedside maneuver to test for occult exposed bone in the base of a foot ulcer or wound. The test is properly performed with a sterile blunt metal probe; if

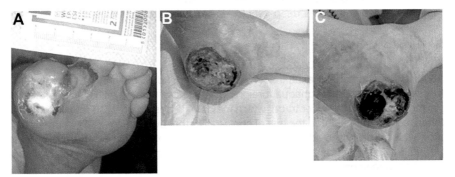

Fig. 2. Diabetic foot ulcers. (*A*) Broad, shallow ulcer associated with prior amputation. (*B, C*) Large, deep undermined foot ulcer showing minor purulent exudate and undermined edges and demonstrating very slow healing. (Photos courtesy of Elly Huang, DPM.)

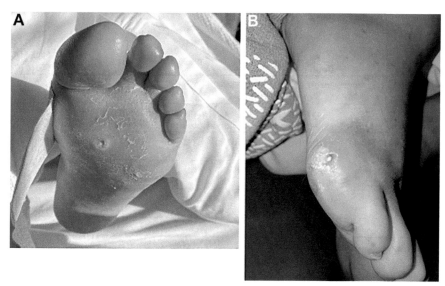

Fig. 3. Minor (class 2) DFIs. (*A*) Small plantar foot ulcer with nonpurulent cellulitis. (*B*) Small ulcer or abscess over metatarsal head with purulence. (Photos courtesy of Elly Huang DPM.)

a probe is not available, a closed Kelly clamp or the wooden end of a sterile cotton-tipped applicator can be used. Feeling a hard, gritty surface constitutes a positive test. The test is typically performed in conjunction with a plain x-ray (see later discussion). In a meta-analysis, pooled sensitivity and specificity of the probe to bone test were 0.9 and 0.8, respectively. However, posttest probability of osteomyelitis will depend on pretest likelihood, which is estimated based on features such as size and chronicity of the associated ulcer and x-ray results.

Differential Diagnosis

A list of other processes that can cause lower extremity pain and inflammation in a patient with diabetes are listed in **Table 3**. Occult fracture (lacking a clear history of trauma) is perhaps the most frequent infection mimic, underscoring the importance of routine x-rays. Otherwise, it is usually possible to distinguish DFI from other causes of foot and leg symptoms without the need for advanced diagnostic tests. Duplex sonography may be needed if deep venous thrombosis is a significant concern.

DIAGNOSTIC TESTS
Imaging

If a DFI is suspected on examination, plain x-rays should generally be obtained to assess for fracture, radio-opaque foreign body, signs of osteomyelitis, and soft tissue gas (beyond that in the ulcer tract), which indicates a possible NSTI (**Fig. 6**). Contrast-enhanced CT is considered the test of choice to further evaluate for NSTI; in the setting of DFI, this modality should be strongly considered when infection extends proximal to the ankle. Diagnostic findings include gas adjacent to fascia, fascial edema, and fascial enhancement.[31]

Plain x-ray signs of osteomyelitis include cortical erosion, periosteal new bone formation, focal medullary osteopenia, bone destruction, and sequestrum (devitalized separated bone).[30,32] Focal findings will typically occur near the base of the ulcer tract

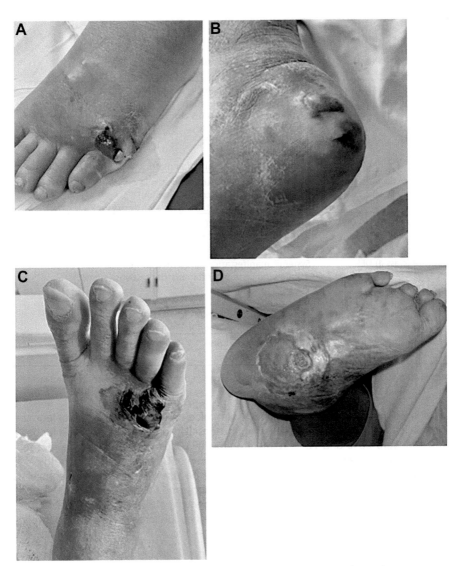

Fig. 4. Moderate or severe (class 3 or 4) DFIs. (Exact categorization depends on presence of systemic signs.) (*A*) Small ulcer over metatarsal head with purulent drainage and cellulitis. (*B*) Infection, abscess, and localized necrosis over calcaneus. (*C*) Infected ulcer with associated necrosis and cellulitis. (*D*) Deep chronic midfoot ulcer; with pressure, purulence and gas could be expressed the distal portion. (Photos [*A–C*] courtesy of Elly Huang, DPM.)

or in conjunction with soft tissue swelling (see **Fig. 6**). X-ray changes take 2 to 3 weeks to occur. A systematic review of plain x-ray alone to diagnose osteomyelitis reported summary positive and negative LRs for of 2.3 and 0.63, indicating that x-ray is somewhat more useful when positive than negative.[30] Current guidelines recommend that when x-rays are positive and consistent with clinical and laboratory findings, no further imaging is usually needed to confirm osteomyelitis.[12] When needed, MRI is generally

Table 2 IWGDF/IDSA diabetic foot infection classification[12]	
Uninfected (class 1) foot ulcer	No local or systemic signs of infection
Infected	2 or more of the following local signs: Local swelling or induration Erythema >0.5 cm or > 0.5 cm from wound Local pain or tenderness Local increased warmth Purulent drainage No other cause of local inflammatory response (eg, fracture)
Mild infection (class 2) DFI	Involves skin and subcutaneous tissue only (no deeper tissue) Erythema extends ≤2 cm from wound No systemic manifestations (see later discussion)
Moderate (class 3) DFI	Involves deeper tissue (tendon, muscle, joint, bone) involved, or Erythema extends >2 cm from wound No systemic manifestations
Severe (class 4) DFI	Systemic manifestations present; 2 or more of the following systemic inflammatory response signs: T > 38°C or < 36°C HR > 90 RR > 20 or $Paco_2$ < 32 mm Hg WBC >12,000/mm³ or < 4000/mm³ Bands!
Osteomyelitis (add "O" to class 2–4)	Infection involves bone

Abbreviation: International Working Group on Diabetic Foot/Infectious Disease of America.

considered the advanced imaging study of choice to further evaluate for osteomyelitis.[31] In a 2017 meta-analysis, the summary sensitivity and specificity of MRI for osteomyelitis were 93% and 75%, respectively, with specificity limited by the fact that reactive marrow edema can also occur with trauma or Charcot neuroarthropathy.[12,33] Nuclear medicine imaging modalities that can be used to diagnose osteomyelitis include labeled white blood cell (WBC) scintigraphy and flourine-18 flouro-D-glucose positron emission tomography /computed tomography (18F-FDG-PET/CT) scanning, but rarely if ever would these imaging modalities be ordered by an emergency provider.[33]

Inflammatory Markers

Guidelines and reviews emphasize that the assessment of whether a foot ulcer is infected, and infection severity, should be based primarily on physical examination findings. Inflammatory markers play a greater role in identifying osteomyelitis (see later discussion). Nonetheless, inflammatory markers have been studied both for their ability to distinguish infected from uninfected foot ulcers and their correlation with DFI outcomes. While the primary literature consists only of small studies which use different test cutoff values, recent systematic reviews concluded that WBC count, erythrocyte sedimentation rate (ESR), c-reactive protein (CRP), and procalcitonin all perform similarly, with generally limited ability to distinguish an uninfected foot ulcer from infection.[34,35] A normal WBC occurs in 56% of DFIs; therefore, it is not reliable to identify whether an ulcer is infected.[34,36] Nonetheless, WBC should be obtained routinely when evaluating DFI severity, since it is a component of the IWGDF/IDSA DFI classification scheme, in that WBC greater than 12,000 mm³, less than 4000 mm³ or bands greater than 10%

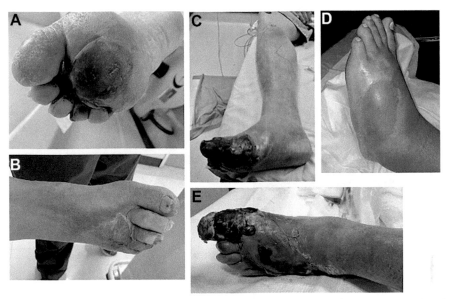

Fig. 5. Diabetic NSTIs of the foot. (*A, B*) Dusky appearance extending from plantar to dorsal surface of the distal foot and toes 2 to 4, which proved grossly infected and devitalized on operative debridement. (*C*) Ischemic and superimposed infected necrosis, with infection extending to the knee, requiring below knee amputation; **Fig. 6**A shows associated plane x-ray. (*D*) hemorrhagic bullae, a classic NSTI "hard sign." (*E*) Ischemic and superimposed infected necrosis.

are considered systemic inflammatory response syndrome (SIRS) criteria (see **Table 2**). Among the other inflammatory markers, a recent meta-analysis concluded that CRP was slightly superior to ESR and PCT, based on summary area under the receiver operator curve, with a CRP value of 22.5 mg/L maximizing sensitivity and specificity.[35]

Table 3
Differential diagnosis of foot and leg pain and inflammation in a diabetic

Process	Comments
Sensory neuropathy alone	Bilateral; minimal inflammatory signs
PAD alone	Claudication; See text for examination findings
Diabetic (Charcot) neuroarthropathy	Typical x-ray findings
Fracture	Trauma history or acute localized tenderness may be absent owing to sensory neuropathy
Foreign body (eg, pin or tack)	Suggestive history may be lacking owing to sensory neuropathy
Stasis dermatitis	Often bilateral, chronic edema, maximum inflammation above the ankle, hyperpigmentation (brawny edema), warmth redness and tenderness may occur without infection
Gout	Recurrent episodes, first MTP involvement (or history of), pain with minor joint movement
Venous thrombosis	Unilateral edema, often without prominent inflammatory signs

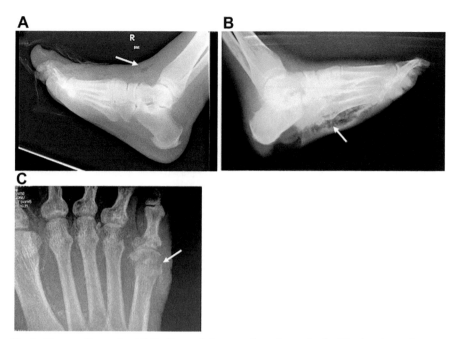

Fig. 6. Plane radiographs. (*A*) Radiograph from patient shown in **Fig. 5C**, showing soft gas at the level of the ankle (*arrow*). (*B*) Extensive soft tissue gas (*arrow*) along plantar fascia, associated with large hind foot ulcer. (*C*) Osteomyelitis around the fifth metatarsal phalangeal joint, showing cortical erosion and sequestrum (*arrow*).

A 2016 meta-analysis evaluating the performance of biomarkers for the diagnosis of osteomyelitis found that ESR had the highest summary area under the curve, with typical ESR cutoff values in individual studies ranging from 45 to 65 mm/h.[37] The 2019 DFI guidelines promote ESR as the preferred, widely available biomarker for osteomyelitis diagnosis, pointing out that a highly elevated ESR (>70 mm/h) is indicative of bone infection rather than soft tissue infection alone.[12] On the other hand, a 2022 meta-analysis focusing on recent literature found that procalcitonin had the highest summary area under the curve for osteomyelitis diagnosis, with a value of 0.33 ng/mL maximizing sensitivity and specificity, though CRP, ESR, and WBC performed similarly.[35]

The correct and expeditious diagnosis of NSTI relies upon maintaining a high index of suspicion followed by findings present upon immediate operative debridement. "Hard signs" (see earlier discussion) present on physical examination, and imaging results, are likely more important than laboratory findings. Nonetheless, severe hyperglycemia, acidosis—from elevated ketones and/or lactate—and acute kidney injury, should all raise concern for severe DFI, including NSTI. The laboratory risk indicator for necrotizing fasciitis (LRINEC) score was derived and initially touted for its ability to differentiate NSTI from less severe skin and soft tissue infections[38] (**Table 4**). However, a systemic review of subsequent studies (with an unclear proportion of DFI-related cases) found a score of 6 or greater had a summary sensitivity of just 68% and specificity of 84% for NSTI.[31] The only study of the LRINEC score limited to DFIs found that a score of 5 or greater (chosen post-hoc) had sensitivity of 69% and specificity of 52% in predicting the need for amputation—suggesting that LRINEC has a limited role in identifying NSTIs among DFIs.[39]

Table 4
Antimicrobial-resistant pathogens often implicated in DFI, their clinical features, and antimicrobials that are typically active against them

Pathogen/Class of Pathogen	Clinical Features	Active Antimicrobials
MRSA (note, more likely when features that predict *S aureus* are present)	Purulent drainage, abscess, prior MRSA isolation, high local MRSA prevalence, and recent hospitalization	TMP-SMX PO Doxycycline PO Linezolid PO or IV Vancomycin Daptomycin
Pseudomonas aeruginosa risk	Prior *P aeruginosa* isolation, macerated wound/ulcer, chronic moisture exposure, and topical climate/latitude	Ciprofloxacin PO or IV Ceftazidime Piperacillin-tazobactam Imipenem-cilastatin Meropenem
MDR gram-negative bacteria, for example, ESBL-producing *E coli*	Broad spectrum antibiotic therapy or hospitalization in prior 90 d, high prevalence region such as South Asia	Imipenem-cilastatin Meropenem Piperacillin-tazobactam
Obligate anaerobic bacteria, for example, *Bacteroides* sp	Necrotic ulcer, deep or chronic ulcer, fetid odor, and limb ischemia with gangrene	Amoxicillin-clavulanate PO Clindamycin PO or IV Moxifloxacin PO or IV Metronidazole PO or IV Ampicillin-sulbactam Piperacillin-tazobactam Imipenem-cilastatin Meropenem

Abbreviations: MRSA, methicillin-resistant *S aureus*; TMP-SMX, trimethoprim-sulfamethoxazole.

Microbiologic Sampling

Guidelines recommend obtaining a specimen for Gram stain and culture in the "great majority" of DFIs that will undergo antibiotic treatment.[12] In many cases, this responsibility will fall upon the emergency provider, particularly in mild (class 2) infections, where patients are often discharged and started on oral treatment prior to seeing a surgical consultant. The superiority of tissue specimen cultures, as compared to simple swab cultures, has been demonstrated in multiple studies, including a pragmatic outpatient study that showed tissue cultures yielded more true pathogens and more often led to a change in antibiotic treatment.[12,13] In the procedure, after cleansing the surface, a small tissue sample is taken from the wound or ulcer base using sterile forceps and a scalpel, then placed in a sterile container and sent immediately to a microbiology laboratory.[40] For suspected osteomyelitis, it is strongly recommended that surgical or percutaneous bone culture be obtained aseptically by a trained foot surgeon, as soon as possible from the onset of antimicrobial therapy. While preoperative empiric antibiotics are expected to have a limited effect on bone culture yield, whether or not to delay empiric antimicrobials until after bone biopsy in selected cases remains controversial.[12,41]

TREATMENT
Antimicrobial Therapy

The microbiological evidence that underlies therapy recommendations is discussed earlier. The following general points tshould be born in mind when considering empiric antimicrobial therapy for DFI. Microbiologic prevalence and resistance patterns differ between geographic regions and hospital systems, suggesting that empiric therapy regimens should be tailored to local antibiogram data, although this concept has not been studied for DFIs.[42] The general approach now recommended in guidelines is to tailor empiric therapy to infection severity, covering the most common pathogens in all cases (methicillin-susceptible S aureus and streptococcal species), with broader parenteral coverage targeting all possible pathogens (MRSA, anaerobes, gram-negative bacteria) reserved for more severe infections.[12] As this practice results in broad-spectrum antibiotic use in many cases, it is critical to obtain proper cultures in the ED to facilitate tailoring of therapy (eg, de-escalation) as soon as possible.

When a true infection is present, systemic antimicrobial therapy is required. Study results do not support the use of topical antimicrobial therapy for foot ulcers or mild DFIs.[12,42,43] There have been only 3 prospective treatment trials with an oral antimicrobial arm.[11,18,44] However, the preference for empiric parenteral therapy both in studies and in practice is not supported by pharmacodynamics; oral cephalosporins, linezolid, quinolones, and other classes are well absorbed and expected to reach effective tissue levels.[9,45] Unfortunately, no studies of nonsevere DFIs have been published yet directly comparing empiric narrow spectrum therapy (oral or parenteral) to broader initial therapy targeting gram negatives and anaerobes.[12] Most of the 21 studies comparing parenteral antimicrobials for DFI have been industry sponsored, comparing various broad-spectrum agents in relatively severe infections, using a noninferiority design. Almost all trials found equivalence, in terms of both safety and efficacy, between the treatment arms. Moreover, meta-analyses have not been able to discern, with a few exceptions, which agents or regimens might be superior.[42,46] At least 9 trials included patients with osteomyelitis and reported osteomyelitis-specific outcomes. Most cases underwent surgical debridement and duration of antimicrobial therapy ranged between 6 and 42 days. Outcomes in these osteomyelitis subgroups also tended to be

Table 5
Recommended empiric antimicrobial regimens according to infection severity

		Antimicrobial Choice	Antimicrobial Choice if Confirmed PCN or Beta-lactam Allergy	Other Recommended Agents/Regimens	Comments
Mild (class 2) DFI—oral therapy generally recommended	Nonpurulent	[a]Cephalexin Weight <60 kg: 500 mg PO qid Weight 60–80 kg: 1000 mg PO tid Weight >80 kg: 1000 mg PO qid	[a]Levofloxacin 750 mg PO qid	Dicloxacillin [a]Amoxicillin-clavulanate	Duration 7–14 d
	Purulent/MRSA risk factors	ADD: [a]TMP-SMX 1–2 DS PO bid OR Doxycycline 100 mg PO bid	ADD: [a]TMP/SMX 1–2 DS PO bid OR Doxycycline 100 mg PO bid	Linezolid	
Moderate (class 3) DFI—IV therapy usually required initially	Nonpurulent	[a]Ampicillin-sulbactam 1.5 g IV q 6 h	[a]Levofloxacin 750 mg IV q 24 h PLUS Metronidazole 500 mg IV q 8 h	Moxifloxacin	Obtain tissue culture (see Microbiologic Sampling) If oral therapy, duration 14 d
	Purulent/MRSA risk factors	ADD: [a]Vancomycin 20 mg/kg IV loading dose, then 15 mg/kg q 12 h (renal adjustment)	ADD: [a]Vancomycin 20 mg/kg loading dose, then 15 mg/kg q 12 h (renal adjustment)	Linezolid [a]Daptomycin	
	Oral therapy	[a]Amoxicillin-clavulanate 750 mg PO bid × 14 d; for purulent/MRSA risk factors, add TMP-SMX OR doxycycline, as above		[a]Ciprofloxacin PLUS clindamycin	

(continued on next page)

Table 5
(continued)

	Antimicrobial Choice	Antimicrobial Choice if Confirmed PCN or Beta-lactam Allergy	Other Recommended Agents/Regimens	Comments
Severe (class 4) DFI—immediate IV broad-spectrum antibiotics	[a]Piperacillin-tazobactam 4.5 g IV q 6 h PLUS [a]Vancomycin IV as above	[a]Levofloxacin PLUS metronidazole PLUS [a]vancomycin, as above	[a]Imipenim-cilastin [a]Meropenem [a]Ciprofloxacin OR [a]ceftazidime PLUS metronidazole To all the above, add [a]vancomycin OR linezolid OR [a]daptomycin	Strongly consider immediate surgical consultation for urgent debridement and source control

[a] Renal dosage adjustment may be required.

equivalent between antimicrobial treatment arms, with no clear preferred agent emerging from the meta-analyses.[42,46]

DFI guidelines published in 2020 use the IWGDF/IDSA classification (see **Table 2**) to define severity and guide empiric antimicrobial selection. Additionally, guidelines and most experts recommend considering various clinical factors not contained in the IWGDF/IDSA classification, which may predict the risk of resistant pathogens; these are listed in **Table 4**. Unfortunately, since there is little trial evidence supporting one antimicrobial agent over another for DFIs, the guidelines lack specific empiric antimicrobial therapy recommendations. **Table 5** lays out a guideline-concordant approach, with one set of empiric antimicrobial choices presented in detail.

Surgical Treatment

Assessing the need for surgical treatment and source control should go hand in hand with antimicrobial selection. Most DFIs will require some surgical treatment, ranging from minor bedside debridement or incision and drainage of a purulent collection—which can be performed by emergency providers—to major operative procedures such as bone resection, amputation, or revascularization. Guidelines recommend immediate surgical consultation for severe limb ischemia, extensive ischemic gangrene, deep abscess, or compartment syndrome and suspected NSTI. In selected cases, it is appropriate to delay the procedure up to 72 hours so that it can be performed in an operating room or surgical specialty clinic. For severe DFIs, there is evidence that early (within 8–72 hours) surgical drainage, debridement, or limited amputation leads to a lower rate of eventual major amputation.[47,48]

In the case of suspected NSTI, numerous studies involving all types of NSTIs have demonstrated that survival and limb salvage are improved in patients who are taken to the operating room within 6 to 24 hours. While there is limited evidence on diabetic foot NSTIs specifically, experience gained from large, single-center case series suggests

Table 6 Factors suggesting that hospitalization is required	
Comorbid factors	PAD with severe ischemia
	Severe venous insufficiency
	Associated surgical or accidental/traumatic foreign body
Associated systemic illness factors	Rapidly progressive symptoms
	Fever, hypotension, and confusion
	Market hyperglycemia, acidosis, and acute kidney injury
	Marked leukocytosis
	Markedly elevated inflammatory markers (ESR, CRP, procalcitonin; see Inflammatory Markers)
Local wound and infection characteristics	Rapid progression of swelling and inflammation
	Extensive cellulitis (>2 cm from ulcer or wound)
	Lymphangitis
	Wound penetration to fascia, tendon, muscle, joint, and bone
	Signs of infectious necrosis: severe pain, crepitus, bullae, and discoloration (see text)
	Tissue gas located beyond ulcer on x-ray
Additional factors	Need for urgent surgical or diagnostic test not available as outpatient
	Failure of outpatient management
	Unable to take oral antibiotics
	Difficult wound care/dressing changes
	Complicating psychosocial factors

that "early and aggressive" surgical treatment reduces mortality and need for major amputation and limb loss.[48] DFI guidelines recommend that when NSTI is suspected, surgical exploration and debridement or amputation be "urgent" or within 48 hours.[16,29]

Interestingly, the need for routine surgical debridement (vs antimicrobial therapy alone) for osteomyelitis is controversial. Three small studies seem to show that surgical removal of infected bone is not routinely required for nonischemic, forefoot osteomyelitis.[42]

Disposition

Most moderate and all severe DFIs require hospitalization and intravenous antimicrobial therapy. Factors to consider in deciding on disposition are listed in **Table 6**. If the patient will not be admitted directly to a surgical service, consultation with a foot (podiatric, orthopedic, or general) surgeon is mandatory. If there is no other decompensated comorbid illness, mild DFIs can usually be discharged on oral antibiotic therapy. Close follow up—usually within 48 hours—preferably with a foot surgeon, is strongly advised.

CLINICS CARE POINTS

- A careful, well-lit inspection of the feet is mandatory in diabetics presenting with foot pain, unexplained hyperglycemia or unexplained fever or sepsis.
- Infection severity can be assessed using the IWGDF/IDSA classification scheme, based on infection depth and systemic inflammatory signs.
- A critical goal of the physical examination in DFI is to detect signs of a rapidly progressive, limb-threatening NSTI.
- Diabetic osteomyelitis is assessed with the probe to bone test in combination with plain x-ray and inflammatory markers, such as ESR.
- Empiric antimicrobial therapy should be tailored to infection severity; choose oral antimicrobials active against *S aureus* and *Streptococcus* for superficial infections without systemic signs, and a parenteral regimen active against MRSA, gram-negative bacteria, and anaerobes for severe infections.
- Surgical debridement and source control is usually required for an effective treatment of severe DFIs.

DISCLOSURE

Dr B.W. Frazee has no relevant commercial or financial conflict of interest or funding source.

REFERENCES

1. Skrepnek GH, Mills JL, Sr , et al. A Diabetic Emergency One Million Feet Long: Disparities and Burdens of Illness among Diabetic Foot Ulcer Cases within Emergency Departments in the United States, 2006-2010. PLoS One 2015;10(8): e0134914.
2. Armstrong DG, Boulton AJM, Bus SA. Diabetic Foot Ulcers and Their Recurrence. N Engl J Med 2017;376(24):2367–75.
3. Ndosi M, Wright-Hughes A, Brown S, et al. Prognosis of the infected diabetic foot ulcer: a 12-month prospective observational study. Diabet Med 2018;35(1):78–88.

4. Tan T-W, Shih C-D, Concha-Moore KC, et al. Disparities in outcomes of patients admitted with diabetic foot infections. PLoS One 2019;14(2):e0211481.
5. Lavery LA, Hunt NA, Ndip A, et al. Impact of chronic kidney disease on survival after amputation in individuals with diabetes. Diabetes Care 2010;33(11):2365–9.
6. Gardner SE, Hillis SL, Heilmann K, et al. The Neuropathic Diabetic Foot Ulcer Microbiome Is Associated With Clinical Factors. Diabetes 2013;62(3):923–30.
7. Johani K, Fritz BG, Bjarnsholt T, et al. Understanding the microbiome of diabetic foot osteomyelitis: insights from molecular and microscopic approaches. Clin Microbiol Infect 2019;25(3):332–9.
8. Lavery LA, Armstrong DG, Wunderlich RP, et al. Diabetic foot syndrome: evaluating the prevalence and incidence of foot pathology in Mexican Americans and non-Hispanic whites from a diabetes disease management cohort. Diabetes Care 2003;26(5):1435–8.
9. Uçkay I, Aragón-Sánchez J, Lew D, et al. Diabetic foot infections: what have we learned in the last 30 years? Int J Infect Dis 2015;40:81–91.
10. Lew DP, Waldvogel FA. Osteomyelitis. Lancet 2004;364(9431):369–79.
11. Lipsky BA, Pecoraro RE, Larson SA, et al. Outpatient management of uncomplicated lower-extremity infections in diabetic patients. Arch Intern Med 1990;150(4):790–7.
12. Lipsky BA, Senneville E, Abbas ZG, et al. Guidelines on the diagnosis and treatment of foot infection in persons with diabetes (IWGDF 2019 update). Diabetes Metab Res Rev 2020;36(Suppl 1):e3280.
13. Nelson A, Wright-Hughes A, Backhouse MR, et al. CODIFI (Concordance in Diabetic Foot Ulcer Infection): a cross-sectional study of wound swab versus tissue sampling in infected diabetic foot ulcers in England. BMJ Open 2018;8(1):e019437.
14. Senneville E, Melliez H, Beltrand E, et al. Culture of Percutaneous Bone Biopsy Specimens For Diagnosis of Diabetic Foot Osteomyelitis: Concordance With Ulcer Swab Cultures. Clin Infect Dis 2006;42(1):57–62.
15. Zenelaj B, Bouvet C, Lipsky BA, et al. Do diabetic foot infections with methicillin-resistant Staphylococcus aureus differ from those with other pathogens? Int J Low Extrem Wounds 2014;13(4):263–72.
16. Lipsky BA. Medical Treatment of Diabetic Foot Infections. Clin Infect Dis 2004;39(Supplement_2):S104–14.
17. Uckay I, Gariani K, Pataky Z, et al. Diabetic foot infections: state-of-the-art. Diabetes Obes Metab 2014;16(4):305–16.
18. Graham DR, Talan DA, Nichols RL, et al. Once-daily, high-dose levofloxacin versus ticarcillin-clavulanate alone or followed by amoxicillin-clavulanate for complicated skin and skin-structure infections: a randomized, open-label trial. Clin Infect Dis 2002;35(4):381–9.
19. Lipsky BA, Armstrong DG, Citron DM, et al. Ertapenem versus piperacillin/tazobactam for diabetic foot infections (SIDESTEP): prospective, randomised, controlled, double-blinded, multicentre trial. Lancet 2005;366(9498):1695–703.
20. Hatipoglu M, Mutluoglu M, Turhan V, et al. Causative pathogens and antibiotic resistance in diabetic foot infections: A prospective multi-center study. J Diabetes Complications 2016;30(5):910–6.
21. Rastogi A, Sukumar S, Hajela A, et al. The microbiology of diabetic foot infections in patients recently treated with antibiotic therapy: A prospective study from India. J Diabetes Complications 2017;31(2):407–12.
22. Varaiya AY, Dogra JD, Kulkarni MH, et al. Extended-spectrum beta-lactamase-producing Escherichia coli and Klebsiella pneumoniae in diabetic foot infections. Indian J Pathol Microbiol 2008;51(3):370–2.

23. Charles PG, Uçkay I, Kressmann B, et al. The role of anaerobes in diabetic foot infections. Anaerobe 2015;34:8–13.
24. Rayman G, Vas PR, Baker N, et al. The Ipswich Touch Test: a simple and novel method to identify inpatients with diabetes at risk of foot ulceration. Diabetes Care 2011;34(7):1517–8.
25. Edelson GW, Armstrong DG, Lavery LA, et al. The acutely infected diabetic foot is not adequately evaluated in an inpatient setting. Arch Intern Med 1996;156(20): 2373–8.
26. Ince P, Abbas ZG, Lutale JK, et al. Use of the SINBAD classification system and score in comparing outcome of foot ulcer management on three continents. Diabetes Care 2008;31(5):964–7.
27. Monteiro-Soares M, Russell D, Boyko EJ, et al. Guidelines on the classification of diabetic foot ulcers (IWGDF 2019). Diabetes Metab Res Rev 2020;36(Suppl 1): e3273.
28. Ince P, Game FL, Jeffcoate WJ. Rate of healing of neuropathic ulcers of the foot in diabetes and its relationship to ulcer duration and ulcer area. Diabetes Care 2007;30(3):660–3.
29. Lipsky BA, Berendt AR, Cornia PB, et al. 2012 Infectious Diseases Society of America clinical practice guideline for the diagnosis and treatment of diabetic foot infections. Clin Infect Dis 2012;54(12):e132–73.
30. Butalia S, Palda VA, Sargeant RJ, et al. Does this patient with diabetes have osteomyelitis of the lower extremity? JAMA 2008;299(7):806–13.
31. Fernando SM, Tran A, Cheng W, et al. Necrotizing Soft Tissue Infection: Diagnostic Accuracy of Physical Examination, Imaging, and LRINEC Score: A Systematic Review and Meta-Analysis. Ann Surg 2019;269(1):58–65.
32. Mandell JC, Khurana B, Smith JT, et al. Osteomyelitis of the lower extremity: pathophysiology, imaging, and classification, with an emphasis on diabetic foot infection. Emerg Radiol 2018;25(2):175–88.
33. Lauri C, Tamminga M, Glaudemans A, et al. Detection of Osteomyelitis in the Diabetic Foot by Imaging Techniques: A Systematic Review and Meta-analysis Comparing MRI, White Blood Cell Scintigraphy, and FDG-PET. Diabetes Care 2017;40(8):1111–20.
34. Senneville É, Lipsky BA, Abbas ZG, et al. Diagnosis of infection in the foot in diabetes: a systematic review. Diabetes Metab Res Rev 2020;36(Suppl 1):e3281.
35. Sharma H, Sharma S, Krishnan A, et al. The efficacy of inflammatory markers in diagnosing infected diabetic foot ulcers and diabetic foot osteomyelitis: Systematic review and meta-analysis. PLoS One 2022;17(4):e0267412.
36. Armstrong DG, Perales TA, Murff RT, et al. Value of white blood cell count with differential in the acute diabetic foot infection. J Am Podiatr Med Assoc 1996;86(5): 224–7.
37. Victoria van Asten SA, Geradus Peters EJ, Xi Y, et al. The Role of Biomarkers to Diagnose Diabetic Foot Osteomyelitis. A Meta-analysis. Curr Diabetes Rev 2016; 12(4):396–402.
38. Wong CH, Khin LW, Heng KS, et al. The LRINEC (Laboratory Risk Indicator for Necrotizing Fasciitis) score: a tool for distinguishing necrotizing fasciitis from other soft tissue infections. Crit Care Med 2004;32(7):1535–41.
39. Sen P, Demirdal T. Predictive ability of LRINEC score in the prediction of limb loss and mortality in diabetic foot infection. Diagn Microbiol Infect Dis 2021;100(1): 115323.
40. Nelson EA, Backhouse MR, Bhogal MS, et al. Concordance in diabetic foot ulcer infection. BMJ Open 2013;3(1).

41. van der Merwe M, Rooks K, Crawford H, et al. The effect of antibiotic timing on culture yield in paediatric osteoarticular infection. J Child Orthop 2019;13(1): 114–9.
42. Peters EJG, Lipsky BA, Senneville É, et al. Interventions in the management of infection in the foot in diabetes: a systematic review. Diabetes/Metabolism Research and Reviews 2020;36(S1).
43. Dumville JC, Lipsky BA, Hoey C, et al. Topical antimicrobial agents for treating foot ulcers in people with diabetes. Cochrane Database Syst Rev 2017;6(6): Cd011038.
44. Lipsky BA, Itani K, Norden C. Treating foot infections in diabetic patients: a randomized, multicenter, open-label trial of linezolid versus ampicillin-sulbactam/ amoxicillin-clavulanate. Clin Infect Dis 2004;38(1):17–24.
45. Li HK, Agweyu A, English M, et al. An unsupported preference for intravenous antibiotics. PLoS Med 2015;12(5):e1001825.
46. Selva Olid A, Solà I, Barajas-Nava LA, et al. Systemic antibiotics for treating diabetic foot infections. Cochrane Database Syst Rev 2015;2015(9):Cd009061.
47. Faglia E, Clerici G, Caminiti M, et al. The role of early surgical debridement and revascularization in patients with diabetes and deep foot space abscess: retrospective review of 106 patients with diabetes. J Foot Ankle Surg 2006;45(4): 220–6.
48. Tan JS, Friedman NM, Hazelton-Miller C, et al. Can aggressive treatment of diabetic foot infections reduce the need for above-ankle amputation? Clin Infect Dis 1996;23(2):286–91.

Tick-Borne Diseases

Check for updates

Wesley Eilbert, MD*, Andrew Matella, DO

KEYWORDS

- Tick borne diseases • Tick borne illnesses • Vector borne illnesses • Lyme disease
- Rocky Mountain spotted fever • Babesiosis • Tularemia • Ehrlichiosis

KEY POINTS

- Most TBDs can be prevented by early removal of the tick.
- Know what TBDs are present in your geographic area of practice and the initial signs and symptoms of those TBDs.
- Many diagnostic tests for TBDs have limited sensitivity early in the disease course.
- Initiate empiric treatment when clinical presentation and geographic location are consistent with a TBD.

While mosquitoes are responsible for the majority of vector-borne illnesses worldwide, ticks are the main vector in the United States, responsible for 95% of vector-borne diseases.[1] The number of reported tick-borne disease (TBD) cases in the United States has more than doubled since 2004, with 50,865 reported in 2019.[2] Between 2004 and 2016, 7 new TBDs were reported in the United States.[3] Tick populations are increasing and their geographic ranges are expanding,[4] a phenomenon attributed to the effects of climate change.[5] Although TBDs exist throughout the continental United States, they occur predominantly in the eastern part of the country.[3] The geographic distribution of TBDs reported to public health departments in the United States is illustrated in **Box 1**. Mandated reporting of TBDs to public health agencies varies by disease and state.

It is essential that emergency providers be well versed in the diagnosis and management of TBD, as well as be able to counsel patients who present with concerns following a tick bite. US emergency departments (EDs) see a large number of visits for tick bites and suspected TBD annually, with an incidence of 49 tick bite-related visits per 100,000 ED visits.[6] The incidence is as high as 110 per 100,000 visits in the Northeast, though just 13 per 100,000 in the Western region. Syndromic surveillance (based on chief complaint) reveals that the number of tick bite-related ED visits is much greater than the number of suspected TBD cases reported to public health

Department of Emergency Medicine, University of Illinois Chicago, College of Medicine, Room 469, COME, 1819 West Polk Street, Chicago, IL 60612, USA
* Corresponding author.
E-mail address: weilbert@uic.edu

Emerg Med Clin N Am 42 (2024) 287–302
https://doi.org/10.1016/j.emc.2024.01.004
0733-8627/24/© 2024 Elsevier Inc. All rights reserved.
emed.theclinics.com

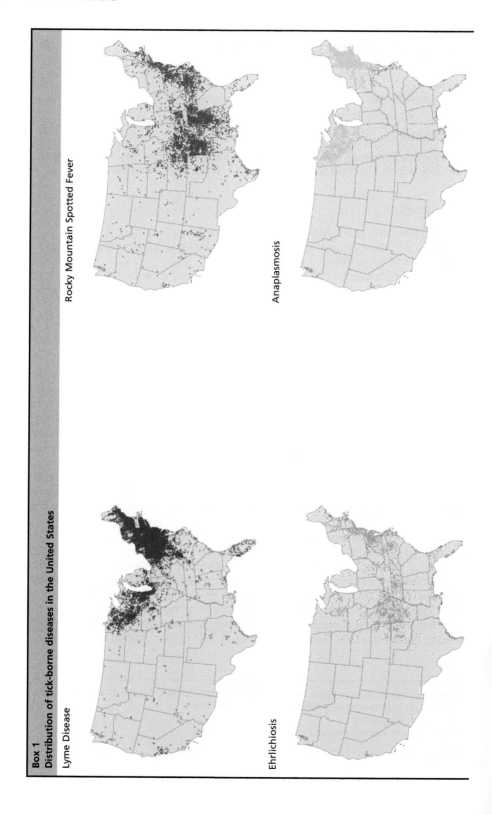

Box 1
Distribution of tick-borne diseases in the United States

Lyme Disease

Rocky Mountain Spotted Fever

Ehrlichiosis

Anaplasmosis

Babesiosis

Tularemia

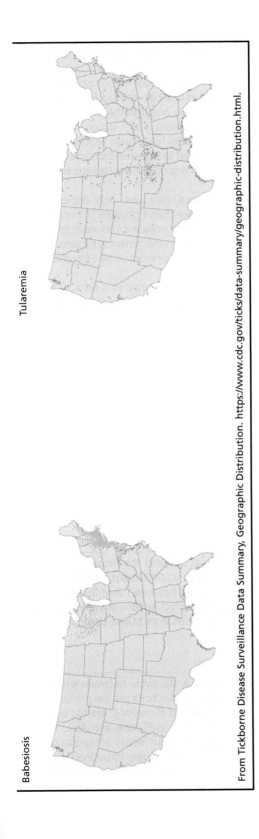

From Tickborne Disease Surveillance Data Summary, Geographic Distribution. https://www.cdc.gov/ticks/data-summary/geographic-distribution.html.

departments.[7] Such visits are particularly common in children less than 10 year old and patients older than 60.

Most TBDs occur between April and October, when outdoor human activity and tick activity are at their peaks.[8] A distinct early peak in tick bite-related ED visits occurs from April through July.[6] A small percentage of TBDs occur in the winter months as many ticks are not killed by cold weather.[8] While most TBDs occur in individuals with recent outdoor activities in wooded areas, TBDs have been reported in urban areas and in individuals who have not recently traveled to high-risk locations.[9] Patients may bring a tick for analysis after a bite, though there is no current recommended role for such testing.[10]

Ticks can transmit bacterial, parasitic, and viral diseases, and depending on geographic location, the same tick may transmit more than 1 disease.[11] Transmission occurs when pathogens harbored in the tick's saliva are released into the host during a blood meal. In general, between 24 and 48 hours of tick attachment is required for disease transmission to occur,[12] so most illnesses can be prevented by early removal of the tick.

In addition to TBDs, tick bites may result in localized allergic reactions, and rarely anaphylaxis.[13] Tick paralysis is a unique phenomenon caused by a toxin present in the salivary glands of various species of ticks.[14] The typical presentation is that of an acute symmetric flaccid paralysis that evolves over hours to days.[14] The definitive treatment of tick paralysis is simply to remove the tick attached to the patient's body.[14]

TBDs occur more often than is generally recognized.[8] This is due, in part, to their nonspecific signs and symptoms such as fever, myalgias, headache, and vomiting. It is not surprising that many patients with TBDs are initially misdiagnosed with other more common viral illnesses such as gastroenteritis, streptococcal pharyngitis, or viral syndromes.[15] Furthermore, only 50% to 70% of patients with a TBD recall being bitten by a tick.[11] Fortunately, most TBDs are easily treated when diagnosed early. Since many diagnostic tests are limited by poor sensitivity early in the disease course, empiric treatment should be initiated when the patient's clinical presentation and geographic location suggest a TBD (see **Box 1**).

LYME DISEASE
Epidemiology

First recognized in 1976,[16] Lyme disease (LD) has become the most commonly reported vector-borne infection in North America, with 30,000 cases reported annually in the United States.[17] The actual number of cases has been estimated to be 10-fold higher.[18] LD has been reported in all 50 states, with over 96% of cases diagnosed in people living in northeastern and mid-Atlantic states from Maine to Virginia, and in Wisconsin, Minnesota, and Michigan.[19]

Microbiology and Pathophysiology

The Borrelia spirochete is maintained in a natural sylvatic cycle between small mammals and its arthropod vector. In the United States, Ixodes ticks are the primary vector for LD, and 2 Borrelia species, Borrelia burgdorferi and B mayonii, are the causative pathogens.[20,21] Other spirochete species predominate in Europe and Asia. Borrelia infection and the initial human immune response first occur locally at the site of inoculation, but within days to weeks, Borrelia disseminates widely throughout the host. Subsequent stages of infection and disease manifestations may depend on low-level persistence of the spirochete in tissues such as joints and the central nervous system, its ability to activate versus evade the immune response, and on antimicrobial treatment.

History and Physical Examination

Lyme disease typically presents in 3 stages. *Stage 1 (early localized LD)* can be recognized by the presence of an expanding erythematous skin lesion known as erythema migrans (EM). EM is the most common sign of LD and is the presenting manifestation in approximately 75% of cases.[22] EM usually begins as an erythematous macule or papule that appears at the site of the tick bite 1 or 2 weeks later.[23] The lesion then expands over the next 3 to 4 weeks to an area more than 5 cm in diameter[17] as the spirochete migrates out from the site of inoculation.[24] (**Fig. 1**) EM lesions may occur anywhere on the body, though are most commonly found on the legs, groin, waist, back, and, in children, the head and neck.[23] Although classically described as having a bull's-eye appearance, approximately two-thirds of EM lesions are uniform in appearance or have only enhanced central erythema.[23] EM may be accompanied by malaise, fatigue, headache, myalgias, fever, and regional lymphadenopathy.[25] If untreated, EM lesions typically resolve in less than 30 days (see **Fig. 1**).[17]

If EM is not treated, the *second stage of Lyme disease, also known as early disseminated infection*, begins within days to weeks as the spirochete begins to spread hematogenously.[24] During this stage, up to one-half of infected individuals develop multiple secondary annular skin lesions that resemble the appearance of the primary EM lesion.[26] The majority of patients will have associated systemic symptoms, such as fever, malaise, and headache.[26] During this stage, approximately 10% of patients will develop neurologic symptoms, known as Lyme neuroborreliosis.[27] The most common clinical features of Lyme neuroborreliosis are lymphocytic meningitis with fever and headache, peripheral neuropathy, and cranial neuropathy.[17] The facial nerve is the cranial nerve affected in approximately three-fourths of cases, with the condition being bilateral up to 25% of the time.[28] Also during the second stage of untreated Lyme disease, up to 4% of patients will develop Lyme carditis.[29] The manifestations of the carditis may include myocarditis with myocardial dysfunction and characteristic electrocardiographic changes, as well as atrioventricular (AV) nodal conduction abnormalities.[29] Patients with AV nodal disease can have a fluctuating pattern of heart block ranging from first-degree to complete heart block.[30] AV blocks are a transient phenomenon and typically resolve in 1 to 6 weeks.[29]

The *third stage of Lyme disease, referred to as late or persistent infection*, occurs in untreated individuals on average 6 months after the appearance of the EM lesion.[31]

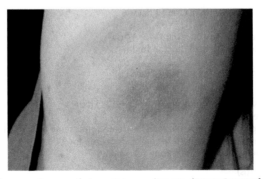

Fig. 1. Classic erythema migrans of stage 1 Lyme disease. (From Center for Disease Control and Prevention.)

The primary manifestation of this stage is a recurrent monoarthritis or oligoarthritis occurring in approximately 60% of patients.[31] The knee is the most commonly affected joint.[24]

Approximately 10% of patients with EM and likely a higher percentage of patients with Lyme neuroborreliosis will develop subjective symptoms such as fatigue, musculoskeletal pain, and cognitive dysfunction starting within 6 months of diagnosis and persisting for at least 6 months after completing antibiotic therapy.[32] These symptoms have been referred to as post-treatment Lyme disease syndrome (PTLDS)[27,32] Treatment of PTLDS is controversial and several randomized clinical trials have failed to find substantive benefit from prolonged antibiotic therapy as treatment.[33]

Diagnosis and Treatment

Detection of borrelial infection by laboratory testing is required for reliable diagnosis of Lyme disease, except when skin lesions suspicious for EM are present. In an individual with a potential tick exposure in a Lyme disease endemic area, a rash consistent with EM is all that is necessary for a clinical diagnosis.[34] For diagnosis of second and third stages of Lyme disease, serum antibody testing is preferred since polymerase chain reaction (PCR) testing is not well standardized.[17,34] In patients suspected of Lyme neuroborreliosis, antibody testing of cerebrospinal fluid should be obtained if a lumbar puncture is performed.[34] If arthrocentesis is performed in those patients with possible Lyme arthritis, PCR testing of the synovial fluid should be obtained.[34]

Prophylactic antibiotic therapy is indicated within 72 hours of removal of an identified high-risk tick bite.[34] A tick bite is considered high risk if the following 3 criteria are met: the bite was from an identified *Ixodes* species tick, the tick was attached for more than 36 hours, and the bite occurred in a highly endemic area.[34] If the tick bite cannot be confirmed as being high risk, a wait-and-see approach is recommended.[34] **Box 2** lists the recommended treatments for the various Lyme disease stages and manifestations.[17,32,34]

Box 2
Treatment of Lyme disease

Post-bite prophylaxis
  Adult: Doxycycline 200 mg once
  Child: Doxycycline 4.4 mg/kg once

Stage 1 (Erythema migrans)
  Adult: Doxycycline 100 mg BID for 10 days
    Or
    Amoxicillin 250 to 500 mg TID for 14 days
    Or
    Cefuroxime axetil 250 to 500 mg BID for 14 days
  Child: Doxycycline 1 to 2 mg/kg BID for 10 days
    Or
    Amoxicillin 25 to 50 mg/kg TID for 14 days

Stage 2
  If only cutaneous manifestations, treat the same as Stage 1
  Lyme neuroborreliosis
    Cranial or peripheral neuropathies can be treated that same as Stage 1
    Meningitis: admission and ceftriaxone or cefotaxime for 14 days
  Lyme carditis: admission and ceftriaxone for 14 days

Stage 3 (Lyme arthritis)
  Treat the same as Stage 1, but for 28 days

ROCKY MOUNTAIN SPOTTED FEVER
Epidemiology

Rocky Mountain spotted fever (RMSF) is the most lethal TBD in the United States with an overall mortality of 5% to 10%.[35] Approximately 2000 cases of RMSF are reported in the United States every year,[9] with an increase in cases over the past 20 years.[36] RMSF has been reported in most of the continental 48 states, with over half of the reported cases occurring in North Carolina, South Carolina, Tennessee, Oklahoma, and Arkansas.[37] See **Box 1.**

Microbiology and Pathophysiology

There are 3 identified tick vectors for RMSF in the United States, with *Dermacentor* sp. ticks responsible for most human transmissions.[38] The gram-negative obligate intracellular spirochete *Rickettsia rickettsii* is the causative pathogen.[38] Transmission to humans may occur with as little as 6 hours of tick attachment. Upon entry into the body from the tick bite, the bacteria infect the endothelial cells of blood vessels, multiply, and then spread to other areas of the body via the bloodstream. Most of the signs and symptoms of RMSF are caused by infiltration of small blood vessels with resultant vasculitis.

History and Physical Examination

Symptoms of RMSF typically appear 3 to 12 days after the tick bite,[35] with an average of 7 days.[38] Initial symptoms include sudden onset of fever, severe headache, malaise, and myalgias.[35,36] Abdominal pain, vomiting, and diarrhea may be present.[39] A total of 90% of individuals will develop a rash, which typically appears 2 to 5 days after the onset of the fever.[39] The classic rash of RMSF starts as blanching macules on the wrists and ankles, then spreads centripetally to the trunk, and may involve the palms and soles.[39] **(Fig. 2)** The rash may become maculopapular with central petechiae.[35,38,39] The classic triad of rash, fever, and headache is present in only 3% of patients within the first 3 days of the illness, though it may be present in up to 70% of patients by 2 weeks.[38] Severe late stage manifestations of RMSF include acute renal failure, adult respiratory distress syndrome, meningoencephalitis, arrhythmias, disseminated intravascular coagulation, and cutaneous necrosis.

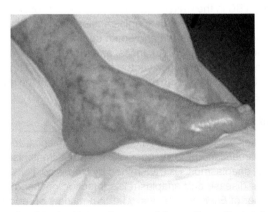

Fig. 2. The classic rash of Rocky Mountain spotted fever. (From Center for Disease Control and Prevention.)

Diagnosis and Treatment

Ideally, RMSF can be diagnosed early in the disease course, since treatment within the first 5 days of the illness significantly reduces disease severity and the probability of death. Clues to the correct diagnosis on standard laboratory studies include thrombocytopenia, elevated liver amino transaminase levels, elevated creatinine kinase, and abnormal coagulation studies.[38,39] Hyponatremia (sodium < 130) is present in 20% to 50% of cases.[39] Indirect fluorescent antibody (IFA) testing is the current criterion standard for detection of spotted fever rickettsial diseases, though antibody levels are typically undetectable until 7 to 10 days after disease onset.[38] A presumptive diagnosis of RMSF should be made clinically, and antibiotic therapy initiated, while awaiting laboratory confirmation of the illness.[10-12,38-40]

Tetracyclines and chloramphenicol are the only antibiotics proven to be effective in humans for the treatment of RMSF. Doxycycline is the antibiotic of choice for all patients regardless of age and pregnancy status.[10,12,35,38] The recommended dose for doxycycline for treatment of RMSF is 100 mg twice daily orally or intravenously (IV).[35] For children less than 45 kg, the dose is 2.2 mg/kg.[41] Emergency providers need to maintain a very low threshold for provisional diagnosis and treatment of RMSF, meaning a suggestive presentation in the appropriate epidemiologic setting should prompt immediate empiric therapy in the ED. Oral therapy is appropriate for those in the early stage of disease, with IV therapy indicated for more severely ill patients requiring hospitalization. The duration of therapy should be at least for 5 to 7 days, and should be continued until the patient has been afebrile for at least 3 days.[35,38]

The American Academy of Pediatrics and Centers for Disease Control both recommend doxycycline as the treatment of choice for RMSF in children regardless of age.[42,43] Previous concerns about teeth staining in children less than 8 years arose from experience with older tetracyclines that bind more readily to calcium than the newer tetracyclines, such as doxycycline.[44] Doxycycline use at the recommended dose and duration for RMSF in children less than 8 years, even after multiple courses, has not been found to result in teeth staining.[45]

EHRLICHIOSIS AND ANAPLASMOSIS
Epidemiology

Ehrlichiosis and anaplasmosis are related tick-borne diseases caused by intracellular rickettsial bacteria that grow within leukocytes. Considered together, they are the second most common TBD in the United States.[39] The mortality of ehrlichiosis is approximately 1%,[46] and significantly less for anaplasmosis.[47] The geographic distribution of ehrlichiosis is along the southeastern and south central United States, with Missouri, Mississippi, Oklahoma, Tennessee, Arkansas, and Maryland with the highest rates of infection.[48] As a result of a shared tick vector, the geographic distribution of anaplasmosis is similar to Lyme disease, with most cases occurring in the northeastern region of the United States and the upper Midwest.[39] See **Box 1**.

Microbiology and Pathophysiology

There are several tick vectors for ehrlichiosis in North America, though the lone star tick (*Amblyomma americanam*) is responsible for most transmission to humans.[48] Like Lyme disease, anaplasmosis is transmitted by *Ixodes* sp. ticks.[48] For this reason, simultaneous Lyme disease and anaplasmosis infection may occur.[35] Ehrlichiosis is caused by a number of *Ehrlichia* species, with the majority of reported cases due to *E. chaffensis*. Anaplasmosis is caused by the bacterium *Anaplasma phagocytophilum*.[49] Both *E. chaffenis* and *A phagocytophilum* are obligate intracellular bacteria that multiply in the cytoplasm of host leukocytes in clusters of bacteria called morulae, hence the technical disease names of human monocyte ehrlichiosis and human granulocyte anaplasmosi.[48] It is the host inflammatory response, rather than the direct effect of the pathogens, that is thought to be the mechanism of tissue damage with ehrlichiosis and anaplasmosis.

History and Physical Examination

Symptoms typically appear 5 to 14 days after the tick bite.[35] Both ehrlichiosis and anaplasmosis present with nonspecific flu-like symptoms. Fever is present in the vast majority of cases, with headache and myalgias reported in most cases.[48,49] Gastrointestinal symptoms, including vomiting and diarrhea are present in a minority of cases.[48,49] Approximately one-third of patients with ehrlichiosis will develop a rash, usually occurring approximately 5 days after illness onset.[35] The rash may be maculopapular or petechial, and usually present on the trunk and extremities.[50] Children are more likely than adults to develop a rash with ehrlichiosis.[48] Rash is less common in patients with anaplasmosis, occurring in less than 10% of cases.[49]

While anaplasmosis is a self-limiting illness in most cases,[35] ehrlichiosis is more severe, with up to 62% of cases requiring hospitalization.[48] The elderly and patients with compromised immune systems are at increased risk for severe disease.[35] Up to 20% of patients with ehrlichiosis will have central nervous system involvement, including meningitis or meningoencephalitis.[48]

Diagnosis and Treatment

Common laboratory findings with ehrlichiosis and anaplasmosis include leukopenia, thrombocytopenia, and elevated hepatic transaminases.[35,49] If available, PCR testing is the most sensitive and specific method to diagnose ehrlichiosis and anaplasmosis in the first 1 to 2 weeks of illness.[4] The value of PCR *testing significantly diminishes after the second week of symptoms*.[4] Serologic testing by IFA assay is considered the reference standard for diagnosing ehrlichiosis and anaplasmosis, though this test is of limited utility in the first week of illness.[4]

Since disease severity is significantly reduced by early antibiotic therapy, patients suspected of having ehrlichiosis or anaplasmosis should be treated without waiting for confirmatory testing.[48] Doxycycline given orally or IV is the treatment of choice for ehrlichiosis and anaplasmosis.[35] The dosing and duration is the same as when given for treatment of RMSF. Rifampin may be used in patients not able to tolerate doxycycline,[12,50] though it is not well studied in this setting.[35] The dose of rifampin is 300 mg twice daily for 7 days in adults and 10 mg/kg twice daily for 7 days in children.[35]

BABESIOSIS
Epidemiology

First described in humans in 1957,[51] babesiosis is caused by *Babesia* sp. protozoa and share many similar clinical features with *Plasmodium* malaria parasites, including reproduction in mammalian red blood cells.[1] Babesiosis is the only TBD caused by protozoa in the United States.[11] The incidence of babesiosis has increased significantly over the past 20 years,[4] with over 2400 cases reported in the United States in 2019.[52] Since *Babesia* sp. are intraerythrocytic parasites, babesiosis may also be transmitted by transfusion of blood products.[53] With the same tick vector as *Borrelia* sp., the geographic distribution of babesiosis is similar to that of Lyme disease in the United States.[39] Because of the same tick vector, between 6% and 23% of patients diagnosed with babesiosis in endemic areas will have concurrent Lyme disease.[41]

Microbiology and Pathophysiology

Ixodes ticks, primarily *Ixodes scapularis*, are the vector for babesiosis in the United States.[50] While several different species of *Babesia* may cause infection in humans, the overwhelming majority of cases in the United States are caused by *Babesia microti*.[53] *B microti*, in the trophozoite stage, are transmitted from the gastrointestinal tract of the nymph tick into the human dermis, where they then migrate to the bloodstream and replicate as merozoites within erythrocytes. The resulting hemolysis is responsible for many of the disease manifestations. Severe disease is significantly more common in individuals with asplenia, advanced age, immunosuppression, and medical comorbidities.[54]

History and Physical Examination

Babesiosis has a variable clinical presentation, ranging from asymptomatic to multiorgan failure. It is estimated that approximately one-half of children and one-fifth of adults with babesiosis will be asymptomatic.[55] In symptomatic patients, symptoms typically begin 1 to 4 weeks after the tick bite.[54] Similar to malaria, intermittent fever, as high as 40°C, is the most common initial symptom along with chills, anorexia, headache, and myalgias.[54] Other symptoms that may occur include abdominal pain, vomiting, conjunctival injection, arthralgias, hyperesthesia, shortness of breath, and dark urine.[39,53,54] Physical examination findings include fever, splenomegaly, hepatomegaly, pallor, and splinter hemorrhages.[53,54] More severe cases may present with symptoms of anemia, acute respiratory distress syndrome, disseminated intravascular coagulation, congestive heart failure, and coma.[39,53,54] Splenic rupture may occur.[54] Fatality rates of 6% to 9% have been reported in patients requiring hospitalization, and in 21% of patients who are immunosuppressed.[53]

Diagnosis and Treatment

The diagnosis of babesiosis should be considered in any patient with an unexplained febrile illness who has lived in or traveled to an endemic area in the previous 2 months.[53] Clues to the diagnosis which may be found on standard laboratory testing include evidence of a mild to moderate hemolytic anemia, such as a low hemoglobin level, elevated reticulocyte count, and elevated lactate dehydrogenase level, as well as thrombocytopenia, elevated liver enzymes, proteinuria, and elevated blood urea nitrogen and serum creatinine.[53,54]

Definitive diagnosis can be made by microscopic identification of the parasites within the red blood cells seen on Giemsa or Wright-stained peripheral thin blood smear. Unfortunately, up to 25% of cases will have a false-negative peripheral smear.[10] Also, *Babesia* can be confused with malaria parasites on thin peripheral smear.[4] Serum antibody testing may be used to aid in diagnosis though may be negative in the early stages of infection.[4] PCR assay is highly sensitive and specific for the detection of the *Babesia* in blood.

The combination of atovaquone and azithromycin is the treatment of choice for immunocompetent patients with mild to moderate disease. (**Box 3**)[4,53] Intravenous clindamycin combined with quinine is recommended for patients with severe disease.[4,53] Exchange transfusion may also be performed in patients with severe disease.[53,54]

TULAREMIA
Epidemiology

First identified in 1911,[56] tularemia is a bacterial illness transmitted to humans through arthropod bites, direct contact with infected animals, inhalation or conjunctival

> **Box 3**
> **Treatment of babesiosis[a]**
>
> Immunocompetent patients with mild to moderate disease
>   Adult: Atovaquone 750 mg BID
>   Azithromycin 500 mg on day 1 and 250 mg daily thereafter
>   Child: Atovaquone 20 mg/kg BID
>   Azithromycin 10 mg/kg on day 1 and 5 mg/kg daily thereafter
>
> Patients with severe disease
>   Adult: Clindamycin 300 to 600 mg IV QID
>   Quinine 650 mg TID or QID
>   Child: Clindamycin 7 to 10 mg/kg IV TID or QID
>   Quinine 8 mg/kg TID
>
> [a]Antibiotic therapy should be administered for 7 to 10 days.

exposure to aerosols, and ingestion of contaminated food or water.[57] While tularemia may present in several different forms, depending on the mode of transmission, ticks are responsible for the majority of cases in the United States. where approximately 200 cases of vector-borne tularemia are reported each year.[3,58] Tularemia cases are most common in the south-central region of the United States., clustered in Oklahoma, Arkansas, Missouri, and Kansas.[12] Before the antibiotic era, the mortality rate of some forms of tularemia approached 60%, with the current rate being less than 2%.[59] Because of its high transmissibility, including via aerosols, potential to cause severe disease, and lack of an available effective vaccine, tularemia is classified as a List A agent of most severe concern for bioterrorism by the US Department of Health and Human Services.[56]

Microbiology and Pathophysiology

The main tick vectors for tularemia in the United States are the dog tick (*Dermacentor variabilis*), the wood tick (*Dermacentor andersoni*), and the lone star tick (*Amblyomma Americanum*).[60] The highly infectious gram-negative bacteria *Francisella tularensis* is the causative pathogen.[57] There are multiple disease forms of tularemia, determined by the route of inoculation. Ulceroglandular tularemia is the most common form of infection (75% to 90% of cases), resulting from of transmission through the skin,

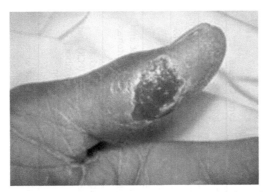

Fig. 3. A cutaneous ulcer caused by tularemia. (From Center for Disease Control and Prevention.)

Table 1
Clinical features of the main tick-borne diseases in North America

	Lyme Disease	Rocky Mountain Spotted Fever	Ehrlichiosis	Anaplasmosis	Babesiosis	Tularemia
Tick Vector	Ixodes sp.	Dermacentor sp.	Amblyomma americanam	Ixodes sp.	Ixodes sp.	Ixodes sp.
Pathogen(s)	Borrelia burgdorferi, Borrelia mayonii	Rickettsia rickettsii	Ehrlichia sp.	Anaplasma phagocytophilum	Babesia sp.	Francisella tularensis
US reported yearly cases	30,000	2000	2000	5700	2400	200
Key clinical features	Rash, neurologic and cardiac symptoms, arthritis	Fever, headache, rash	Fever, headache, rash	Fever, headache, rash	Fever, headache, hemolytic anemia	Fever, headache, skin ulcer, lymphadenopathy
Diagnostic tests	Polymerase chain reaction (PCR) and serum antibody detection	Serum antibody detection	PCR and serum antibody detection	PCR and serum antibody detection	Thin blood smear, PCR, and serum antibody detection	F. tularensis detection in tissues (culture, PCR, DFA) and serum antibody detection
Antimicrobials	Doxycycline or amoxicillin or cephalosporins	Doxycycline or chloramphenicol	Doxycycline or rifampin	Doxycycline or rifampin	Atovaquone plus azithromycin or clindamycin plus quinine	Doxycycline or ciprofloxacin or aminoglycosides

usually from a tick bite.[61] Pneumonic tularemia occurs through inhalation of infected aerosols. Oropharyngeal tularemia is caused by ingestion of contaminated food or water. Conjunctival exposure may cause oculoglandular tularemia. Typhoidal tularemia is a systemic form of the disease, most commonly occurring in immunocompromised patients. Glandular tularemia is characterized by lymphadentitis without an obvious mode of transmission.

History and Physical Examination

Tick-borne tularemia results in ulceroglandular disease.[50] Symptoms typically begin 3 to 5 days after the tick bite, with a range of 1 to 21 days.[10] Flu-like symptoms appear first, including fever, headache, cough, vomiting, and diarrhea. After these initial symptoms, a painful papule develops at the site of the tick bite. The papule usually evolves into a painful ulcer with an elevated border.[56] (**Fig. 3**) Lymph nodes near the ulcer enlarge as the bacteria disseminates through the lymphatics. The involved lymph nodes may become fluctuant, and draining suppuration may be noted in the areas of lymphadenopathy.[11] Left untreated, ulceroglandular tularemia lasts an average of 32 days.[56] Typically, this form of tularemia is not fatal.[50]

Diagnosis and Treatment

A characteristic skin ulcer, as described earlier, with associated lymphadenopathy, in the setting of possible tick exposure, should lead to suspicion of ulceroglandular tularemia. Definitive diagnosis is made by isolation of the organism in a clinical specimen or by serologic testing. Detection of *F tularensis* in specimens obtained from skin ulcers or lymph node biopsy or drainage may be performed by culture, PCR testing, or direct fluorescent antibody testing.[10,50] A serologic diagnosis may be made by an elevated serum antibody titer.[56]

Treatment of suspected ulceroglandular tularemia should not be delayed by confirmatory testing.[11] Antibiotic therapy should be continued for 10 to 21 days depending on the severity of illness. Mild infection can be treated with ciprofloxacin 750 mg orally twice daily or doxycycline 100 mg orally twice daily.[56] In children, the dosing of doxycycline should be the same as that used for RMSF.[8] More severe infections should be treated with an aminoglycoside, such as streptomycin 1 g IV twice daily or gentamicin 5 mg/kg IV once or twice daily.[56] In children, streptomycin 15 mg/kg IV twice daily or gentamicin 2.5 mg/kg IV 3 times a day can be used.[56]

The clinical features of each main TBD in North America are summarized in **Table 1**.

CLINICS CARE POINTS

- Ticks are responsible for the majority of vector-borne illnesses in the United States.
- The number of reported tick-borne disease cases has more than doubled since 2004.
- Ticks can transmit bacterial, parasitic, and viral illnesses.
- Between 24 and 48 hours of tick attachment is required for transmission of most TBDs, so illnesses can be prevented by early removal of the tick.
- TBDs present a challenge to emergency providers: immediate empiric therapy based on clinical diagnosis is generally recommended (and is critical in the case of RMSF), yet signs and symptoms are vexingly nonspecific, and TBDs are often initially misdiagnosed as viral illnesses.
- Only 50% to 70% of patients with a tick-borne disease recall being bitten by a tick.

DISCLOSURE

The authors have no commercial or financial conflicts to disclose. The authors received no funding used in the preparation of this article.

REFERENCES

1. Rochlin I, Toledo A. Emerging tick-borne pathogens of public health importance: a mini review. J Med Microbiol 2020;69(6):781–91.
2. Centers for Disease Control and Prevention. Tickborne disease surveillance data summary. Available at: https://www.cdc,gov/ticks/data-summary/index.html. [Accessed 16 September 2022].
3. Rosenberg R, Lindsey NP, Fisher M, et al. Vital signs: trends in reported vector-borne disease cases - United States and territories, 2004 - 2016. MMWR Morb Mortal Wkly Rep 2018;67(17):496–501.
4. Madison-Antenucci S, Kramer LD, Gebhardt LL, et al. Emerging tick-borne diseases. Clin Microbiol Rev 2020;33(2). 000833-e118.
5. Beard C, Eisen R, Barker C, et al. The impacts of climate change on human health in the United States: a scientific assessment. Available at: https://health2016.globalchange.gov/vectorborne-diseases#. [Accessed 17 September 2022].
6. Marx G, Spillane M, Beck A, et al. Emergency Department Visits for Tick Bites – United States January 2017-December 2019. MMWR (Morb Mortal Wkly Rep) 2021;70(17):612–6.
7. Daly E, Fredette C, Mathewson A, et al. Tick bite and Lyme disease-related emergency department encounters in New Hampshire, 2010-2014. Zoonoses Public Health 2017;64:655–61.
8. Mukkada S, Buckingham SC. Recognition of and prompt treatments for tickborne infections in children. Inf Dis Clin N Am 2015;29(3):539–55.
9. Salgo MP, Telzak EE, Curie B, et al. A focus of Rocky Mountain spotted fever within New York City. N Engl J Med 1988;318(21):1345–8.
10. Pace EJ, O'Reilly M. Tickborne diseases: diagnosis and management. Am Fam Physician 2020;101(9):530–40.
11. Werner SL, Banda BK, Burnsides CL, et al. Zoonosis: update on existing and emerging vector-borne illnesses in the USA. Curr Emerg Hosp Med Rep 2019;7(3):91–106.
12. Pujalte GGA, Marbarry ST, Libertin CR. Tick-borne illnesses in the United States. Prim Care 2018;45(3):379–91.
13. Van Wye JE, Hsu YP, Terr AI, et al. Anaphylaxis from a tick bite. N Engl J Med 1991;324(11):777–8.
14. Edlow JA, McGillicuddy DC. Tick paralysis. Infect Dis Clin N Am 2008;22(3):397–413.
15. Buckingham SC. Tick-borne diseases of the USA: 10 things clinicians should know. Infect Dis Clin North Am 2015;29(3):539–55.
16. Steere AC, Malawista SE, Snydman DR, et al. Lyme arthritis: an epidemic of oligoarticular arthritis in children and adults in three Connecticut communities. Arthritis Rheum 1977;20(1):7–17.
17. Schoen RT. Lyme disease: diagnosis and treatment. Curr Opin Rheumatol 2020;32(3):247–54.
18. Kuehn BM. CDC estimates 300,000 US cases of Lyme disease annually. JAMA 2013;310(11):1110.
19. Mead PS. Epidemiology of Lyme disease. Infect Dis Clin North Am 2015;29(2):187–210.

20. Applegren ND, Kraus CK. Lyme disease: Emergency department considerations. J Emerg Med 2017;52(6):815–24.
21. Schwartz AM, Hinckley AF, Mead PS, et al. Surveillance for Lyme disease - United States, 2008 - 2015. MMWR Surveill Summ 2017;66(22):1–12.
22. Steere AC Sikand VK. The presenting manifestations of Lyme disease and outcomes of treatment. N Engl J Med 2003;348(24):2472–4.
23. Shapiro ED. Clinical practice. Lyme disease. N Engl J Med 2014;370(18): 1724–31.
24. Bush LM, Vasquez-Pertejo MT. Tick borne illness – Lyme disease. Dis Mon 2018; 64(5):195–212.
25. Wormser GP. Clinical practice. Early Lyme disease. N Engl J Med 2006;354(26): 2794–801.
26. Steere AC, Bartenhagen NH, Craft JE, et al. The early clinical manifestations of Lyme disease. Ann Intern Med 1983;99(1):76–82.
27. Kullberg BJ, Vrijmoeth HD, van de Schoor F, et al. Lyme Borreliosis: diagnosis and management. BMJ 2020;369:m1041.
28. Halperin JJ. Nervous system lyme disease: diagnosis and treatment. Curr Treat Options Neurol 2013;15(4):454–64.
29. Robinson ML, Kobayashi T, Higgins Y, et al. Lyme carditis. Infect Dis Clin North Am 2015;29(2):255–68.
30. Steere AC, Batsford WP, Weinberg M, et al. Lyme carditis: cardiac abnormalities of Lyme disease. Ann Intern Med 1980;93(1):8–16.
31. Steere AC, Schoen RT, Taylor E. The clinical evolution of Lyme arthritis. Ann Intern Med 1987;107(5):725–31.
32. Steere AC, Strle F, Wormser GP, et al. Lyme borreliosis. Nat Rev Dis Primers 2016; 2:16090.
33. Marques A. Persistent symptoms after treatment of Lyme disease. Infect Dis Clin N Am 2022;36(3):621–38.
34. Lantos PM, Rumbaugh J, Bockenstedt LK, et al. Clinical practice guidelines by the Infectious Diseases Society of America, American Academy of Neurology, and American College of Rheumatology: 2020 guidelines for the prevention, diagnosis, and treatment of Lyme disease. Neurology 2021;96(6):262–73.
35. Biggs HM, Behravesh CV, Bradley KK, et al. Diagnosis and management of tick-borne rickettsial diseases: Rocky Mountain spotted fever and other spotted fever group Rickettsioses, Ehrlichioses, and Anaplasmosis - United States. MMWR Recomm Rep (Morb Mortal Wkly Rep) 2016;65(2):1–44.
36. Centers for Disease Control and Prevention. Rocky Mountain spotted fever. Epidemiology and statistics. Available at: https://www.cdc.gov/rmsf/stats/index.html. [Accessed 15 October 2022].
37. McFee RB. Tick borne illnesses Rocky mountain spotted fever. Dis Mon 2018; 64(5):185–94.
38. Gottlieb M, Long B, Koyfman A. The evaluation and management of Rocky mountain spotted fever in the emergency department: a review of the literature. J Emerg Med 2018;55(1):42–50.
39. Liu A. Tickborne illnesses. Pediatr Ann 2021;50(9):e350–5.
40. Jay R, Armstrong PA. Clinical characteristics of Rocky Mountain spotted fever in the United States: A literature review. J Vector Borne Dis 2020;57(2):114–20.
41. Diuk-Wasser MA, Vannier E, Krasue PJ. Coinfection by tick-borne pathogens Babesia microti and Borrelia burgdorferi: ecologic, epidemiologic and clinical consequences. Trends Parasitol 2016;32(1):30–42.

42. Chapman AS, Bakken JS, Folk SM, et al. Diagnosis and management of tick-borne rickettsial diseases: Rocky Mountain spotted fever, ehrlichioses, and anaplasmosis - United States: a practical guide for physicians and other health-care and public health professionals. MMWR Recomm Rep (Morb Mortal Wkly Rep) 2006;55(RR-4):1–27.

43. American Academy of Pediatrics, Committee on Infectious Diseases. Rickettsial diseases. In: Kimberlin DW, Long SS, Brady MT, et al, editors. Red book: 2015 report of the committee on infectious diseases. 30th edition. Elk Grove Village, IL: American Academy of Pediatrics; 2015. p. 677–80.

44. Schach von Wittenau M. Some pharmacokinetic aspects of doxycycline metabolism in man. Chemotherapia 1968;13(Suppl 1):41–50.

45. Todd SR, will Dahlgren FS, Traeger MS, et al. No visible dental staining in children treated with doxycycline for suspected Rocky Mountain spotted fever. J Pediatr 2015;166(5):1246–51.

46. Centers for Disease Control and Prevention. Ehrlichiosis. Epidemiology and statistics. Available at: https://www.cdc.gov/ehrlichiosis/stats/index.html. [Accessed 25 October 2022].

47. Centers for Disease Control and Prevention. Anaplasmosis. Epidemiology and statistics. Available at: https://www.cdc.gov/anaplasmosis/stats/index.html. [Accessed 25 October 2022].

48. Ismail N, McBride JW. Tick-borne emerging infections: Ehrlichiosis and anaplasmosis. Clin Lab Med 2017;37(2):317–40.

49. Bakken JS, Dummler JS. Human granulocytic anaplasmosis. Infect Dis Clin N Am 2015;29(2):341–55.

50. Rodino KG, Theel ES, Pritt BS. Tick-borne diseases in the United States. Cli Chem 2020;66(4):537–48.

51. Skrabalo A, Deanovic A. Piroplasmosis in man: Report on a case. Doc Med Geogr Trop 1957;9(1):11–6.

52. Centers for Disease Control and Prevention. Babesiosis. Epidemiology and statistics. Available at: https://www.cdc.gov/parasites/babesiosis/resources/Surveillance_Babesiosis_US_2019.pdf. [Accessed 3 November 2022].

53. Vannier E, Krause PJ. Human babesiosis. N Engl J Med 2012;366(25):2397–407.

54. Krause PJ. Human babesiosis. Int J Parasitol 2019;49(2):165–74.

55. Vannier EG, Duik Wasser MA, Ben Mamoun C, et al. Babesiosis. Infect Dis Clin North Am 2015;29(2):357–70.

56. Troha K, Bozanic Urbancic N, Korva M, et al. Vector-borne tularemia: a re-emerging cause of cervical lymphadenopathy. Trop Med Infect Dis 2022;7(8):189.

57. Orbaek M, Lebech AM, Helleberg M. The clinical spectrum of tularemia - Two cases. IDCases 2020;21:e00890.

58. Zellner B, Huntley JF. Ticks in tularemia: Do we know what we don't know? Front Cell Infect Microbiol 2019;9:146.

59. Tarnvik A, Chu MC. New approaches to diagnosis and therapy of tularemia. Ann N Y Acad Sci 2007;1105:378–404.

60. Centers for Disease Control and Prevention. Tularemia. Transmission. Available at: https://www.cdc.gov/tularemia/transmission/index.html. [Accessed 28 December 2022].

61. Kukla R, Kracmarova R, Ryskova L, et al. Francisella tularensis caused cervical lymphadenopathy in little children after a tick bite: Two case reports and a short literature review. Ticks Tick Bourne Dis 2022;13(2):101893.

Fever and Rash

Check for updates

Richard Diego Gonzales Y Tucker, MD[a,b,*],
Aravind Addepalli, MD[a]

KEYWORDS

- Rash • Fever • Emergency medicine • Exanthem • Toxic shock syndrome
- Rocky Mountain spotted fever • Arbovirus • Meningococcemia

KEY POINTS

- When evaluating fever and rash, an exhaustive history and head-to-toe skin examination are cornerstones of diagnosis.
- Fever with rash can herald life-threatening infection and imminent clinical decompensation.
- Particular attention should be directed toward identifying petechiae and bullae.
- Many life-threatening causes of infectious fever and rash remain clinical diagnoses, and laboratory confirmation should not delay life-saving antimicrobial therapy and supportive care.
- The differential diagnosis for fever and rash differential also includes life-threatening, noninfectious causes and indolent infectious diseases.

INTRODUCTION

Emergency department (ED) visits for rash comprise up to 8% of annual ED visits.[1] Timely outpatient visits to a primary care physician or dermatologist are particularly difficult to obtain for underinsured patients in the United States, requiring ED evaluation for what is often a benign skin condition.[2,3] However, cutaneous manifestations of infection can carry higher risk, with up to 18% of ED patients requiring dermatology consultation also needing hospital admission.[1] Rash plus fever poses even greater concern; the combination may herald life-threatening infectious disease and imminent hemodynamic collapse.[4–6] Many of these infections can cause fatal illness long before laboratory confirmation, highlighting the need for a fundamental knowledge of the most dangerous cutaneous diagnoses and a well-developed clinical gestalt. The importance of rapid management is highlighted by increased mortality when appropriate antibiotics and supportive therapy is delayed.[7,8] Emergency providers additionally play a critical role in the fight against communicable diseases; prompt recognition, isolation, and disease reporting can prevent outbreaks in the community as well among ED staff.

[a] Department of Emergency Medicine, University of California San Francisco, Box 0209, 505 Parnassus Avenue, San Francisco, CA 94143, USA; [b] Department of Emergency Medicine, Alameda Health System - Wilma Chan Highland Hospital, 1411 E 31st Street, Oakland, CA 94602, USA
* Corresponding author.
E-mail addresses: rtucker@alamedahealthsystem.org; richard.tucker@ucsf.edu

Emerg Med Clin N Am 42 (2024) 303–334
https://doi.org/10.1016/j.emc.2024.01.005
0733-8627/24/© 2024 Elsevier Inc. All rights reserved.

emed.theclinics.com

The differential for fever and rash is enormous, contributing to the diagnostic challenge of distinguishing benign, self-limited disease from life-threatening infection. This review article provides a basic approach to fever and rash in the ED and focuses on several infectious causes of fever and rash associated with significant morbidity and mortality.

DEFINITIONS, MORPHOLOGY, AND PATHOPHYSIOLOGY

Fluency in rash morphology and terminology is essential both to create an algorithmic differential and communicate effectively with consultants (**Table 1**).[9,10]

Maculopapular (also referred to as morbilliform, meaning "measles-like") rashes comprise the most common cutaneous manifestation of infection. Maculopapular rashes are usually generalized and thought to result from local or diffuse perivascular lymphocytic infiltration into the dermis, usually without capillary leak, as virus infects various cellular components of skin.[11–13] Maculopapular rashes are most commonly caused by one of the numerous childhood viruses (the so-called viral exanthems) (**Table 2**).[10,14,15] This is also the main type of arbovirus rash since skin is the primary site of viral replication in arbovirus infection.[11,14]

Erythroderma is a generalized "sunburn" like rash. When infectious, it corresponds to the diffuse nature of the responsible toxin or bacteremia, superantigens, and

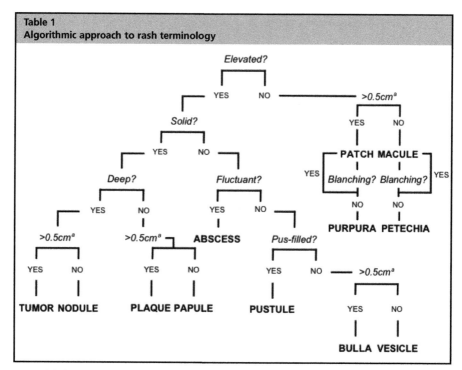

Table 1
Algorithmic approach to rash terminology

General definitions of rashes based on descriptive factors broken into an algorithmic approach.
[a]Diameter of lesion.

Data from Walls RM, Hockberger RS, Gausche-Hill M. Rosen's emergency medicine: concepts and clinical practice. Ninth edition. ed. Elsevier; 2018:2 volumes (xxviii, 2443, I-88 pages); and Santistevan J, Long B, Koyfman A. Rash Decisions: An Approach to Dangerous Rashes Based on Morphology. J Emerg Med. Apr 2017;52(4):457-47.

Table 2
Distributions of febrile versus afebrile maculopapular rash

	Central	Peripheral

Febrile	Lyme disease (erythema migrans)
	Viral exanthem
		Meningococcemia
		RMSF
		Syphilis
		Lyme disease (erythema migrans)
		Targetoid
		   Stevens-Johnson Syndrome
		   Erythema multiforme

Afebrile	Drug reaction Pityriasis	Psoriasis Scabies Eczema

Maculopapular exanthem body distribution in the setting of febrile versus afebrile rash (excluding diffuse rashes).
Data from Refs.[10,14,15]

immune-mediated cytokine release.[6] This leads to a generalized capillary dilation, endothelial dysfunction, and extravasation of blood components into interstitial tissue, as seen in toxic shock syndrome (TSS).[16,17]

Vesiculobullous rash results from fluid accumulation between the dermis and epidermis, manifesting as vesicles, which can coalesce to bullae and eventually desquamate.[16,18] This process is secondary to a compromised dermal–epidermal junction, often from toxin-mediated cleavage of junctional proteins.

Petechiae are small, 0.5 cm red–brown lesions that do not blanch when pressure is applied.[10,18] They can be flat or palpable. Petechiae often coexist with maculopapular rashes, representing further endothelial dysfunction, capillary leak, and microvascular dysfunction.[19,20] Petechiae can be toxin-mediated or from direct bacterial invasion of vascular endothelium and smooth muscle cells, causing mononuclear cell infiltration, vasculitis, capillary leak, coagulation dysfunction, and platelet consumption (**Fig. 1**).[21,22] Petechiae can increase in size and coalesce, resulting in *purpura*.

INITIAL EVALUATION
History

A careful and thorough history is the cornerstone for correct rash diagnosis. Questions about health habits and travel should include outdoor activity, geographic location of any recent travel, urban versus rural travel, routine and travel-related vaccination status, travel-related chemoprophylaxis and adherence, contact with fresh or saltwater, livestock contact, and types of foods eaten.[23,24] A sexual history is mandatory as many sexually transmitted infections (STIs) have cutaneous manifestations (**Table 3**).[25–31] Questions about past medical history should focus on comorbidities that affect immunocompetence, including HIV, diabetes, complement deficiency, and use of chemotherapeutic and immunomodulating agents.[32–34] Medication history is critical since new medications are frequent triggers of serious and potentially fatal noninfectious rashes, which can be accompanied by fever (**Table 4**).[35–39]

The emergency provider must elicit a specific history of the fever and rash, including their temporal relationship with one another.[40,41] They should create a historical narrative of rash morphology, location, migration, and evolution. Categorize location and evolution as local versus generalized and centripetal versus centrifugal.

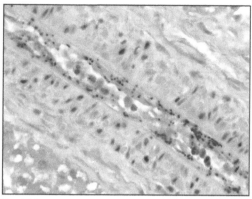

Photo/CDC

Fig. 1. Immunohistochemical staining of invading *R rickettsii* (*red*) in endothelial cells of blood vessels. (Biggs HM, Behravesh CB, Bradley KK, et al. Diagnosis and Management of Tickborne Rickettsial Diseases: Rocky Mountain Spotted Fever and Other Spotted Fever Group Rickettsioses, Ehrlichioses, and Anaplasmosis - United States. *MMWR Recomm Rep.* 2016;65(2):1-44. Published 2016 May 13. https://doi.org/10.15585/mmwr.rr6502a1. Fig. 20 in series.)

Note whether it is pruritic or painful.[42] Other prodromal and associated symptoms can help differentiate between infections with similar morphology, particularly maculopapular rashes.[10,13,14,43] In the case of travel, determine the possible incubation period from exposure to fever and rash onset.

Physical Examination

A head-to-toe dermatologic examination is an essential part of the evaluation. Patients must be fully undressed in a hospital gown, and placed in a well-lit examination room. Visually inspect all body locations systematically, including the palms, soles, axilla, intertriginous areas, and flexor and extensor surfaces.[16] Note rash morphology and location, whether it involves extremities (acral vs central), sun-exposed areas, and dermatomes. Examine for involvement of ocular, oropharyngeal, and genital mucosal surfaces (termed enanthem).

Palpation follows visual inspection. Use a gloved hand to palpate whether lesions are flat or raised. The "glass test" provides a window to assess whether lesions blanch with pressure or maintain color as with petechiae (**Fig. 2**).[5] Interrogate vesicles or bullae with a gloved hand, assessing for the Nikolsky sign, in which superficial skin shears easily from underlying layers with lateral pressure, signifying dermal–epidermal junction lysis and higher morbidity.[18]

Providers must maintain a particular awareness of skin of color and its effect on correct diagnosis. Several studies have highlighted the tendency to feature photographs of lighter skin in medical education and dermatology literature.[44,45] Research has demonstrated providers' difficulty identifying life-threatening pathology such as Rocky Mountain spotted fever (RMSF) and meningococcemia in darker-skinned patients.[7,46,47]

Laboratory Testing

Laboratory testing can be used to assess illness severity and evolution and prognosticate patient deterioration and organ failure.[13,41,48,49] Appropriate initial laboratory

Table 3
Cutaneous manifestations of sexually transmitted infections

STI	Description	Pain/Pruritus	Lymph Nodes
Disseminated gonococcal infection	Very nonspecific, need high index of suspicion based on history. Erythematous, 1–2 mm pustules, fluctuant furuncle-like nodules, indurated abscesses, shallow erosions, indurated ulcers of varying size.	No	Rarely
Syphilis	Primary syphilis: a 1–2 cm ulcer with raised indurated margins called a chancre. Secondary syphilis: can be almost any form so high index of suspicion required but classically a diffuse symmetric macular or papular eruption involving trunk and extremities that does NOT spare the palms and soles. May present as pustular. Atypical presentations common with concomitant AIDS. Tertiary syphilis/individuals with HIV: gummas may present as ulcers or granulomatous lesions with round, irregular, or serpiginous shape.	Usually painless	Firm, nontender, regionally enlarged lodes
Herpes	Multiple small grouped ulcers, erythematous base. Vesicles can be open and form ulcers/erosions that coalesce.	Usually painful	Reactive, painful nodes
Scabies	Multiple small, erythematous papules often excoriated. Distribution is key to diagnosis: interdigital spaces, skinfolds including wrists, elbows, axilla, waist, knee, buttocks.	Pruritic	Uncommon
Primary HIV	Erythematous maculopapular eruption, over the trunk, collar, face and sometimes the palms and soles. May become confluent. May include oral/genital lesions.	Unusual	Nontender adenopathy often present
Mpox	Progresses through stages. Macules to papules, vesicles, then umbilicated pseudo-pustules (so named due to containing cell debris rather than pus or fluid). Eventually crust and fall off. Found in anogenital, perioral areas as well as sometimes acral/truncal.	Often painful and pruritic	Uncommon

Cutaneous manifestations of common sexually transmitted infection.
Data from Refs.[25,26,28–31]

Table 4
Emergent noninfectious causes of fever and rash

Name	Pathophysiology	Rash Morphology
DRESS	T-cell-mediated hypersensitivity reaction generally due to an immune response to an offending drug. Incompletely understood.	Maculopapular eruption progressing to a coalescing erythema with purpura, infiltrated plaques, pustules, exfoliative dermatitis, and target-like lesions. Symmetrically distributed on trunk and extremities. Facial edema, mild mucosal involvement present in majority of cases. Skin detachment uncommon.
SJS/TEN	Suggestions of a cell-mediated cytotoxic reaction against keratinocytes both directly and indirectly. Incompletely understood. SJS is a less severe condition (>30%).	Coalescing, erythematous macules with target lesions,[a] blisters, erosions, skin detachment, and severe mucosal involvement in multiple sites of body
Graft-versus-host disease	Immune cells transplanted from a nonidentical donor recognize transplant recipient as foreign, causing an immune reaction in recipient.	First clinical manifestation often maculopapular rash. Involves neck, ears, shoulders, palms of hand, and soles of feet and can spread to whole integument. Classically described as a sunburn, pruritic, and painful. Severe forms involve formation of bullous lesions similar to TEN.
Pemphigus vulgaris	Acantholysis due to binding of autoantibodies to epithelial cell surface antigens due to both genetic and environmental factors.	Mucosal, often oral, blisters which are painful and rupture easily with resultant bleeding. Nikolsky sign positive.
Erythema multiforme	Cell-mediated immune process against pathogen (viral [often HSV]/drug) antigens deposited in skin. Generally transient condition. Incompletely understood.	Cutaneous lesions in a symmetric distribution on extensor surfaces of extremities, spreads centripetally. Classically target lesions: a dusky central area or blister with a pale ring of edema and finally an erythematous halo on periphery of lesion. Can involve mucosa.
Kawasaki disease	Likely inflammatory cell infiltration into vascular tissues often triggered by transmissible agents. Incompletely understood.	1 of 5 diagnostic criteria are a polymorphous rash. Begins as perineal erythema and desquamation, then macular, morbilliform lesions of trunk and extremities. Children can develop diffuse erythema of palms/soles.

Fatal and emergent noninfectious etiologies of fever and rash.
Abbreviations: DRESS, drug reaction eosinophilia and systemic symptoms; HSV, herpes simplex virus; SJS, Stevens–Johnson syndrome; TEN, toxic epidermal necrolysis; GVHD, graft versus host disease.
[a] See erythema multiforme for description.
Data from Refs.[35–39]

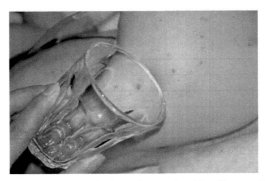

Fig. 2. An example of the glass test, which can be used to identify petechiae. Current image from a patient with meningococcemia. (https://doi.org/10.1016/S0140-6736(07)61016-2 Reprinted with permission from Elsevier. The Lancet, 2007;369(9580):2196-2210.)

studies include complete blood count (CBC) with differential, CMP, erythrocyte sedimentation rate (ESR)/C-reactive protein (CRP), coagulation studies, and creatine kinase (CK). Troponin, kidney function and liver function tests, and indicators of disseminated intravascular coagulation (DIC), can indicate organ system failure and coagulation disruption.

While laboratory tests and infectious etiologic testing can help establish diagnosis and prognosis, they should not delay expeditious antibiotic treatment when indicated. Rapid treatment has been associated with improved outcomes and decreased mortality in many infections that present with rash.[7,50] While blood, urine, and body fluid Gram stain and cultures should be obtained, providers must recognize their sensitivity may be limited, particularly in toxin-mediated exanthem.[6,17,41,51,52] Polymerase chain reaction (PCR) viral testing offers high sensitivity and specificity for viral etiologies, though it may take days to return.[43,53,54] On occasion, skin biopsy of lesions or petechiae may reveal dermal bacterial invasion.[55,56]

DIFFERENTIAL DIAGNOSIS

The differential diagnosis for fever and rash is intimidatingly long, encompassing the entire gamut of infectious, toxic, metabolic, vascular, and autoimmune pathology. Within this long differential are several life-threatening but noninfectious causes, which must always be considered given their potential high mortality, worsened by diagnostic delay (see **Table 4**).[35–39] While this article focuses specifically on rapidly progressive infections, it is important to recognize the numerous indolent but important infections that manifest with fever and rash (**Table 5**).[57,58]

ROCKY MOUNTAIN SPOTTED FEVER
Epidemiology, Transmission, and Pathophysiology

First identified in 1896 in Western Montana, RMSF is the most common rickettsial illness in the United States with an incidence of 8.9 per million cases.[4,21,59] Since 2000, RMSF has increased in incidence, peaking in 2017.[21] This increase is in part due to change in nomenclature and creation of the larger, generally less fatal spotted fever group rickettsiosis (SFGR) categorization. The case fatality rate for confirmed RMSF, however, remains high at 5% to 10%.[21] This is higher for specific populations, including children, which comprise two-thirds of total cases, Latino, and Native American populations.[4,60–62]

Table 5 Indolent causes of fever and rash	
Disease	**Incubation Period**
Syphilis	9–90 d
Blastomyces	30–45 d
Coccidioides	7–21 d
Disseminated gonococcal infection	7 d to mo
Epstein–Barr virus (EBV)	30–50 d
Human immunodeficiency virus (HIV)	28–180 d
Infective endocarditis	7–90 d

General time course of indolent causes of fever and rash.
From Sanders CVN, L.T. The Skin and Infection: A Color Atlast and Text. Williams & Wilkins; 1995:325; and N'Guyen Y, Duval X, Revest M, et al. Time interval between infective endocarditis first symptoms and diagnosis: relationship to infective endocarditis characteristics, microorganisms and prognosis. Ann Med. Mar 2017;49(2):117-125. https://doi.org/10.1080/07853890.2016.1235282.

While RMSF occurs throughout the United States, 60% of cases occur in the Southeast.[21] RMSF is transmitted predominantly through *Dermacentor variabilis* and *Dermacentor andersoni* ticks. It is highly seasonal, with 90% of cases occurring between April and September, when up to 3% of ticks can be infected in endemic areas.[4] However, with recent identification of *Rhipicephalus sanguineus* as a potential vector in the Southwestern United States and Central America, infections have been increasingly observed throughout the year in these regions.[61,63]

RMSF is caused by the spirochete *Rickettsia rickettsii*, an obligate, intracellular, gram-negative spirochete. Ticks act as the primary vector with humans an incidental host.[21] Upon initiating feeding, ticks can transmit rickettsial species within 4 to 6 hours of attachment. Transmission can also occur through tick fluids, feces, and handling of crushed tissue.[4,21,64] The spirochete has a tropism for endothelial capillary cells, which spreads centripetally from the inoculation site, causing direct cellular damage and subsequent vascular injury and endothelial permeability.[65]

Signs and Symptoms

The RMSF initial incubation period ranges from 3 to 12 days, followed by fever, headache, myalgias, conjunctival injection, and photophobia. Fever is a hallmark symptom, present in 80% to 94% of patients, and included in the Centers for Disease Control and Prevention (CDC) case definition.[4,21,63,66] Abrupt illness onset and headache are classically described. In a report on American tribal land outbreaks, a myriad of nonspecific symptoms were also observed, potentially leading to confusion with other viral illnesses.[63] Children are more likely to present with initial abdominal pain and periorbital edema.[14,21,67] Other manifestations include meningitis, myocarditis, pneumonitis, muscle necrosis, rhabdomyolysis, and kidney injury.[21]

Rash in Rocky Mountain Spotted Fever

RMSF produces a generalized rash in up to 95% of patients. In the classic presentation, which may occur in only 58%, rash appears 2 to 5 days after fever onset as a blanching, several millimeter macular rash on the wrist and ankles, and can also include the palms and soles.[4,42,65,66] Other peripheral sites of rash presentation have been described.[4,42,67] The rash then travels centripetally toward the neck, torso, and back. It may take on a papular appearance, with subsequent central petechia as endothelial dysfunction commences (**Fig. 3**). By day 5 to 6, the rash develops a petechial predominance, echoing further endothelial dysfunction and coagulation cascade disturbance, with purpura fulminans in the end stages.[4,64] Microvascular thrombosis depletes coagulation factors and consumes platelets, leading to tissue necrosis and extremity ischemia.[7,66]

Diagnosis

Because treatment delay is associated with higher mortality and definitive diagnostic testing may take days to return, RMSF requires a high index of suspicion and low threshold for empirical treatment.[4,21] Misdiagnosis remains high, with up to 75% of patients misdiagnosed on initial physician encounter.[67] The triad of fever, headache, and rash manifests in only 3% of patients by day 3 and must be abandoned as a requisite for ED diagnosis.[4,21] While over 90% of individuals manifest a rash, only 50% produce a characteristic exanthem by day 3.[68] Known tick exposures, found in only 50%, cannot be relied on for diagnosis.[68] Providers must consider geographic location, time of year, and the patient's behavioral risk for tick exposure. In the right epidemiologic setting, a provisional diagnosis of RMSF may be appropriate if there is fever without rash or known tick bite.

Laboratory evaluation has a limited role in initial diagnosis of RMSF, though certain findings may provide important diagnostic clues and assist in gauging severity of disease. Appropriate initial laboratories include CBC, comprehensive metabolic panel (CMP), prothrombin time, International normalized ratio (PT/INR), liver function tests (LFTs), CK, and blood cultures. Thrombocytopenia and hyponatremia with normal white blood cell count (WBC) count has been classically described, though can be absent early in disease.[21,64] If lumbar puncture is performed, cerebrospinal fluid (CSF) can show pleocytosis with lymphocytic predominance, normal glucose, and elevated protein.[21,64]

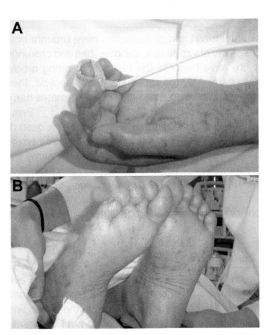

Fig. 3. (*A, B*) Rocky Mountain spotted fever petechial rash with involvement of palms and soles. (Courtesy of Dr. Amina Ahmed, Professor, Wake Forest University School of Medicine and Atrium Health.)

Formal testing options include enzyme-linked immunoassay (ELISA) and antibody immunoglobulin G, immunoglobulin M (IgG/IgM) testing. These take weeks to return, do not distinguish from other species in the spotted fever group *Rickettsia* (SFGR), and should not delay appropriate treatment.[21]

Treatment

Immediate treatment with antimicrobials is critical in RMSF. Doxycycline provides effective therapy, reducing mortality from 23% to 6% when given within 5 days of symptom onset.[4,7,21] Early treatment has additionally been associated with reduced risk of permanent neurologic sequelae.[60] Yet rates of delayed doxycycline administration remain high, with studies reporting just 44% of cases being treated by day 5, despite being seen by a physician prior to diagnosis in 90%.[7] Another study found only 35% of physicians would correctly prescribe doxycycline when tested on RMSF clinical scenarios.[69] A primary reason for prescription avoidance is the pervasive myth that doxycycline is contraindicated in children.[70] Association with tooth discoloration has been disproven, and doxycycline therapy is currently recommended by the American Association of Pediatrics for RMSF treatment.[21,71]

Prognosis and Prevention

Despite improved outcomes with early antibiotic therapy, RMSF mortality remains at 5% to 10%.[21,67] Patients at higher risk for complications include those less than 8 years or more than 40 year old, those with glucose-6-phosphate dehydrogenase (G6PD) deficiency, alcohol use disorder, and Native Americans.[4,63] Currently, no vaccines exist for SFGR, and disease prevention focuses on tick avoidance and protection.[4,21]

DENGUE, ZIKA, AND CHIKUNGUNYA
Introduction

Increased intercontinental travel and globalization have brought novel mosquito-borne illness to the Americas. A trio of viral fevers, dengue, Zika and chikungunya, which constitute a disease triptych, have become the fastest spreading arboviruses of the New World.[13,43,53,72] Initially carried by the mosquito *Aedes aegypti*, these viruses are now found in *Aedes albopictus,* whose tolerance for colder climates has expanded the species' habitat to nearly half of the United States (**Fig. 4**).[43,73–75] Previously seen only in returning travelers, US autochthonous transmission has now been described.[43,53,76–78] The majority of US outbreaks occur in Caribbean and Pacific territories with infection peaks from June to October.[78,79] Since the trio shares the same mosquito vector and the initial clinical presentation of each is almost indistinguishable, the diagnosis of dengue, Zika, and chikungunya should be simultaneously considered (**Table 6**).[54] While only dengue carries a significant risk of mortality in adults, Zika is linked to devastating teratogenicity and chikungunya can lead to debilitating chronic arthropathy.

DENGUE
Epidemiology and Transmission

With descriptions dating back to the third century, "Breakbone Fever," or dengue, has become a global hemorrhagic fever responsible for significant mortality.[80,81] Dengue is the most common and fastest growing arbovirus in the world, with up to 100 million cases and 20,000 deaths per year worldwide, and 2.4 million cases in the Americas in 2015.[13,80] A total of 2016 US cases of dengue were reported to the CDC in 2022, the majority in returning travelers, but with autochthonous infection (acquired in the geographic location where the patient lives) in US island territories, Florida, and Arizona.[79]

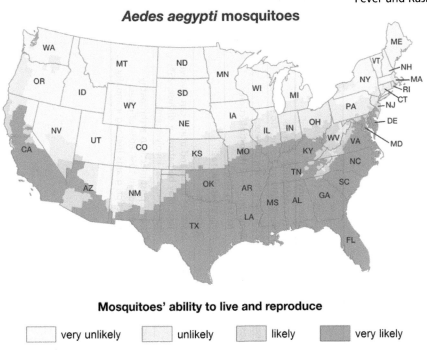

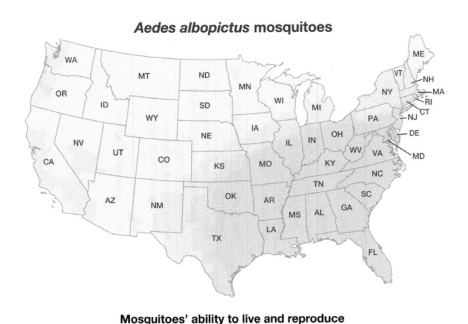

Fig. 4. Estimated potential range of *A aegypti* and *A albopictus* in the United States, 2017. (https://www.cdc.gov/zika/pdfs/Zika-mosquito-maps.pdf ESTIMATED potential range of Aedes aegypti and Aedes albopictus in the United States, 2017*. Retrieved from: https://www.cdc.gov/zika/pdfs/zika-mosquito-maps.pdf.)

Table 6
Characteristics of arboviral infections

	Dengue	Zika	Chikungunya
Transmission	Vector: mosquito. Can be vertical/blood-borne. No sexual.	Vector: mosquito. Can be vertical/blood-borne/sexual.	Vector: mosquito. Can be vertical/blood-borne. No sexual.
Symptomatic postinfection?	20% manifesting disease.	20% manifesting disease.	85% manifesting disease.
Incubation	Symptoms 2–7 d postinfection	Symptoms 3–12 d postinfection	Symptoms 1–12 d postinfection, most by day 3
Rash morphology	Maculopapular and morbilliform rash	Generally papular NOT macular rash	Maculopapular rash
Pruritic	Sometimes	Often	Sometimes
Rash distribution	Starts on dorsum of hands and feet, spreads centripetally; 30% with mucosal involvement.	Mostly face, upper limbs, and trunk.	Starts on limbs and trunk, can involve face, may be patchy or diffuse; 25% with mucosal involvement.
Sequelae	Prior infection predisposes to more severe future infection	Severe neonatal teratogenicity if vertical transmission occurs	Chronic postinfectious arthropathy common in 10%–60% of cases. Infection grants lifelong immunity.

General characteristics of mosquito-borne arboviral infections.
From Refs.[12,13,19]

Four serotypes of dengue exist, labeled DENV1-4, all carrying potential for severe disease, and transmitted via the aforementioned *Aedes* mosquito vectors, with potential for vertical and blood-borne transmission.[32,82] Sexual transmission has not been described.[43,79] Most infections remain asymptomatic, with approximately 20% causing symptomatic disease.[32,43,80]

Signs and Symptoms

Dengue is divided into 3 phases: febrile, critical, and recovery. Febrile phase occurs 2 to 7 days after infection, with high fever, myalgias, headache, nausea, vomiting, and a diffuse maculopapular rash.[80] Dengue critical phase occurs in 5% of febrile phase individuals, usually by day 4 to 5. Critical phase is characterized by diffuse endothelial dysfunction, leading to hypotension from distributive shock, pulmonary edema, ascites, and multiorgan system failure. Concurrent coagulation pathway disruption occurs, leading to hemorrhagic complications.[80] Using preexisting risk factors along with characteristic warning signs, the CDC has developed an algorithm to guide providers in predicting progression to the critical phase (**Fig. 5**). One such physical examination finding, the tourniquet test, provides an effective method to differentiate dengue from Zika and chikungunya (**Fig. 6**).[83] Recovery phase manifests as resorption of fluids and normalization of the coagulation pathway. This period may manifest as sudden pulmonary edema and congestive heart failure if IV fluid resuscitation was excessive during critical phase.[80]

Rash in Dengue Fever

Dengue rash occurs during the febrile phase, between days 2 and 7 of illness, developing in 30% to 80% of cases, and more commonly in young patients.[19,33,84] It is characterized by a pruritic, dense, diffuse maculopapular, or morbilliform rash, described as an "isles of white on a sea of red" appearance (**Fig. 7**).[19,85] Thirty percent of individuals will display mucosal involvement, including aphthous ulcers, posterior oropharyngeal erythema, and petechiae.[19,84] Patients who progress to the critical phase are more likely to have petechiae, reflecting endothelial dysfunction and coagulation disturbance.[80]

Diagnosis

The initial provisional diagnosis of dengue, Zika, or chikungunya relies on recognition of typical symptoms and signs in individuals residing in or traveling from an endemic area. Dengue is further identified and risk stratified by the high-risk physical examination and laboratory findings included in the CDC algorithm, which predict progression to the critical phase (see **Fig. 5**). Characteristic laboratory findings include elevated hematocrit, leukopenia, and thrombocytopenia, with leukopenia being unique to dengue as compared to Zika or chikungunya.[19,80] Increased liver function tests and ferritin have been associated with severe disease.[19]

Definitive diagnostic tests will depend on the time from symptom onset, cost and availability considerations, and the need to also test for Zika. In the first 7 days of symptoms, molecular tests (nucleic acid antigen tests and PCR) are preferred and highly accurate.[48,86] A viral antigen test can also be used in this time period. Beyond 7 days, IgM serologic testing is preferred and can remain positive for months. However, the results can be complicated by previous dengue infection, and false positives may result from other flavivirus infections.[48,80] In most cases, testing for both dengue and Zika is performed together. The CDC has additionally introduced a multiplex PCR assay for all 3 viruses, for use in areas with habitat overlap.[87] Since testing decisions

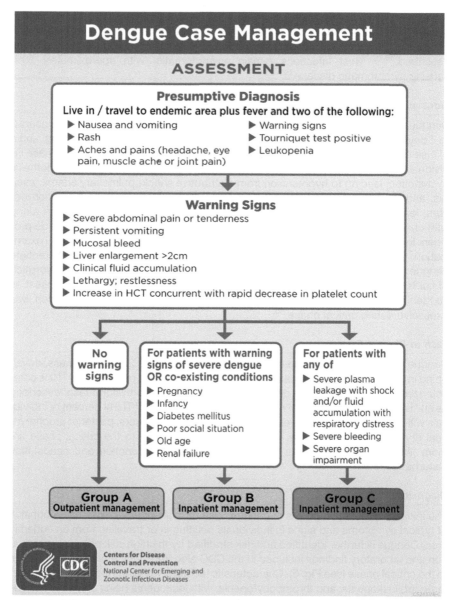

Fig. 5. http://www.cdc.gov/dengue/resources/DENGUE-clinician-guide_508.pdfDengue Case Management. Retrieved from: https://www.cdc.gov/dengue/resources/DENGUE-clinician-guide_508.pdf.

can be complex, US emergency providers should generally consult an infectious disease or public health officer for assistance.

Treatment, Prognosis, and Prevention

Dengue treatment remains supportive. Given the potential for dengue-induced coagulation disturbance and thrombocytopenia, non-steroidal anti-inflammatory

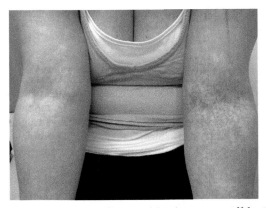

Fig. 6. The tourniquet test is done by inflating a blood pressure cuff for 5 minutes, halfway between the systolic and diastolic pressures. A petechial rash below the cuff (as seen in the patient's left arm) defines a positive test. Notice the maculopapular, morbilliform rash on the contralateral arm, characteristic of dengue. (Feder HM Jr, Plucinski M, Hoss DM. Dengue with a morbilliform rash and a positive tourniquet test. JAAD Case Rep. 2016 Nov 9;2(5):422-423. https://doi.org/10.1016/j.jdcr.2016.07.010. PMID: 27872891; PMCID: PMC5107725.)

drugs (NSAIDs) should be avoided while dengue fever is being considered.[80,88] Early recognition of warning signs, with appropriate hospitalization and use of intensive care, can reduce mortality from 20% to under 1% in patients proceeding to critical phase. In general, mortality has steadily decreased since 2010.[33,80]

Risk factors for increased mortality include underlying diabetes and hypertension.[33] Prior dengue infection also increases the risk of severe disease and mortality.[80] Termed the dengue antibody-dependent enhancement hypothesis, this phenomena is thought to be due to preexisting antibodies binding new viral particles, causing upregulated phagocytosis and accelerated viral replication,[82] with increased risk of progression to critical phase. A history of prior infection is thus important when considering the need for hospitalization or vaccination.

A CDC and FDA-approved vaccine became available in 2022. Dengvaxia, a tetravalent dengue vaccine for all 4 dengue serotypes, is currently available to children and

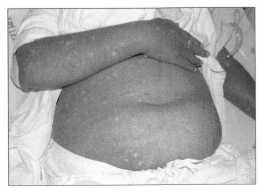

Fig. 7. "Isles of white on a sea of red" characteristic appearance of morbilliform dengue rash. (Printed, with permission, from: Thomas EA, John M, Kanish B. Mucocutaneous manifestations of dengue fever. Indian J Dermatol. 2010;55(1):79-85. https://doi.org/10.4103/0019-5154.60359.)

adolescents ages 9 to 16 years who have laboratory-confirmed previous dengue infection and live in dengue-endemic US territories.[86]

ZIKA
Epidemiology and Transmission

Identified in 1947, Zika remained a sporadic disease in Africa and Asia until sustained transmission was recorded in 2007.[13] After reaching the Americas in 2015, Zika distribution exploded to 89 countries. US cases peaked in 2017 with cases of autochthonous spread described in Florida and Texas.[89–91] Despite its extremely low mortality rate, among pregnant mothers, Zika virus carries a risk of devastating neurocognitive teratogenicity.[92]

Zika virus is predominantly vector-borne, with most US infections occurring in returning travelers from endemic areas.[93] However, sexual transmission in the United States has been described.[13,54,78]

Signs and Symptoms

Like dengue, the majority of Zika infections remain asymptomatic, with only 20% of individuals manifesting disease.[54] The incubation period lasts 3 to 14 days.[13,91] Symptoms are generally nonspecific, including low-grade fever, arthralgias, dysesthesias, conjunctivitis, and rash (**Fig. 8**).[13,94–96]

Zika Rash

A pruritic, generalized, papular rash is the hallmark of Zika infection, occurring in up to 98% of symptomatic patients, and is included in the WHO case definition.[40,91,97,98] Eruption occurs within 48 hours of symptom onset, can last up to 6 days, and may be the only significant symptom.[11,95,99] Areas most frequently affected include the face, upper limbs, and trunk, followed by abdomen and lower limbs, covering on average 45% of total body surface area (**Fig. 9**).[13] Zika rash may involve palms and soles and about one-half exhibit acral edema.[94,95] A dengue-like macular rash with petechiae has been described, but should not result in a positive tourniquet test.[94]

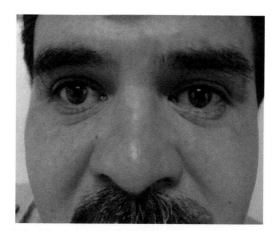

Fig. 8. Conjunctivitis in Zika. Notice the associated faint maculopapular facial rash. (*Borrowed from* Martinez JD, Garza JAC, Cuellar-Barboza A. Going Viral 2019: Zika, Chikungunya, and Dengue. Dermatol Clin. 2019;37(1):95-105. https://doi.org/10.1016/j.det.2018.07.008)

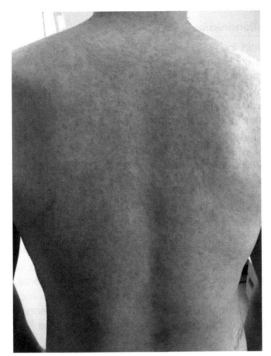

Fig. 9. Maculopapular rash in Zika. (*Borrowed from* Martinez JD, Garza JAC, Cuellar-Barboza A. Going Viral 2019: Zika, Chikungunya, and Dengue. *Dermatol Clin.* 2019;37(1):95-105. https://doi.org/10.1016/j.det.2018.07.008.)

Diagnosis

Given its similarity to other arbovirus infections, Zika diagnosis on clinical grounds is difficult. Simultaneous testing for Zika and dengue, and sometimes also for chikungunya, should be undertaken together. Tests and testing strategies are similar as described earlier for dengue. Pregnant patients who may have been infected or with suggestive symptoms should undergo both molecular and serologic testing as soon as possible.

Treatment, Prognosis, and Prevention

Treatment of Zika is supportive. NSAIDs should be avoided until dengue has been ruled out or symptoms resolve. Mortality remains extremely low, well under 1%.[32] The seriousness of Zika virus infection lies primarily in its teratogenicity. The US Zika Pregnancy and Infancy Registry reports a 6.1% rate of brain and eye disorders among infants born to women with laboratory-confirmed Zika. Given that two-thirds of maternal cases report no symptoms, prevention involves a combination of education, avoidance of mosquito exposure, and isolation strategies in individuals desiring pregnancy.[92]

Zika infection in adults carries 2.4/10,000 risk of neurologic sequelae occurring within 6 days of symptom onset, including encephalitis, transverse myelitis, Guillain–Barré syndrome, and chronic inflammatory demyelinating polyneuropathy.[100] Currently, there are no approved Zika vaccines, though multiple vaccine trials are in progress.[101]

CHIKUNGUNYA
Epidemiology and Transmission

Identified in Tanzania in 1953, chikungunya translates to "that which bends up," describing the arthralgias and chronic arthropathy associated with infection.[102] Like other New World arboviruses, reports of chikungunya were confined to Africa until explosive outbreaks occurred in India and Southeast Asia in the 2000s.[43] Chikungunya reached the Americas in 2013, with 2 million total cases reported from 44 countries in 2020, and an increase in associated mortality reported in 2023.[72] As with dengue and Zika, US autochthonous transmission has recently been described.[43,103]

Infections are predominantly *Aedes* mosquito vector-borne, with occasional cases reported from blood donation.[12,104] Vertical transmission, which carries serious neonatal risk, occurs most frequently at time of delivery.[105]

Signs and Symptoms

Unlike other arboviruses, infection with chikungunya infection is usually symptomatic, with up to 85% of infected individuals developing symptoms 1 to 12 days after infection and usually by day 3.[12,43,53,74,106] Symptoms include fever, headache, myalgias, and vomiting.[107–109] The hallmark of chikungunya infection is a severe, usually symmetric, polyarthralgia syndrome, which occurs in 80% of patients.[74,107]

The risk of neonatal infection from an acutely infected mother is as high as 50%.[105,106] Infection will manifest 3 to 7 days after birth as neonatal encephalopathy, with eventual cerebral palsy or other neurocognitive sequelae.[110]

Rash in Chikungunya

Chikungunya rash develops in 25% to 90% of individuals.[43,74,107–109,111] Rash is more common in younger patients, occurring in 100% of infected infants.[112] Typically, it is a fine maculopapular exanthem that appears about 48 hours after fever onset.[108,109,113] It may start at the site of inoculation, followed by generalized spread, eventually covering up to 90% of total body surface area and involving the palms and soles.[43] It is pruritic in 80% of patients.[108,109,113] Twenty-five percent of patients develop perianal, genital, or oral mucosal involvement.[108] Vesiculobullous transformation has been described in infants.[114] Unique to chikungunya is delayed development of a hyperpigmented, predominantly malar rash in the days to weeks after infection.[108]

Diagnosis

Chikungunya infection remains a largely clinical diagnosis, with laboratories helpful in distinguishing it from dengue and Zika. Lymphopenia has been described, though it is neither sensitive nor specific for diagnosis.[115] Definitive diagnosis is considered less critical than for dengue and Zika, and testing for chikungunya should generally be coupled with dengue and Zika testing. Both molecular and serologic tests for chikungunya are available, including the multiplex PCR test for all 3 arboviruses.[13]

Treatment, Prognosis, and Prevention

As with dengue and Zika, the initial treatment is supportive, with avoidance of NSAIDs until dengue has been excluded. Most infections are self-limited, ending within 7 to 10 days.[53] While mortality from chikungunya remains under 0.1%, rare cases of myocarditis and encephalitis, with high associated mortality, have been described.[116] However, morbidity from a postinfectious, sometimes chronic arthropathy, can be significant. This occurs in 10% to 60% of cases, more commonly in elderly patients, those with immunosuppression, and diabetes.[117,118] Unlike dengue, chikungunya infection grants lifelong immunity. Several vaccine studies are in Phase III trials as of December 2022.[119]

STAPHYLOCOCCAL TOXIC SHOCK SYNDROME
Introduction, Epidemiology, and Pathophysiology

TSS is a rapidly-progressive, toxin-mediated syndrome of hypotension and organ dysfunction caused by *Staphylococcus aureus* and invasive Group A Strep infections. The 2 forms of TSS differ. Streptococcal TSS occurs in the setting of invasive soft tissue infection, pregnancy-related infection, or respiratory infection, often with associated bacteremia, and carries high mortality. Streptococcal TSS rash is uncommon. Staphylococcal TSS has a lower rate of associated bacteremia and lower—albeit significant—mortality and it is distinguished by an erythroderma rash, which may later desquamate.[16] This discussion focuses primarily on staphylococcal TSS.

Staphylococcal TSS was first described in 1978 by Todd and colleagues, and awareness of it increased after cases were described associated with superabsorbent tampon use in the early 1980s.[41,120] Current TSS incidence is 6.65 per million persons, with both streptococcal and staphylococcal cases increasing in recent years.[121,122] Warnings were issued by the CDC in 2022 for streptococcal TSS in Minnesota and Colorado pediatric populations.[122] Risk factors for the disease include female sex, Asian race, and extremes of age (<5 years and >65 years).[121]

S aureus infection and subsequent TSS occur after staphylococcal entry through a compromised epidermal or mucosal barrier.[17] Cases have been associated with post-surgical and postpartum wound infections, burns, cutaneous and oropharyngeal abscess, insect bites, implanted prosthetics, breast augmentation, abdominoplasty, and liposuction.[17,123–125] Recurrent TSS has been described.[126,127] Increasing vaginal pH during menstruation and changes in local oxygen and carbon dioxide levels with tampon introduction contribute to menstruation staphylococcal TSS. This form carries a unique risk profile and is separately categorized in case definition as menstruation-associated TSS.[121,128]

In staphylococcal TSS, the production of exotoxins, which act as superantigens, plays an important role in pathogenesis. These exotoxins include staphylococcal toxic shock syndrome toxin-1 (TSST-1) and enterotoxin. These result in direct *t*-cell activation, leading to diffuse cytokine release, further recruitment of immune cells, and a subsequent feedback loop resulting in the syndrome's rapidly progressive capillary leak, hypotension, shock, and multiorgan system failure.[16,129]

Signs and Symptoms

TSS poses a diagnostic challenge, with initially nonspecific symptoms that can rapidly progress to fulminant disease. Chesney describes a 24 to 48 hour symptom progression with initial high fever and severe myalgias found in all patients, vomiting in 90%, diarrhea in 80%, odynophagia and arthralgias in 83%, with altered mentation in nearly 60%, respectively.[41,126] Symptoms quickly decompensate to distributive shock, tissue ischemia, fulminant liver failure, acute kidney injury, cardiac dysfunction, and average time from symptom onset to mortality is 48 hours.[41,126,130]

Rash in Toxic Shock Syndrome

The rash of staphylococcal TSS is definitive, found in all patients, incorporated into the CDC case definition, and present as inclusion criteria in most studies.[121,131–133] The rash is described as a diffuse "sunburn" erythroderma, with a fine, confluent macular or scarlatiniform presentation.[10,16,111,126] The rash can have flexural accentuation when involving extremities, may involve the palms and soles, and has a predilection for the trunk in hypotensive patients.[16,111,120] TSS rash presents early in disease onset, usually within 24 hours of illness presentation, and 2 to 4 days in cases associated with postoperative infections.[17,126,127] Mucosal involvement has been described, though appears later in disease presentation.[41] Tissue desquamation is a late finding in survivors of TSS and should not be used in initial diagnostic criteria.[6,41]

Diagnosis

Because of potential for rapid progression and significant mortality when treatment is delayed, TSS remains a clinical diagnosis, relying heavily on a history of surgical, menstrual, or other infectious risk factors. Physical examination should include the vagina and other body cavities, searching for a potential infection nidus. Cross-sectional imaging should be considered.

Laboratory testing is used to assess for organ dysfunction and identification of DIC. Associated abnormalities include azotemia, lymphopenia, hypocalcemia, hypoalbuminemia, disruption of coagulation studies, elevated liver function tests, and elevated creatine kinase.[41] The white blood cell count may be normal.[130] In a largely toxin-mediated disease, blood cultures are rarely positive in staphylococcal TSS.[17,41,130,134] Skin and wound cultures may be obtained and can be helpful, but reports have described minimal or no purulent drainage at operative wound sites.[130] The CDC has created diagnostic criteria for TSS, which are used for research and not for initial diagnosis.[135,136]

Treatment and Prognosis

Considerations in selecting empirical antibiotic therapy include the following: streptococcal and staphylococcal TSS may be difficult to discern early in disease; methicillin-resistant S aureus has been implicated in TSS, an agent that reduces toxin production may be beneficial; and most cases will initially warrant treatment for sepsis of unclear cause.[137,138] Given these considerations, the combination of vancomycin, clindamycin, and a broad-spectrum beta-lactam is reasonable.[6,139] Clindamycin and linezolid reduce toxin production within hours of administration, and clindamycin has been associated with improved outcomes in both staphylococcal and invasive streptococcal TSS.[140,141] Meta-analysis suggest that there is mortality benefit with intravenous immunoglobulin (IVIG) administration in streptococcal TSS.[140,142]

Mortality remains high for staphylococcal TSS at approximately 10%.[121,130] Associations with mortality include coagulopathy, significant hepatic dysfunction, elderly age, and respiratory failure.

MENINGOCOCCEMIA
Introduction, Epidemiology, Transmission, and Pathophysiology

Neisseria meningitidis, a gram-negative diplococcus that colonizes human respiratory mucosa, is responsible for invasive meningococcal disease (IMD). IMD manifests primarily as 2 diseases: meningitis and the less common meningococcemia, with hematogenous spread resulting in the classic presentation of petechial rash and shock. This discussion will focus primarily on meningococcemia, though much of the epidemiology and treatment is similar. With its rapid progression from symptom onset to fulminant disease and high rate of misdiagnosis, meningococcemia requires early recognition by emergency providers, followed by immediate antibiotic treatment, resuscitation and supportive care, appropriate patient isolation, and close contact notification.[8]

IMD incidence was 0.11/100,000 cases in the United States in 2020.[143] However, IMD remains a more common cause of epidemic infection in Africa, where rates can reach 1/1000 during peak epidemics.[144] Within the United States, infection occurs most commonly in the winter months of January to March, disproportionately affecting infants, adolescents age 16 to 23 years, and elderly over 80 years of age.[143,145]

N meningitidis colonizes approximately 10% of the human population, which can increase to 25% during active epidemics.[5,146,147] Any social behavior that increases population density increases carriage rate, including the first week of university and annual Hajj Mecca pilgrimage, with rates as high as 71% reported in military dormitories.[148–150] N meningitidis is divided into 13 serogroups, categorized by individual polysaccharide characteristics, 6 producing fatal disease.[51] These serogroups are important in geographic and infection trends and population-targeted vaccine campaigns.[51,143] Serogroups B, C, W, and Y are most commonly found in the United States.[143,144]

Transmission occurs through close or intimate contact with carriers through saliva and respiratory secretions, followed by colonization and replication in the upper respiratory mucosa.[22] Factors that increase colonization include dry air, smoking, concurrent upper respiratory tract infections, cocaine, and methamphetamine use.[5,151] Risk factors for progression to disease include waning maternal immunity in infants, genetic complement deficiency or impaired complement formation, and asplenia.[46,148,152] HIV results in a 10-fold increased infection risk.[34]

Many of the devastating manifestations of meningococcemia result from lipo-oligosaccharide endotoxin embedded in the bacterial capsule. Hematogenous spread, rapid bacterial division, activation of host immune cells by the endotoxin, and production of pro-inflammatory cytokines all result in an explosive inflammatory cascade, widespread endothelial dysfunction, and vascular collapse.[153]

Signs and Symptoms

Time from colonization to disease manifestation takes 1 to 14 days.[22] Initial symptoms that herald the onset of meningococcemia are vexingly nonspecific, including fevers, myalgias, headache, and upper respiratory infection symptoms. Young children exhibit a more characteristic early presentation of abdominal pain, leg pain, abnormal skin color, and cold hands and feet.[8,154] The patient can deteriorate within 24 hours, with onset of shock, hemodynamic collapse, and tissue ischemia.[5,155]

Meningococcemia Rash

Rash develops in 28% to 77% of patients with meningococcemia and is more common in pediatric patients. Time from symptom onset to rash is 9 to 16 hours, with earlier onset in younger patients.[8] Up to 11% of children presenting to the ED with a nonblanching rash may have meningococcemia.[5,156,157] The exanthem begins as faint macules measuring less than 5 mm, evolving within hours to palpable petechiae, which coalesce into purpura, an indicator of poor prognosis (**Fig. 10**).[5,20,47] End-stage cutaneous manifestations include desquamation and purpura fulminans.[5,155] Petechiae are not invariably present, with 15% of cases showing only maculopapular findings.[155] Petechiae may be few, with 71% of patients having less than 12 petechiae on initial presentation, underscoring the need for a thorough head-to-toe skin examination.[155] Petechiae isolated to the distribution of the superior vena cava (upper chest, neck, and face) are negatively associated with meningococcemia.[156]

Diagnosis

Given the short time between symptom onset and shock, the emergency provider must maintain a high index of suspicion for IMD and meningococcemia. Unfortunately, only about half of patients with meningococcemia are sent to the ED after initial

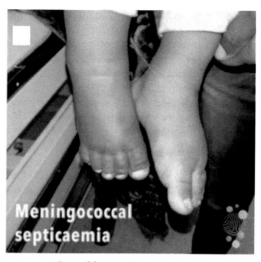

Fig. 10. Subtle violaceous mottling of foot, with early necrosis on dorsum of toe in an infant with meningococcemia. (*Borrowed from* Shanmugavadivel D, Liu JF, Buonsenso D, Davis T, Roland D. Assessing Healthcare Professionals' Identification of Pediatric Dermatologic Conditions in Darker Skin Tones. Children (Basel). 2022 Nov 15;9(11):1749. https://doi.org/10.3390/children9111749. PMID: 36421198; PMCID: PMC9688675.)

outpatient physician contact, and median time to hospital admission from symptom onset was 19 hours in one study.[8]

Diagnostic tests can aid in meningococcal identification, particularly laboratory findings indicating DIC (elevated PT, low platelet count, and low fibrinogen) with prolonged PT associated with higher mortality.[157] Blood culture sensitivity ranges from 50% to 92%, depending in part on whether antibiotics were given before cultures were drawn.[144,158] Suspected meningococcemia is an instance where administration of empirical antibiotics should precede obtaining blood cultures. Skin biopsy and Gram stain of petechial lesions can aid in diagnosis.[55,56] Meningococcal PCR testing has high sensitivity and is unaffected by antibiotic administration.[159]

Treatment, Prognosis, and Prevention

Early antibiotic therapy, at the time of first physician encounter, has been repeatedly shown to reduce mortality, with reductions from 80% to 15% with effective antimicrobials.[8,14,144,160] Penicillin and fluoroquinolone-resistant strains of *N meningitides* have been identified in the United States, and ceftriaxone remains the first-line agent.[143] The early administration of ceftriaxone increases bacterial doubling time, and plasma endotoxin levels drop within 2 hours of antibiotic delivery. However, one-third of patients do not receive antibiotic therapy before laboratory-confirmed diagnosis.[160–162]

Despite significant reductions in mortality through early diagnosis, antibiotic treatment, and vaccination, mortality remains nearly 14%.[5,145,157] The predictors of poor outcome include extremes of age, meningococcemia without meningitis, decreased mental status, hypotension, leukopenia, thrombocytopenia, and evidence of DIC. The progression of rash to purpura fulminans imparts poor prognosis.[20]

Chemoprophylaxis is recommended for individuals who have had close contact with the patient from 1 week before symptom onset until 24 hours after antibiotic administration. This includes health care providers with oral secretion exposure (such as performing intubation).[20,51,52] A single dose of oral ciprofloxacin or intramuscular ceftriaxone reduces the risk of illness by 89% and is most effective when given within 24 hours of identification of a confirmed case.[163]

N meningitidis vaccination campaigns have reduced the incidence of IMD worldwide. In the United States, MenACWY vaccines have resulted in a nearly 90% decline in IMD incidence among adolescents since being introduced in 2005.[143,145] In 2014, a MenB vaccine was also introduced. The current CDC guidelines recommend vaccination for adolescents ages 12 to 18 years as well as for certain other high-risk populations, including: military recruits, asplenic patients, HIV-positive patients, or those working with *N meningitides* in laboratories.[143,145] Recent IMD outbreaks in communities of men who have sex with men in the United States highlight the persistent risk of this infection and the importance of public health surveillance and targeted vaccination in high-risk cohorts as recommended by the CDC.[164]

CLINICS CARE POINTS

- ED physicians must develop a framework for discerning life-threatening from benign exanthems, which comprise the majority of ED presentations.
- Comprehensive history and physical examination are essential for diagnoses of emergent fever and rash so as to not delay antimicrobial and supportive care.
- Rocky Mountain spotted fever is the most common rickettsial illness in the United States; it is frequently misdiagnosed and doxycycline remains the choice antimicrobial in both adults and pediatrics.
- Dengue, Zika, and chikungunya are now endemic arboviruses to the Americas with similar symptomatic presentation; all 3 must be simultaneously considered with a focus on assessment of dengue given higher risk of mortality. Triple PCR testing exists through the CDC.
- Early antimicrobial coverage is necessary for treatment and reduced mortality for the rapidly progressive staphylococcal TSS; 100% of patients will present with erythroderma.
- Meningococcemia poses high risk to targeted populations and areas of concentrated human congregation. Reduced infection rates are successful through vaccination campaigns and early chemoprophylaxis.

REFERENCES

1. Jack AR, Spence AA, Nichols BJ, et al. Cutaneous Conditions Leading to Dermatology Consultation in the Emergency Department. West J Emerg Medicine Integrating Emerg Care Popul Heal 2011;12(4):551–5.
2. McKenzie SA, Seivright JR, Hakopian S, et al. Geospatial analysis of access to dermatology care in Los Angeles County: a cross sectional study. Dermatology Online J 2023;29(1).
3. Kilic D, Yigit O, Kilic T, et al. Epidemiologic characteristics of patients admitted to emergency department with dermatological complaints; a retrospective cross sectional study. Archives Acad Emerg Medicine 2019;7(1):e47.
4. Gottlieb M, Long B, Koyfman A. The Evaluation and Management of Rocky Mountain Spotted Fever in the Emergency Department: a Review of the Literature. J Emerg Medicine 2018;55(1):42–50.
5. Stephens DS, Greenwood B, Brandtzaeg P. Epidemic meningitis, meningococcaemia, and Neisseria meningitidis. Lancet 2007;369(9580):2196–210.

6. Lappin E, Ferguson AJ. Gram-positive toxic shock syndromes. Lancet Infect Dis 2009;9(5):281–90.

7. Kirkland KB, Marcom PK, Sexton DJ, et al. Rocky Mountain spotted fever complicated by gangrene: report of six cases and review. Clin Infect Dis 1993;16:629–34.

8. Thompson MJ, Ninis N, Perera R, et al. Clinical recognition of meningococcal disease in children and adolescents. Lancet 2006;367(9508):397–403.

9. Walls R.M., Hockberger R.S., Gausche-Hill M., Rosen's emergency medicine: concepts and clinical practice. Ninth edition. Elsevier; 2018:2 (xxviii, 2443, I-88)

10. Santistevan J, Long B, Koyfman A. Rash Decisions: An Approach to Dangerous Rashes Based on Morphology. J Emerg Medicine 2017;52(4):457–71.

11. Atzori L, Ferreli C, Mateeva V, et al. Clinicopathologic features among different viral epidemic outbreaks involving the skin. Clin Dermatol 2022;40(5):573–85.

12. Campion EW, Weaver SC, Lecuit M. Chikungunya virus and the global spread of a mosquito-borne disease. New Engl J Medicine 2015;372(13):1231–9.

13. Martinez JD, Garza JAC de la, Cuellar-Barboza A. Going Viral 2019 Zika, Chikungunya, and Dengue. Dermatol Clin 2019;37(1):95–105.

14. Muzumdar S, Rothe MJ, Grant-Kels JM. The rash with maculopapules and fever in adults. Clin Dermatol 2019;37(2):109–18.

15. Kang JH. Febrile illness with skin rashes. Infect Chemother 2015;47:155–66.

16. Kang S., Amagai M., Bruckner A.L., et al., Contributors. 2019. Available at: accessmedicine.mhmedical.com/content.aspx?aid=1160946748. Accessed April 3, 2023.

17. ArthurL R, KathrynN S, BruceB D, et al. Toxic-Shock Syndrome not associated with menstruation. A Review of 54 cases. Lancet 1982;319(8262):1–4.

18. Schlossberg D. Fever and rash. Infect Dis Clin N Am 1996;10(1):101–10.

19. Huang HW, Tseng HC, Lee CH, et al. Clinical significance of skin rash in dengue fever: A focus on discomfort, complications, and disease outcome. Asian Pac J Trop Med 2016;9(7):713–8.

20. Baxter P, Priestley B. Meningococcal Rash. Lancet 1988;331(8595):1166–7.

21. Biggs HM, Behravesh CB, Bradley KK, et al. Diagnosis and management of tickborne rickettsial diseases: rocky mountain spotted fever and other spotted fever group rickettsioses, ehrlichioses, and anaplasmosis - United States. MMWR Recomm Rep 2016;65:1–44.

22. Tzeng YL, Stephens DS. Epidemiology and pathogenesis of Neisseria meningitidis. Microbes Infect 2000;2(6):687–700.

23. Freedman DO, Weld LH, Kozarsky PE, et al. Spectrum of disease and relation to place of exposure among ill returned travelers. N Engl J Med 2006;354:119–30.

24. House HR, Ehlers JP. Travel-Related Infections. Emerg Med Clin N Am 2008; 26(2):499–516.

25. Rosen T, Brown TJ. Cutaneous manifestations of sexually transmitted diseases. Med Clin North Am 1998;82:1081–104, vi.

26. HJC de V. Skin as an indicator for sexually transmitted infections. Clin Dermatol 2014;32:196–208.

27. Schmid GP. Approach to the patient with genital ulcer disease. Med Clin North Am 1990;74:1559–72.

28. Tindall B, Cooper DA. Primary HIV infection: host responses and intervention strategies. AIDS 1991;5:1–14.

29. Lapins J, Gaines H, Lindbäck S, et al. Skin and mucosal characteristics of symptomatic primary HIV-1 infection. AIDS Patient Care STDS 1997;11:67–70.

30. Prasad S, Casas CG, Strahan AG, et al. A dermatologic assessment of 101 mpox (monkeypox) cases from 13 countries during the 2022 outbreak: Skin lesion morphology, clinical course, and scarring. J Am Acad Dermatol 2023; 88:1066–73.
31. Català A, Clavo-Escribano P, Riera-Monroig J, et al. Monkeypox outbreak in Spain: clinical and epidemiological findings in a prospective cross-sectional study of 185 cases. Br J Dermatol 2022;187:765–72.
32. Simmons CP, Farrar JJ, van Nguyen VC, et al. Dengue. N Engl J Med 2012;366: 1423–32.
33. Guo C, Zhou Z, Wen Z, et al. Global Epidemiology of Dengue Outbreaks in 1990–2015: A Systematic Review and Meta-Analysis. Front Cell Infect Mi 2017;7:317.
34. Harris CM, Wu HM, Li J, et al. Meningococcal Disease in Patients With Human Immunodeficiency Virus Infection: A Review of Cases Reported Through Active Surveillance in the United States, 2000-2008. Open Forum Infect Dis 2016;3: ofw226.
35. Kano Y, Shiohara T. The variable clinical picture of drug-induced hypersensitivity syndrome/drug rash with eosinophilia and systemic symptoms in relation to the eliciting drug. Immunol Allergy Clin North Am 2009;29:481–501.
36. Venugopal SS, Murrell DF. Diagnosis and clinical features of pemphigus vulgaris. Immunol Allergy Clin North Am 2012;32:233–43, v-vi.
37. Schwartz RA, McDonough PH, Lee BW. Toxic epidermal necrolysis: Part I. Introduction, history, classification, clinical features, systemic manifestations, etiology, and immunopathogenesis. J Am Acad Dermatol 2013;69. 173.e1-13; [quiz 185-186].
38. Vargas-Díez E, García-Díez A, Marín A, et al. Life-threatening graft-vs-host disease. Clin Dermatol 2005;23:285–300.
39. Burns JC, Mason WH, Glode MP, et al. Clinical and epidemiologic characteristics of patients referred for evaluation of possible Kawasaki disease. United States Multicenter Kawasaki Disease Study Group. J Pediatr 1991;118:680–6.
40. Derrington SM, Cellura AP, McDermott LE, et al. Mucocutaneous Findings and Course in an Adult With Zika Virus Infection. Jama Dermatol 2016;152(6):691.
41. Chesney PJ, Davis JP, Purdy WK, et al. Clinical manifestations of toxic shock syndrome. JAMA 1981;246:741–8.
42. Jay R, Armstrong P. Clinical characteristics of Rocky Mountain spotted fever in the United States: A literature review. J Vector Dis 2020;57(2):114.
43. Patterson J, Sammon M, Garg M. Dengue, Zika and Chikungunya: Emerging Arboviruses in the New World. West J Emerg Medicine Integrating Emerg Care Popul Heal 2016;17(6):671–9.
44. Syder NC, Elbuluk N. Racial and Ethnic Disparities in Research and Clinical Trials. Dermatol Clin 2023;41:351–8.
45. Hooper J, Shao K, Feng H. Racial/ethnic health disparities in dermatology in the United States, part 1: Overview of contributing factors and management strategies. J Am Acad Dermatol 2022;87:723–30.
46. Stephens DS, Hajjeh RA, Baughman WS, et al. Sporadic Meningococcal Disease in Adults: Results of a 5-Year Population-Based Study. Ann Intern Med 1995;123(12):937.
47. Shanmugavadivel D, Liu JF, Buonsenso D, et al. Assessing Healthcare Professionals' Identification of Paediatric Dermatological Conditions in Darker Skin Tones. Children (Basel) 2022;9. https://doi.org/10.3390/children9111749.
48. Muller DA, Depelsenaire ACI, Young PR. Clinical and Laboratory Diagnosis of Dengue Virus Infection. J Infect Dis 2017;215(suppl_2):S89–95.

49. O'Loughlin RE, Roberson A, Cieslak PR, et al. The Epidemiology of Invasive Group A Streptococcal Infection and Potential *Vaccine* Implications: United States, 2000–2004. Clin Infect Dis 2007;45(7):853–62.
50. Hahné SJM, Charlett A, Purcell B, et al. Effectiveness of antibiotics given before admission in reducing mortality from meningococcal disease: systematic review. BMJ 2006;332:1299–303.
51. Rosenstein NE, Perkins BA, Stephens DS, et al. Meningococcal disease. N Engl J Med 2001;344:1378–88.
52. Deuren M van, Brandtzaeg P, Meer JWM van der. Update on Meningococcal Disease with Emphasis on Pathogenesis and Clinical Management. Clin Microbiol Rev 2000;13(1):144–66.
53. Mourad O, Makhani L, Chen LH. Chikungunya: An Emerging Public Health Concern. Curr Infect Dis Rep 2022;24(12):217–28.
54. Sharp TM, Fischer M, Muñoz-Jordán JL, et al. Dengue and Zika Virus Diagnostic Testing for Patients with a Clinically Compatible Illness and Risk for Infection with Both *Viruses*. Mmwr Recomm Rep 2019;68(1):1–10.
55. Arend SM, Lavrijsen APM, Kuijken I, et al. Prospective controlled study of the diagnostic value of skin biopsy in patients with presumed meningococcal disease. Eur J Clin Microbiol Infect Dis 2006;25:643–9.
56. Staquet P, Lemee L, Verdier E, et al. Detection of Neisseria meningitidis DNA from skin lesion biopsy using real-time PCR: usefulness in the aetiological diagnosis of purpura fulminans. Intensive Care Med 2007;33:1168–72.
57. Sanders C.V. and Nesbitt L.T., The skin and infection: a color Atlas and Text. Williams & Wilkins, Available at: https://books.google.com/books?id=hOJsAAAAMAAJ. Accessed April 3, 2023.
58. N'Guyen Y, Duval X, Revest M, et al. Time interval between infective endocarditis first symptoms and diagnosis: relationship to infective endocarditis characteristics, microorganisms and prognosis. Ann Med 2017;49:117–25.
59. Spencer R. Rocky Mountain Spotted Fever. J Infect Dis 1929;44:257–76.
60. Drexler NA, Close R, Yaglom HD, et al. Morbidity and Functional Outcomes Following Rocky Mountain Spotted Fever Hospitalization—Arizona, 2002–2017. Open Forum Infect Dis 2022;9(10). ofac506.
61. Kjemtrup AM, Padgett K, Paddock CD, et al. A forty-year review of Rocky Mountain spotted fever cases in California shows clinical and epidemiologic changes. Plos Neglect Trop D 2022;16(9):e0010738.
62. Holman RC, McQuiston JH, Haberling DL, et al. Increasing incidence of Rocky Mountain spotted fever among the American Indian population in the United States. Am J Trop Med Hyg 2009;80:601–5.
63. Traeger MS, Regan JJ, Humpherys D, et al. Rocky Mountain Spotted Fever Characterization and Comparison to Similar Illnesses in a Highly Endemic Area—Arizona, 2002–2011. Clin Infect Dis 2015;60(11):1650–8.
64. Thorner AR, Walker DH, Petri WAJ. Rocky mountain spotted fever. Clin Infect Dis 1998;27:1353–9 [quiz 1360].
65. Lacz N, Schwartz R, Kapila R. Rocky Mountain spotted fever. J Eur Acad Dermatol 2006;20(4):411–7.
66. Buckingham SC, Marshall GS, Schutze GE, et al. Clinical and Laboratory Features, Hospital Course, and Outcome of Rocky Mountain Spotted Fever in Children. J Pediatrics 2007;150(2):180–4.e1.
67. Usatine RP, Sandy N. Dermatologic emergencies. Am Fam Physician 2010;82:773–80.

68. Helmick CG, Bernard KW, D'Angelo LJ. Rocky Mountain spotted fever: clinical, laboratory, and epidemiological features of 262 cases. J Infect Dis 1984;150:480–8.

69. Mosites E, Carpenter LR, McElroy K, et al. Knowledge, attitudes, and practices regarding Rocky Mountain spotted fever among healthcare providers, Tennessee, 2009. Am J Trop Med Hyg 2013;88:162–6.

70. Zientek J, Dahlgren FS, McQuiston JH, et al. Self-Reported Treatment Practices by Healthcare Providers Could Lead to Death from Rocky Mountain Spotted Fever. J Pediatrics 2014;164(2):416–8.

71. Todd SR, Dahlgren FS, Traeger MS, et al. No visible dental staining in children treated with doxycycline for suspected Rocky Mountain Spotted Fever. J Pediatr 2015;166:1246–51.

72. Epidemiological Alert: Increase in Cases and Deaths from Chikungunya in the Region of the Americas. PAHO/WHO. 2023. Available at: https://www.paho.org/en/documents/epidemiological-alert-increase-cases-and-deaths-chikungunya-region-americas#:~:text=of%20the%20Americas-,Epidemiological%20Alert%3A%20Increase%20in%20cases%20and%20deaths%20from%20chikungunya,the%20Region%20of%20the%20Americas&text=In%202022%2C%20the%20Region%20of,numbers%20reported%20in%20previous%20years. [Accessed 3 April 2023].

73. Potential range of Aedes aegypti and Aedes albopictus in the United States, 2017, Available at: https://www.cdc.gov/mosquitoes/mosquito-control/professionals/range.html, 2020. Accessed March 17, 2023.

74. Burt FJ, Chen W, Miner JJ, et al. Chikungunya virus: an update on the biology and pathogenesis of this emerging pathogen. Lancet Infect Dis 2017;17(4):e107–17.

75. Tsetsarkin KA, Vanlandingham DL, McGee CE, et al. A Single Mutation in Chikungunya Virus Affects Vector Specificity and Epidemic Potential. Plos Pathog 2007;3(12):e201.

76. Ali AA, Bajric B, Isache CL, et al. Mosquito borne illness in a Floridian hiker. Am J Emerg Med 2021;45:681.e1–2.

77. Monaghan AJ, Morin CW, Steinhoff DF, et al. On the Seasonal Occurrence and Abundance of the Zika Virus Vector Mosquito Aedes Aegypti in the Contiguous United States. PLoS Curr 2016;8.

78. Zika - Statistics and Maps. Centers for Disease Control and Prevention. 2023. Available at: https://www.cdc.gov/zika/reporting/index.html. [Accessed 23 April 2023].

79. Statistics and Maps. Dengue. 2023. Available at: https://www.cdc.gov/dengue/statistics-maps/index.html. [Accessed 23 April 2023].

80. Organization WH. In: Dengue: guidelines for diagnosis, treatment, prevention and Control. Geneva, Switzerland: World Health Organization; 2009. p. 157.

81. Bhatt S, Gething PW, Brady OJ, et al. The global distribution and burden of dengue. Nature 2013;496:504–7.

82. Guzman MG, Vazquez S. The Complexity of Antibody-Dependent Enhancement of Dengue Virus Infection. Viruses 2010;2(12):2649–62.

83. Feder HM, Plucinski M, Hoss DM. Dengue with a morbilliform rash and a positive tourniquet test. Jaad Case Reports 2016;2(5):422–3.

84. Azfar NA, Malik LM, Jamil A, et al. Cutaneous manifestations in patients of dengue fever. Journal of Pakistan Association of Dermatologists 2012;22(4):320–4.

85. Thomas EA. Cutaneous manifestations in patients with Dengue Fever. Indian J Dermatol 2010;55(1):79–85.

86. Dengue for Healthcare Providers | CDC. Dengue. 2020. Available at: https://www.cdc.gov/dengue/vaccine/hcp/index.html. [Accessed 23 April 2023].

87. Santiago GA, Vázquez J, Courtney S, et al. Performance of the Trioplex real-time RT-PCR assay for detection of Zika, dengue, and chikungunya viruses. Nat Commun 2018;9(1):1391.

88. Conceição PJP da, Carvalho LR de, Godoy BLV de, et al. Detection of DENV-2 and ZIKV coinfection in southeastern Brazil by serum and urine testing. Med Microbiol Immunol 2023.

89. Adams LE, Martin SW, Lindsey NP, et al. Epidemiology of Dengue, Chikungunya, and Zika Virus Disease in U.S. States and Territories, 2017. Am J Tropical Medicine Hyg 2019;101(4):884–90.

90. McCarthy M. First US case of Zika virus infection is identified in Texas. BMJ 2016;352:i212.

91. Zika epidemiology update - February 2022. World Health Organization. 2022. Available at: https://www.who.int/publications/m/item/zika-epidemiology-update—february-2022. [Accessed 3 April 2023].

92. Roth NM, Reynolds MR, Lewis EL, et al. Zika-Associated Birth Defects Reported in Pregnancies with Laboratory Evidence of Confirmed or Possible Zika Virus Infection - U.S. Zika Pregnancy and Infant Registry, December 1, 2015-March 31, 2018. MMWR Morb Mortal Wkly Rep 2022;71:73–9.

93. Hall V, Walker WL, Lindsey NP, et al. Update: Noncongenital Zika Virus Disease Cases - 50 U.S. States and the District of Columbia, 2016. MMWR Morb Mortal Wkly Rep 2018;67:265–9.

94. Cordel N, Biermbaux X, Chaumont H, et al. Main Characteristics of Zika Virus Exanthema in Guadeloupe. Jama Dermatol 2017;153(4):325.

95. He A, Brasil P, Siqueira AM, et al. The Emerging Zika Virus Threat: A Guide for Dermatologists. Am J Clin Dermatol 2017;18(2):231–6.

96. Duffy MR, Chen TH, Hancock WT, et al. Zika virus outbreak on Yap Island, Federated States of Micronesia. N Engl J Med 2009;360:2536–43.

97. Halani S, Tombindo PE, O'Reilly R, et al. Clinical manifestations and health outcomes associated with Zika virus infections in adults: A systematic review. Plos Neglect Trop D 2021;15(7):e0009516.

98. Cerbino-Neto J, Mesquita EC, Souza TML, et al. Clinical Manifestations of Zika Virus Infection, Rio de Janeiro, Brazil, 2015 - Volume 22, Number 7—July 2016 - Emerging Infectious Diseases journal - CDC. Emerg Infect Dis 2016;22(7):1318–20.

99. Ginier M, Neumayr A, Günther S, et al. Zika without symptoms in returning travelers: What are the implications? Travel Med Infect Dis 2016;14:16–20.

100. Cao-Lormeau VM, Blake A, Mons S, et al. Guillain-Barré Syndrome outbreak associated with Zika virus infection in French Polynesia: a case-control study. Lancet 2016;387:1531–9.

101. Silva JVJ, Lopes TRR, Oliveira-Filho EF de, et al. Current status, challenges and perspectives in the development of vaccines against yellow fever, dengue, Zika and chikungunya viruses. Acta Trop 2018;182:257–63.

102. ROBINSON MC. An epidemic of virus disease in Southern Province, Tanganyika Territory, in 1952-53. I. Clinical features. Trans R Soc Trop Med Hyg 1955;49:28–32.

103. Kendrick K, Stanek D, Blackmore C. Notes from the field: Transmission of chikungunya virus in the continental United States–Florida, 2014. MMWR Morb Mortal Wkly Rep 2014;63:1137.
104. Brouard C, Bernillon P, Quatresous I, et al. Estimated risk of Chikungunya viremic blood donation during an epidemic on Reunion Island in the Indian Ocean, 2005 to 2007. Transfusion 2008;48:1333–41.
105. Contopoulos-Ioannidis D, Newman-Lindsay S, Chow C, et al. Mother-to-child transmission of Chikungunya virus: A systematic review and meta-analysis. PLoS Negl Trop Dis 2018;12:e0006510.
106. Staples EJ, Hils S, Powers A. Chikungunya. In: Nemhauser J, Halsy E, editors. CDC Yellow book 2024: health information for International travel. New York, NY: Oxford University Press; 2023. p. 341–4. Available at: https://wwwnc.cdc.gov/travel/yellowbook/2024/infections-diseases/chikungunya.
107. Kawle AP, Nayak AR, Bhullar SS, et al. Seroprevalence and clinical manifestations of chikungunya virus infection in rural areas of Chandrapur, Maharashtra, India. J Vector Dis 2017;54(1):35–43.
108. Kaleem S, Ghafoor R, Khan S, Admin. Mucocutaneous manifestations of Chikungunya fever, an experience of tertiary care hospital. J Pak Med Assoc 2020;71:1–13, 2(B).
109. Kumar R, Sharma MK, Jain SK, et al. Cutaneous Manifestations of Chikungunya Fever: Observations from an Outbreak at a Tertiary Care Hospital in Southeast Rajasthan, India. Indian Dermatology Online J 2017;8(5):336–42.
110. Ferreira FCP, Silva ASV da, Recht J, et al. Vertical transmission of chikungunya virus: A systematic review. PLoS One 2021;16:e0249166.
111. Drago F, Ciccarese G, Gasparini G, et al. Contemporary infectious exanthems: an update. Future Microbiol 2017;12(2):171–93.
112. Handler MZ, Handler NS, Stephany MP, et al. Chikungunya fever: an emerging viral infection threatening North America and Europe. Int J Dermatol 2017;56(2):e19–25.
113. Kannan M, Rajendran R, Sunish IP, et al. A study on chikungunya outbreak during 2007 in Kerala, south India. Indian J Med Res 2009;129:311–5.
114. Singh N, Chandrashekar L, Konda D, et al. Vesiculobullous viral exanthem due to chikungunya in an infant. Indian Dermatol Online J 2014;5:S119–20.
115. Weaver SC, Lecuit M. Chikungunya virus and the global spread of a mosquito-borne disease. N Engl J Med 2015;372:1231–9.
116. Economopoulou A, Dominguez M, Helynck B, et al. Atypical Chikungunya virus infections: clinical manifestations, mortality and risk factors for severe disease during the 2005-2006 outbreak on Réunion. Epidemiol Infect 2009;137:534–41.
117. Schilte C, Staikowsky F, Couderc T, et al. Chikungunya virus-associated long-term arthralgia: a 36-month prospective longitudinal study. PLoS Negl Trop Dis 2013;7:e2137.
118. Guillot X, Ribera A, Gasque P. Chikungunya-Induced Arthritis in Reunion Island: A Long-Term Observational Follow-Up Study Showing Frequently Persistent Joint Symptoms, Some Cases of Persistent Chikungunya Immunoglobulin M Positivity, and No Anticyclic Citrullinated Peptide Seroconversion After 13 Years. J Infect Dis 2020;222:1740–4.
119. National Institute of Health. Search of: chikungunya - list results. Home - ClinicalTrials.gov, Available at: https://clinicaltrials.gov/ct2/results?cond=chikungunya&term=&cntry=&state=&city=&dist=, 2022. Accessed March 17, 2023.
120. Todd JK. Toxic shock syndrome. Clin Microbiol Rev 1988;1(4):432–46.

121. Strom MA, Hsu DY, Silverberg JI. Prevalence, comorbidities and mortality of toxic shock syndrome in children and adults in the USA. Microbiol Immunol 2017;61(11):463–73.
122. Barnes M, Youngkin E, Zipprich J, et al. Notes from the Field: Increase in Pediatric Invasive Group A Streptococcus Infections - Colorado and Minnesota, October-December 2022. MMWR Morb Mortal Wkly Rep 2023;72:265–7.
123. Lehnhardt M, Homann HH, Daigeler A, et al. Major and Lethal Complications of Liposuction: A Review of 72 Cases in Germany between 1998 and 2002. Plast Reconstr Surg 2008;121(6):396e–403e.
124. Nakamura H, Makiguchi T, Hasegawa Y, et al. Staphylococcal Toxic Shock Syndrome after Autologous Breast Reconstruction: A Case Report and Literature Review. Plastic Reconstr Surg Global Open 2022;10(12):e4710.
125. Liu Z, Zhang W, Zhang B, et al. Toxic shock syndrome complicated with symmetrical peripheral gangrene after liposuction and fat transfer: a case report and literature review. Bmc Infect Dis 2021;21(1):1137.
126. Tofte RW, Williams DN. Clinical and Laboratory Manifestations of Toxic Shock Syndrome. J Urology 1982;128(6):1412.
127. Wolf J, Rabinowitz L. Streptococcal Toxic Shock Syndrome. Zentralblatt Für Bakteriologie 1990;272(3):257–64.
128. Schlievert PM, Case LC, Strandberg KL, et al. Vaginal Staphylococcus aureus Superantigen Profile Shift from 1980 and 1981 to 2003, 2004, and 2005. J Clin Microbiol 2007;45(8):2704–7.
129. Patel T, Quow K, Cardones AR. Management of Infectious Emergencies for the Inpatient Dermatologist. Curr Dermatology Reports 2021;10(4):232–42.
130. Gottlieb M, Long B, Koyfman A. The Evaluation and Management of Toxic Shock Syndrome in the Emergency Department: A Review of the Literature. J Emerg Medicine 2018;54(6):807–14.
131. Toxic shock syndrome (other than streptococcal) (TSS) 2011 case definition. 2021. Available at: https://ndc.services.cdc.gov/case-definitions/toxic-shock-syndrome-2011/. [Accessed 23 March 2023].
132. Cook A, Janse S, Watson JR, et al. Early Release - Manifestations of Toxic Shock Syndrome in Children, Columbus, Ohio, USA, 2010–2017 - Volume 26, Number 6—June 2020 - Emerging Infectious Diseases journal - CDC. Emerg Infect Dis 2020;26(6):1077–83.
133. Morrison V. Postoperative Toxic Shock Syndrome. Arch Surg 1983;118(7):791–4.
134. MURRAY RJ. Recognition and management of Staphylococcus aureus toxin-mediated disease. Intern Med J 2005;35(s2):S106–19.
135. Contou D, Colin G, Travert B, et al. Menstrual Toxic Shock Syndrome: A French Nationwide Multicenter Retrospective Study. Clin Infect Dis 2021;74(2):246–53.
136. Berger S, Kunerl A, Wasmuth S, et al. Menstrual toxic shock syndrome: case report and systematic review of the literature. Lancet Infect Dis 2019;19(9):e313–21.
137. Jamart S, Denis O, Deplano A, et al. Methicillin-resistant Staphylococcus aureus Toxic Shock Syndrome - Volume 11, Number 4—April 2005 - Emerging Infectious Diseases journal - CDC. Emerg Infect Dis 2005;11(4):636–7.
138. Stevens DL, Wallace RJ, Hamilton SM, et al. Successful treatment of staphylococcal toxic shock syndrome with linezolid: a case report and in vitro evaluation of the production of toxic shock syndrome toxin type 1 in the presence of antibiotics. Clin Infect Dis 2006;42:729–30.
139. Silversides JA, Lappin E, Ferguson AJ. Staphylococcal toxic shock syndrome: mechanisms and management. Curr Infect Dis Rep 2010;12:392–400.

140. Laho D, Blumental S, Botteaux A, et al. Invasive Group A Streptococcal Infections: Benefit of Clindamycin, Intravenous Immunoglobulins and Secondary Prophylaxis. Frontiers Pediatrics 2021;9:697938.
141. Babiker A, Li X, Lai YL, et al. Effectiveness of adjunctive clindamycin in β-lactam antibiotic-treated patients with invasive β-haemolytic streptococcal infections in US hospitals: a retrospective multicentre cohort study. Lancet Infect Dis 2021; 21(5):697–710.
142. Amreen S, Brar SK, Perveen S, et al. Clinical efficacy of intravenous immunoglobulins in management of toxic shock syndrome: an updated literature review. Cureus 2021;13(1):e12836.
143. Meningococcal disease surveillance, Available at: https://www.cdc.gov/meningococcal/surveillance/index.html#surveillance-systems, 2023. Accessed April 5, 2023.
144. Takada S, Fujiwara S, Inoue T, et al. Meningococcemia in Adults: A Review of the Literature. Internal Med 2016;55(6):567–72.
145. MacNeil JR, Blain AE, Wang X, et al. Current epidemiology and trends in meningococcal disease—United States, 1996–2015. Clin Infect Dis 2017;66(8): 1276–81.
146. Trotter CL, Gay NJ, Edmunds WJ. The natural history of meningococcal carriage and disease. Epidemiol Infect 2006;134:556–66.
147. Cartwright KA, Stuart JM, Jones DM, et al. The Stonehouse survey: nasopharyngeal carriage of meningococci and Neisseria lactamica. Epidemiol Infect 1987; 99:591–601.
148. Pace D, Pollard AJ. Meningococcal disease: Clinical presentation and sequelae. Vaccine 2012;30. B3-B9.
149. Yazdankhah SP, Caugant DA. Neisseria meningitidis: an overview of the carriage state. J Med Microbiol 2004;53(9):821–32.
150. Wilder-Smith A, Barkham TMS, Earnest A, et al. Acquisition of W135 meningococcal carriage in Hajj pilgrims and transmission to household contacts: prospective study. BMJ 2002;325:365–6.
151. Ridpath A, Greene SK, Robinson BF, et al. Risk Factors for Serogroup C Meningococcal Disease during Outbreak among Men who Have Sex with Men, New York City, New York, USA. Emerg Infect Dis 2015;21:1458–61.
152. McKinnon HD, Howard T. Evaluating the febrile patient with a rash. Am Fam Physician 2000;62(4):804–16.
153. Stephens DS. Biology and pathogenesis of the evolutionarily successful, obligate human bacterium Neisseria meningitidis. Vaccine 2009;27:B71–7.
154. Deghmane AE, Taha S, Taha MK. Global epidemiology and changing clinical presentations of invasive meningococcal disease: a narrative review. Infect Dis 2022;54(1):1–7.
155. Marzouk O, Thomson AP, Sills JA, et al. Features and outcome in meningococcal disease presenting with maculopapular rash. Arch Dis Child 1991; 66(4):485.
156. Wells LC, Smith JC, Weston VC, et al. The child with a non-blanching rash: how likely is meningococcal disease? Arch Dis Child 2001;85(3):218.
157. Bibi S, Gilani SYH, Siddiqui TS, et al. Meningococcemia in children—an under recognized public health problem in Pakistan. J Ayub Medical Coll Abbottabad 2022;34:S699–702, 3 (SUPPL 1.
158. Campsall PA, Laupland KB, Niven DJ. Severe Meningococcal Infection A Review of Epidemiology, Diagnosis, and Management. Crit Care Clin 2013;29(3): 393–409.

159. Bryant PA, Li HY, Zaia A, et al. Prospective study of a real-time PCR that is highly sensitive, specific, and clinically useful for diagnosis of meningococcal disease in children. J Clin Microbiol 2004;42:2919–25.
160. Hahné SJM, Charlett A, Purcell B, et al. Effectiveness of antibiotics given before admission in reducing mortality from meningococcal disease: systematic review. Bmj 2006;332(7553):1299.
161. Barquet N, Domingo P, Caylà JA, et al. Prognostic factors in meningococcal disease. Development of a bedside predictive model and scoring system. Barcelona Meningococcal Disease Surveillance Group. JAMA 1997;278:491–6.
162. Durand ML, Calderwood SB, Weber DJ, et al. Acute bacterial meningitis in adults. A review of 493 episodes. N Engl J Med 1993;328:21–8.
163. McNamara M, Blain A. Meningococcal - vaccine preventable diseases surveillance manual | cdc. 2023. Available at: https://www.cdc.gov/vaccines/pubs/surv-manual/chpt08-mening.html. [Accessed 8 April 2023].
164. Bozio CH, Blain A, MacNeil J, et al. Meningococcal Disease Surveillance in Men Who Have Sex with Men — United States, 2015–2016. Morbidity Mortal Wkly Rep 2018;67(38):1060–3.

Sexually Transmitted Infections in the Emergency Department

Rachel E. Solnick, MD, MSc[a],*, Laura Hernando López, MD[a],
Patricia Mae Martinez, MD[a], Jason E. Zucker, MD[b]

KEYWORDS

- Emergency department • Sexually transmitted infections • Syphilis • Gonorrhea
- Chlamydia • Expedited Partner therapy • Extragenital testing • Mpox

KEY POINTS

- Emergency medicine clinicians must stay updated on STI trends like syphilis resurgence and new pathogens for effective diagnosis.
- Clinicians should adhere to CDC guidelines for testing and treatment, ensuring evidence-based care.
- To best serve their populations, EDs should consider implementing rapid testing, extragenital testing, expedited partner treatment, and novel prophylaxis approaches for comprehensive STI management.

INTRODUCTION
Epidemiology in the United States

Rates of *Neisseria gonorrhoeae* (gonorrhea, GC), *Chlamydia trachomatis* (chlamydia, CT), and *Treponema pallidum* (syphilis), the 3 most common reportable sexually transmitted infections (STIs), continue to increase in the United States, with a reported combined incidence of 2.5 million reported cases.[1,2] Additionally, *Trichomonas vaginalis* (trichomoniasis, TV), the most common non-viral STI, had a prevalence of 2.6 million cases in 2018.[3] The Centers for Disease Control and Prevention (CDC) estimated that approximately 20% of the US population had an STI on any given day in 2018, with an estimated 26.2 million incident and 67.6 million prevalent STI infections.[4] This rise may be due to various factors, including decreasing availability and funding of sexual health clinic services,[5,6] socioeconomics,[7] and social and behavioral changes.[8]

[a] Icahn School of Medicine at Mount Sinai Hospital, Department of Emergency Medicine-Research Division, 555 West 57th Street, 5th Floor Suite 5-25, New York, NY 10019, USA;
[b] Columbia University Vagelos College of Physicians and Surgeons, 630 West 168th Street, Box 82, New York, NY 10032, USA
* Corresponding author.
E-mail address: Rachel.solnick@mountsinai.org

Emerg Med Clin N Am 42 (2024) 335–368
https://doi.org/10.1016/j.emc.2024.02.006
0733-8627/24/© 2024 Elsevier Inc. All rights reserved.

Health and Economic Impacts

STIs cost the US health care system billions of dollars annually and contribute to avoidable morbidity. The total lifetime medical cost of incident STIs is $15.9 billion, primarily due to human immunodeficiency virus (HIV) ($13.7 billion), with $1 billion attributed to gonorrhea and chlamydia combined.[9] In addition to their financial and social costs, STIs can have profound implications for long-term health, particularly female reproductive health. Repeated chlamydia infections can lead to pelvic inflammatory disease and infertility.[10] Re-exposure to an untreated partner may contribute to an estimated 14% rate of chlamydia reinfection in the United States.[11] Furthermore, many STIs, inclusive of TV, can increase the risk of acquiring and transmitting HIV.[3,12,13] Prompt recognition and treatment of STIs is therefore crucial.

Health Disparities

The epidemic of STIs is intricately linked to structural factors that disproportionately burden marginalized groups, including racial and ethnic minorities, sexual and gender minorities, and socioeconomically disadvantaged populations.[14] Research examining how community factors and social determinants of health[15] affect sexual health has found higher rates of CT/GC,[16] TV,[17] and HIV[18] in more socially vulnerable areas. There are higher STI rates during pregnancy in areas with worse racial segregation and income inequality.[19] Additionally, incarceration is associated with higher rates of STIs,[20–22] due to a confluence of the aforementioned structural factors among inmates and STI prevalence in sexual networks.[23,24]

Sexually Transmitted Infections in the Emergency Department

Emergency departments (EDs) have faced increasing rates of STI visits. While this reflects overall trends in health care delivery,[25–27] it is also due to rising rates of positive STI test results among ED patients.[26] When compared to outpatient clinic patients, patients presenting to the ED are more likely to test positive for an STI.[28] With sexual health clinic defunding,[29] there was a 39% increase in US ED visits with an STI diagnosis between 2008 and 2013. This rise significantly outpaced the 2% increase in overall ED visits over the same period. Thus, EDs play a critical and growing role in the prevention, diagnosis, and treatment of the epidemic of STIs.

Heath disparities are also evident in ED STI-related visits, which are more common among marginalized ED patients.[30] Black ED patients are more likely than white patients to receive an STI diagnosis and receive empiric antibiotics.[27] In a study of patients attending an sexually transmitted disease (STD) clinic, black patients were more likely to also use the ED for STI care.[31] Additionally, repeat visits for STIs are common in marginalized groups. A study in St Louis found that 27% of patients had a repeat STI visit over 6 years, and that these patients were more likely young, female, black, and lacking insurance or with public insurance.[32]

Focus of This Review

This review will cover the recognition and diagnosis of both common and less common STIs, highlighting new and underused testing strategies such as extragenital testing, new point-of-care (POC) tests, and STI screening in the ED. We also present current treatment recommendations while highlighting proactive approaches like expedited partner therapy (EPT).

CLINICAL PRESENTATION AND DIAGNOSIS
Discussing Sexual Health with Patients

Taking a sex-positive, nonjudgmental, and respectful sexual history is a crucial skill for emergency clinician and may lead to improved STI risk assessment and diagnosis. When a thorough sexual history is required, use the CDC-endorsed "5 P's" approach, which provides a structured, gender-neutral framework **Box 1**.[33] The evidence-based GOALS (give a preamble that emphasizes sexual health, offer opt-out HIV/STI testing and information, ask an open-ended question, listen for relevant information and fill in the blanks, suggest a course of action) framework recommends focusing on benefits as opposed to risk, normalizing sexuality as part of health care, offering universal opt-out testing, and asking open-ended questions to help identify patient priorities.[34] Technological advances include computerized self-interviews that can assist in the identification of patients for STI testing,[35–37] and brief videos[38] or behavioral interventions[39,40] that encourage safer sex practices.

Asymptomatic Infections

The determination of who should be treated for STIs is challenging because they are so often asymptomatic. In 1 multicenter study of patients rescreened for STIs, 66% of those with CT, GC, or TV had no symptoms.[41] Studies have shown that men with asymptomatic infections account for about half of cases of transmission to women.[42,43] These findings underscore the importance of asking about new partners or exposures, routine EPT, and wider use of STI screening in asymptomatic populations.

Common Clinical Syndromes and Sexually Transmitted Pathogens

Cervicitis

Cervicitis is frequently asymptomatic but may have symptoms of abnormal vaginal discharge or intermenstrual bleeding.[44] Signs of cervicitis include mucopurulent endocervical exudate on speculum examination or friability of the cervical os. Cervicitis frequently has no identifiable etiology, but GC/CT are the pathogens most often identified (**Table 1**). Less common etiologies include TV, herpes simplex virus (HSV)-2, and *Mycoplasma genitalium* (Mgen).

Endocervical or vaginal swabs for nucleic acid amplification test (NAAT) for CT/GC/TV are the preferred means of etiologic diagnosis. For female urogenital CT/GC infections, vaginal swabs are preferred by the CDC to first-void urine, which has a lower sensitivity for CT/GC, as well as TV, due to low urine organism load.[44] Reliance on urine specimens as opposed to vaginal and endocervical swabs will result in ~10% fewer infections identified,[45] and result in many missed infections.[46–48] Patients'

Box 1
Taking a Sexual History (the Centers for Disease Control and Prevention's 5 P's)

- "Partners"—1/multiple and gender of sexual partners
- "Practices"—types of sexual activities the patient engages in (eg, vaginal, oral, anal)
- "Protection from STIs"—use of condoms and consistency of use
- "Past history of STIs"—previous STIs, which may increase susceptibility to future STIs
- "Pregnancy intention"—contraception and preferences regarding childbearing

Abbreviation: STI, sexually transmitted infection.

Table 1
Sexually transmitted infection pathogens: signs, symptoms, and diagnostics

	Genital	Extragenital
Bacterial STIs		
Chlamydia trachomatis (CT) Cervicitis and mucopurulent discharge[57]	*Incubation period:* 7–14 d,[58] up to 6 wk. Testing is best done 2 wk after exposure. *Symptoms:* Mostly asymptomatic. Symptoms could include dysuria, urinary frequency, genital itch. Women: ~80% asymptomatic. Cervicitis, abnormal discharge, intermenstrual bleeding, dyspareunia, abdominal/pelvic pain. Men: ~50% asymptomatic. Urethritis 1–3 wk after exposure with urethral discharge and dysuria. Epididymitis possible. *Diagnostics:* Men: urine NAAT. *Testing:* Vaginal swab NAAT is more sensitive than urine NAAT. Patient-collected vaginal swab are as accurate as clinician-collected. Point-of-care NAAT testing is available, but infrequently used in EDs.[59]	*Pharyngeal and rectal:* Majority are asymptomatic. *Sequelae/complications:* Reactive arthritis, predominantly large joints, 4–10 wk after infection. Premature birth; neonatal conjunctivitis. *Diagnostics:* Some NAATs have FDA clearance for rectal and oropharyngeal sampling; self-collected samples comparable to clinician-collected samples[59]
Neisseria gonorrhoeae (referred to as GC for gonococcal) Disseminated gonorrhea rash[60] Gonococcal lesion[61]	*Incubation period:* 2–5 d,[58] up to 14 d. *Symptoms:* Dysuria, frequency, abnormal discharge. Women: 50% asymptomatic. Cervicitis,[63] pruritus[63] Men: 40% asymptomatic.[64] Urethritis,[62] testicular pain. *Diagnostics:* Men: first-void urine NAAT. *Testing:* Vaginal swab NAAT is more sensitive than urine NAAT. Patient-collected vaginal swabs are as accurate as clinician-collected ones. Point-of-care NAAT testing is available, but infrequently used in EDs.[59]	*Pharynx:* 90% asymptomatic, pharyngitis. *Ocular:* Gonococcal ophthalmia. *Rectal:* Tenesmus, anal/rectal soreness, proctitis is more frequent in MSM.[62] *Disseminated gonococcal infection (DGI):* Undulating fever, polyarthritis, tenosynovitis, skin lesions (papules, pustules or necrosis in acral areas). *Sequelae/complications:* Pregnancy: premature rupture of membrane, premature birth, septic abortion. Neonatal purulent conjunctivitis.[62] *Diagnostics:* Some NAATs have FDA clearance for rectal and oropharyngeal sampling; self-collected samples comparable to clinician-collected samples.[59]

Treponema pallidum (Syphilis)[62,63]

Primary genital syphilis—Chancre[65]

Secondary syphilis—condyloma lata[65]

Primary syphilis: (10–90 d incubation (21 d on average), spontaneous remission of chancre within 2–3 wk)[62,63]
- Genital: painless ulcer (chancres)
- Atypical: painful, multiple lesions, usually rectal[66]
- Extragenital: nontender regional lymphadenopathy

Secondary syphilis: (4–6 wk latency period)
- General/flulike symptoms and lymphadenopathy
- Multiorgan: hepatitis, arthritis, iridocyclitis, meningitis.
- Skin: maculopapular, nonpruritic rash, typically affecting the palms and soles, condylomata lata (wartlike lesions), alopecia.

Tertiary syphilis: (3–10 y of latency period)
- Cardiovascular: aortitis, aortic aneurysm
- Gummatous lesion (gummas) typically on skin, mucosal membrane, liver, testes, bone
- No longer contagious

Neurosyphilis:[67] (can occur at any time)
- Cognitive dysfunction, personality changes
- Ocular syphilis—may result in blindness
- Otic syphilis—may result in deafness
- *Later stages (years):* Tabes dorsalis–dorsal column dysfunction, sensory disturbance and ataxia; Argyll-Robertson pupil constricts w/near focus, not w/light

Pregnancy complications:
- Congenital syphilis can cause bone damage, anemia, meningitis, low-birthweight, pre-term birth, neonatal death

Diagnostics:
- *Reverse sequence algorithm:* Syphilis antibody screening treponemal test (EIA/CIA) followed by quantitative nontreponemal test with titer (RPR/VDRL).
- *Traditional sequence algorithm:* Serologic testing involving both a nontreponemal test (RPR/VDRL) and a treponemal test (TP-PA)
- Neurosyphilis requires serologic testing plus CSF analysis.[68]

(continued on next page)

Table 1
(continued)

	Genital	Extragenital
Lymphogranuloma venereum (LGV); *CT serovars L1,L2, or L3* Inguinal bubo[69]	*Incubation period:* 3 days- 3 wk *Symptoms:* Begins with a painless papule, nodule, pustule, or ulcer; can progress to tender unilateral inguinal-femoral lymphadenopathy. If untreated can cause strictures, fibrosis, fistulae. *Rectal:* Anal pruritis, rectal pain, tenesmus; can lead to proctocolitis,[70] colorectal fistulas, strictures[70] *Complications:* Reactive arthropathy[70] *Diagnostics:* CT NAAT is capable of detecting LGV *Chlamydia trachomatis* strains.[70] Diagnosis usually based on clinical suspicion, prevalence, CT NAAT. Specific serovar PCR test exists but are not widely available.	
Mycoplasma genitalium (Mgen) Urethritis[71]	*Incubation period:* 2–4 wk[62] *Both genders:* Majority asymptomatic and infection can spontaneously clear in some cases, abnormal discharge, urethritis. *Women:* cervicitis, intermenstrual bleeding, dyspareunia, pelvic pain, may lead to PID[62] *Men:* persistent/recurrent urethritis,[62] possible proctitis in MSM[72] *Diagnostics:* urine, urethral, penile meatal, endocervical, or vaginal swab samples may be tested for Mgen NAAT[68]	
Viral STIs		
HIV Maculopapular rash[73]	*Incubation period:* 2–6 wk post-exposure.[74] *Acute HIV infection:* flulike illness, fever, adenopathy, rash and oral ulcers, diarrhea. *Potential laboratory findings:* ↓WBCs, ↓lymphocytes, ↓PLTs, ↑LFTs *Diagnostics:* HIV 1/2 Ag/Ab testing. Oral testing less frequently done in the ED due to higher rate of false positives. If high concern or recent exposure (<2 wk), test HIV RNA viral load	
Genital herpes simplex 1 & 2 HSV-2 outbreak[75]	*Incubation period:* 2–12 d (4 average), ulcers take 2–4 wk to heal *Skin:* Painful blisters, ulcers, sores, crust or itching, and dysuria. *Diagnostics:* Type specific HSV NAAT (HSV-1 vs HSV-2) of genital and mucocutaneous lesions is most sensitive, preferred. Viral culture via swab of lesions is less sensitive option. HSV PCR of the blood is not done unless concerned for disseminated infection. *HSV typing:* HSV-2 infection increases the risk of recurrence and 2-3x higher risk of acquiring HIV.[68] If unable to swab lesion, serology can aid in typing and prognosis.	

Human papillomavirus (HPV) Verruciform xanthoma[76]	*Incubation period:* Genital warts: 1–20 mo (2–3 mo average), HPV-related cancers: 10 y *Genital manifestations:* Genital warts.[77] associated cancers (cervical, anal, vulvar, vaginal, mouth/throat and penile cancers.) *Vaccination:* HPV vaccine is recommended at age 11, (can be started at age 9). It prevents cervical cancer, other genital/head and neck cancers, and genital warts. *Sequelae/complications:* Cancer of cervix, vulva, vagina, penis, anus and oropharynx[78,79] *Diagnostics:* Regular screening with conventional or liquid-based cytologic tests (ie, Pap tests) women ages 21–65 y is recommended, usually in primary care, not ED.
Hepatitis B virus (HBV) Jaundice[80]	*Incubation period:* 60–150 d (90 d average) *Acute infection:* ~50% symptomatic. Flu-like symptoms, abdominal pain, nausea. Liver dysfunction may occur. Most adults clear the infection; 2%–6% of adults become chronically infected.[59] *Diagnostics:* HbsAg, anti-HBs, total anti-HBc[68]
Hepatitis C virus (HCV) Jaundice[80]	*Incubation period:* 4–20 wk (7 wk average) *Acute infection:* Usually asymptomatic (>66%)[81] Can present with jaundice. Fulminant hepatitis very rare[82] *Chronic infection:* 50%–85% develop chronic HCV,[83]. fatigue, abdominal pain, itching[83] Once fibrosis develops, risk of cirrhosis is approximately 10% per year. *Diagnostics:* Anti-HCV = active/resolved infection; false positive screening, HCV RNA NAAT = active infection
Mpox Umbilicated lesions[84]	*Incubation period:* 7–14 d[85] *Most frequent symptoms:* Rash, fever, skin lesions, and lymphadenopathy[85] *Other presentations:* Proctitis, deep-seated umbilicated lesions on the penis, perianal area, anus, anorectal region[85] *Diagnostics:* PCR[86] swabs from skin lesions (blister fluid, skin, crusts) that do not need to be unroofed, but should be collected by vigorous swabbing.[87,88]

(continued on next page)

Table 1
(continued)

	Genital	Extragenital
Parasitic STIs		
Trichomonas vaginalis (TV)[89] Purulent exudate and erythematous cervix[90]	*Incubation period:* 5–28 d[89] *Majority asymptomatic:* 70%–85%[59] *Women:* Fishy odor, yellow-green vaginal discharge, dyspareunia, frequency, dysuria, and/or vulvar pruritus or erythema *Men:* Urethritis symptoms, less common prostatitis and epididymitis[89] *Diagnostics:* Women: TV NAAT on urine, endocervical, or vaginal samples. Much higher sensitivity than "wet prep." Some TV NAATs are cleared for male urine samples. Rapid tests are available[91] but infrequently used in EDs	

Abbreviations: Ag/Ab, antigen/antibody; CIA, chemiluminescence immunoassay; CSF, cerebrospinal fluid; CT, chlamydia; EIA, enzyme immunoassay; ED, emergency department; EPT, expedited partner therapy; FDA, Food and Drug Administration; GC, gonorrhea; HIV, human immunodeficiency virus; HSV, herpes simplex virus; LFTs, liver function tests; MSM, men who have sex with men; NAAT, nucleic acid amplification test; nPEP, non-occupational post-exposure prophylaxis; PCR, polymerase chain reaction; PLTs, platelets; PrEP, pre-exposure prophylaxis; RNA, ribonucleic acid; RPR, rapid plasma reagin; STI, sexually transmitted infection; TP-PA; *Treponema pallidum* particle agglutination; VDRL, venereal disease research laboratory; WBCs, white blood cells self-collected vaginal swabs have comparable sensitivity to clinician-collected endo-cervical swabs,[47,49–52] and have been specifically found to be feasible and non-inferior to clinician-collected swabs in the ED environment.[51,53,54] POC tests are increasingly available (see Point of Care Diagnostics in the following sections)[55,56] For the diagnosis of TV, wet prep or wet mount microscopy is much less sensitive than NAAT.[44] For persistent or recurrent cervicitis, antibiotic-resistant GC and Mgen should be considered, in addition to the possibility of re-exposure. In such cases, consider GC culture and susceptibility testing and testing for Mgen with a Food and Drug Administration (FDA)–cleared NAAT (eg, Aptima Mgen assay). Noninfectious causes to be considered include cervical dysplasia or polyps.

Treatment for the various pathogens that can cause cervicitis is detailed in **Table 2**. The CDC recommends presumptive treatment for GC and CT when follow-up cannot be ensured—which applies to many ED patients—or when NAAT is unavailable. Since most local health departments do not have the capacity for contact tracing for GC and CT infection, expedited partner treatment (EPT) should be considered (see the following EPT section). Patients should abstain from sex until they and their partners have completed treatment. Because of high reinfection rates, retesting in 3 months is recommended.

Urethritis

Symptoms and signs of urethritis in men and women include dysuria, pruritis, and mucopurulent discharge. Discharge may be present on the examination in the absence of symptoms. Urethritis in young men is almost always due to an STI—common etiologies include GC and CT, and less frequently, Mgen (see the following Mgen section). Mgen is increasingly recognized as an etiology in individuals with chronic symptoms. Additional considerations include TV and HSV.

The recommended initial diagnostic approach is to test for GC/CT with a NAAT, using urine in men and vaginal swabs in females. For non-STI bacteria causing urethritis, urinalysis and urine culture should be considered, especially in women and older men. For persistent or recurrent urethritis, consider testing for Mgen. TV should be considered in men with persistent symptoms based on population prevalence or known exposure. Recent TV tests that have received FDA clearance for males in addition to females include GeneXpert TV and Max CTGCTV2 assay (see **Table 1**).

Presumptive or culture-directed treatment mirrors that of cervicitis, as detailed in **Table 2**.

Vulvovaginitis and trichomoniasis

Vulvovaginitis is characterized by pruritis, dysuria, dyspareunia, vaginal soreness, irritation, odor, or abnormal discharge. Potential etiologies include TV, bacterial vaginosis (BV), and vulvovaginal candidiasis (VVC). BV and VVC are not considered STIs, but both are associated with an increased risk of HIV transmission and BV also increases the risk of other STIs and is associated with pelvic inflammatory disease (PID). Cervicitis can also present with abnormal vaginal discharge. Clinicians should ask about pertinent risk factors in the patient's history: new or multiple partners with inconsistent condom use (a risk factor for BV and TV), vaginal douching (a risk factor for VVC and BV), and over-the-counter yeast infection treatments (see **Table 1**).

TV is the most prevalent nonviral STI worldwide, with 2.6 million annual cases in the United States. It is mainly asymptomatic, and untreated infections can last years. In women, it can cause vulvar irritation and abnormal discharge. In men, it may cause dysuria, frequency, or symptoms similar to epididymitis or prostatitis. TV is associated with a 1.5 times increased risk of HIV acquisition, 1.4 times increased likelihood of

Table 2
Medications for specific sexually transmitted infections

Infection	Recommended Regimen	Alternative Regimen	Comments
Bacterial vaginosis	Metronidazole 500 mg PO BID for 7 d OR Metronidazole gel 0.75%, one 5 gm applicator intravaginally 1x/day for 5 d	Clindamycin 300 mg PO BID for 7 d OR Tinidazole 2 gm PO 1x/day for 2 d	Not an STI; however, can be triggered by sexual intercourse
Chlamydia infections	Doxycycline 100 mg PO BID for 7 d	Azithromycin 1gm PO single dose OR Levofloxacin 500 mg PO 1x/day for 7 d	Pregnancy: Azithromycin 1gm PO once
Epididymitis			
Caused by GC/CT	Ceftriaxone 500 mg IM AND Doxycycline 100 mg PO BID for 10 d	N/A	Individuals ≥150 kg, use ceftriaxone 1gm. All suspected cases should be tested for CT and GC
Caused by GC/CT or enteric organisms (ie, MSM w/insertive anal sex)	Ceftriaxone 500 mg AND Levofloxacin 500 mg PO 1x/day for 10 d	N/A	Individuals ≥150 kg, use ceftriaxone 1gm. All suspected cases should be tested for CT and GC
Caused by enteric organisms only	Levofloxacin 500 mg PO 1x/day for 10 d	N/A	
Gonococcal infections			
Infections in cervix, urethra, rectum, pharynx	Ceftriaxone 500 mg IM or IV once. Individuals ≥150 kg, use 1 g	*If cephalosporin allergy:* Gentamicin 240 mg IM AND Azithromycin 2 gm PO once. *If ceftriaxone administration not available (eg, expedited partner therapy):* Cefixime 800 mg PO	Due to difficulty curing pharyngeal gonorrhea, patients should return in 14 d for test of cure. Due to high rates of reinfection/recurrent infection, individuals should be retested for any gonococcal infection at 3 mo.

Conjunctivitis	Ceftriaxone 1g IM or IV once	N/A	Consider 1-time lavage of the infected eye with saline solution
Disseminated gonococcal infections (DGIs)	Ceftriaxone 1g IM or IV every 24 h	Cefotaxime 1 gm by IV every 8 h OR Ceftizoxime 1 gm every 8 h	
Mycoplasma genitalium (Mgen)	Mgen detected by NAAT, but Mgen resistance testing unavailable: Doxycycline 100 mg PO BID for 7 d FOLLOWED BY Moxifloxacin 400 mg 1x/day for 7 d	*For settings with macrolide resistance testing or when moxifloxacin cannot be used:* Doxycycline 100 mg BID for 7 d, FOLLOWED BY Azithromycin 1 gm PO on first day, FOLLOWED BY Azithromycin 500 mg PO 1x/day for 3 d. Test-of-cure 21 d after therapy	Test for Mgen in cases of persistent and recurrent urethritis or cervicitis
Trichomonas	Male: Metronidazole 2 gm PO once Female: Metronidazole 500 mg PO BID for 7 d	Tinidazole 2 gm PO once	
LGV Presumptively treat in cases of proctocolitis, severe inguinal lymphadenopathy with bubo formation, or genital ulcer after ruling out other causes.	Doxycycline 100 mg PO BID for 21 d	Azithromycin 1 gm orally once weekly for 3 wk* OR Erythromycin base 500 mg orally 4x/day for 21 d	Consider test of cure with CT NAAT 4 wk after treatment
Proctitis	Ceftriaxone 500 mg IM in a single dose AND doxycycline 100 mg PO BID for 7 d	Individuals ≥150 kg: use 1 g of Ceftriaxone	Doxycycline should be extended to 100 mg orally BID for 21 d in the presence of bloody discharge, perianal or mucosal ulcers, or tenesmus or positive rectal chlamydia test.

(continued on next page)

Table 2
(continued)

Infection	Recommended Regimen	Alternative Regimen	Comments
Pelvic inflammatory disease (PID)	Oral treatment: Ceftriaxone 500 mg IM single dose AND Doxycycline 100 mg PO BID for 14 d AND Metronidazole 500 mg PO BID for 14 d IV Treatment (hospitalized): Ceftriaxone 1g IV q24 h AND Doxycycline 100 mg IV q12 h AND Metronidazole 500 mg IV q12 h	*Oral Treatment:* Cefoxitin 2 gm IM single dose AND Probenecid 1 gm PO, administered concurrently in a single dose AND Doxycycline 100 mg PO BID for 14 d AND Metronidazole 500 mg PO BID for 14 d *IV Treatment (Hospitalized):* Ampicillin-sulbactam 3 gm IV q6 hs Cefotetan 2g VI q12 h OR cefoxitin 2g IV q 6h rs AND Doxycycline 100 mg IV q12 h	Potential Hospitalization criteria: • Tubo-ovarian abscess • Pregnancy • Severe illness, nausea and vomiting, or oral temperature >38.5°C • Unable to tolerate oral regimen • No improvement with oral therapy • Immunocompromised
Syphilis			
Incubation, primary, secondary, early latent	Benzathine penicillin G 2.4 million units IM single dose	Non-pregnant people with a penicillin allergy (also during penicillin shortages): Doxycycline 100 mg PO BID for 14 d	Patients with early syphilis may experience a Jarisch-Herxheimer reaction (febrile reaction to syphilis therapy) within 24 h of treatment, symptoms may be managed with antipyretics.
Late latent adults (or latent syphilis of unknown duration)	Benzathine penicillin G 7.2 million units total, administered as 3 doses of 2.4 million units IM each at 1-wk intervals	Non-pregnant people with a penicillin allergy (also during penicillin shortages): Doxycycline 100 mg PO BID for 28 d	

Condition	Regimen	Alternative	Notes
Neurosyphilis, ocular syphilis, and otosyphilis	Aqueous crystalline penicillin G 18–24 million units per day, administered as 3–4 million units by IV every 4 h or continuous infusion, for 10–14 d	Procaine penicillin G 2.4 million units IM 1x/day AND Probenecid 500 mg PO 4x/day, both for 10–14 d	Pregnant patients, and those with neuro-, ocular- or otosyphilis, with proven penicillin allergy should undergo desensitization
Genital herpes			
First clinical episode of genital herpes	Valacyclovir 1 gm PO BID for 7–10 d OR Acyclovir 400 mg PO 3x/day for 7–10 d	Famciclovir 250 mg PO 3x/day for 7–10 d	Treatment can be extended if healing is incomplete after 10 d of therapy
Episodic therapy for recurrent HSV-2 genital herpes	Valacyclovir 500 mg PO BID for 3 d OR Acyclovir 800 mg PO BID for 5 d	Valacyclovir 1 gm PO 1x/day for 5 d OR Acyclovir 800 mg PO 3x/day for 2 d OR Famciclovir 1 gm PO BID for 1 d	• Almost all persons with symptomatic HSV-2 will have recurrent episodes of genital lesions • Most effective when started within 1 d of lesion onset or during prodrome • For frequent recurrences, patients may seek daily suppressive therapy, regimens not discussed here
Genital warts (human papillomavirus, HPV)			
External anogenital warts	*Patient-applied:* Imiquimod[6] 3.75% or 5% cream OR Podofilox 0.5% solution or gel OR Sinecatechins 15% ointment	N/A	Persons with external anal warts might have intra-anal warts and might benefit from digital examination of the anal canal. If found, refer to colorectal surgeon.
Urethral, vaginal, cervical, intra-anal warts	Refer to specialist for cryotherapy with liquid nitrogen OR Surgical removal.		

Treatment in accordance with 2021 CDC STI Treatment Guidelines.[44] *Abbreviations:* CT, chlamydia; GC, gonorrhea; HIV, human immunodeficiency virus; IM, intramuscularly; IV, intravenous; LGV, lymphogranuloma venereum; SM, men who have sex with men; NAAT, nucleic acid amplification test; STI, sexually transmitted infection.

preterm birth, premature rupture of membranes, and infants small for gestational age. See **Table 2** for treatment recommendations.

The traditional diagnostic approach to vulvovaginitis involves vaginal fluid microscopy (ie, wet prep or wet mount) for real-time identification of clue cells, suggesting BV, and *Trichomonas* and *Candida* organisms. As noted earlier, NAATs are far more sensitive than wet prep for TV diagnosis. NAATs that identify many of the bacterial species known to be responsible for BV are also available. More recently, tests that combine detection of TV, BV, and VVC from a single specimen have become available (eg, NuSwab Vaginitis Plus, BD Affirm VPIII).

Pelvic inflammatory disease[59]

PID encompasses a range of inflammatory conditions caused by infections affecting the female upper genital tract and is associated with serious potential consequences, including increased risk of ectopic pregnancies and infertility.[59] These conditions may involve various combinations of endometritis, salpingitis, tubo-ovarian abscess (TOA), pelvic peritonitis, perihepatitis, and chronic pain. GC and CT are commonly implicated, though only about half of the patients treated for PID have positive tests for GC/CT. Thus, the absence of GC/CT infection does not exclude PID as a diagnosis. Other etiologic microorganisms include facultative anaerobes (*Gardnerella vaginalis, Haemophilus influenzae,* enteric gram-negative rods, Mgen, *Streptococcus agalactiae),* cytomegalovirus (CMV), TV, *Mycoplasma hominis,* and *Ureaplasma urealyticum.*[92,93]

Due to the difficulty in diagnosing PID and the risks of untreated infection, the CDC recommends maintaining a low threshold for presumptive treatment. PID should be treated in women at risk for STIs with lower abdominal and pelvic pain, no clear alternate cause identified, and at least 1 of 3 criteria on pelvic examination: cervical motion tenderness, uterine tenderness, or adnexal tenderness.

Additional criteria that support the PID diagnosis are shown in **Box 2**. Diagnostic testing can be used to improve the specificity of PID diagnosis and determine the etiology in some cases. Wet prep of cervical discharge showing many white blood cells and blood work showing elevated blood inflammatory markers support the diagnosis. NAATs for CT/GC/TV may be sampled using endocervical or vaginal swabs, but is worth noting that some research has found vaginal swabs detect more cases of STIs than endocervical swabs.[47,94–96] Consider BV testing via NAAT, if available. If TOA is suspected in cases of unilateral tenderness or systemic illness, pelvic

---

Box 2
Signs of pelvic inflammatory disease

- Cardinal signs
  - Cervical motion tenderness
  - Uterine tenderness
  - Adnexal tenderness

- Additional signs may include
  - Temperature greater than 38.3°C
  - Abnormal cervical mucopurulent discharge or cervical friability
  - Significant number of WBCs in microscopy of vaginal fluid (where available)
  - Elevated ESR
  - Elevated CRP
  - Laboratory confirmation of cervical GC or CT

Abbreviations: CRP, C-reactive protein; CT, chlamydia; ESR, erythrocyte sedimentation rate; GC, gonorrhea; STI, sexually transmitted infection; WBCs, white blood cells.

ultrasound or computed tomography should be considered. Women diagnosed with CT/GC PID should undergo retesting 3 months after treatment.

Early administration of recommended antimicrobials can prevent PID complications such as infertility. Preferred outpatient treatment includes ceftriaxone and 14 days of doxycycline and metronidazole. Admission for intravenous (IV) antibiotics and further monitoring should be considered for patients with TOA, pregnancy, failure of outpatient care, or systemic illness (see **Table 2**).

Herpes simplex virus

Genital HSV, the most common infectious cause of genital ulcers, presents as recurrent, painful vesicular, or ulcerative genital lesions. Primary genital infections cause local pain, tender inguinal adenopathy, and lesions that last approximately 12 days and can be associated with headache, fever, malaise, and urinary retention that may precede the rash. Latent HSV persists in neurons in infected individuals throughout life with the potential to reactivate.[97] Recurrent infections last 5 to 10 days without treatment and have a prodrome of local irritation. Neonates and immunocompromised or pregnant individuals are at risk for severe and/or disseminated HSV infection, such as pneumonitis, hepatitis, meningitis, or encephalitis. There are 2 types of HSV: HSV-1 and HSV-2. HSV-2 is responsible for the majority of recurrent genital herpes cases, and infects approximately 11.9% of individuals aged 14 to 49 years.[98] A growing percentage of anogenital herpetic infections among young women and men who have sex with men (MSM) are caused by HSV-1.[99] Generally, HSV-1 causes less frequent symptoms and viral shedding.

If genital lesions are present, a NAAT of the lesions should be obtained to confirm the diagnosis and identify the HSV type. Viral culture is an alternative with lower sensitivity. The vesicle should be unroofed with a sterile needle or scalpel and the swab is rotated on the base of the lesion. Type-specific testing is helpful for patient counseling because recurrence is more frequent with HSV-2. For patients with suspected HSV hepatitis, pneumonitis, or meningitis, signifying dissemination, HSV types 1 and 2 deoxyribonucleic acid polymerase chain reaction (PCR) can be performed on blood or cerebrospinal fluid. HSV-2 serologies have little role in the ED setting. HSV treatment is listed in **Table 2**.

Syphilis[100]

Syphilis, caused by the *T pallidum* spirochete, is re-emerging as an important public health threat in the United States. Between 2017 and 2021, reported cases increased 74% to 176,713.[1] Although MSM account for roughly half of incident cases, syphilis is increasing in all demographics, including females of child-bearing age. In 2022, the CDC reported 3761 cases of congenital syphilis, a 755% increase since 2012.[101]

Syphilis staging is an essential step in determining treatment (**Fig. 1**). Primary syphilis classically presents with a single painless sore known as a chancre. Chancres typically develop 10 to 90 days after transmission and are highly infectious. They are typically firm, round, and painless, and thus are easy to overlook in the genital area, anus, or mouth. However, atypical cases have been described recently with multiple or painful lesions, frequently in or near the rectum.[66] Syphilis antibody tests may return negative at this stage. In some clinics specializing in STIs, dark field microscopy of a swab specimen from the chancre may provide an earlier diagnosis. In the ED, the diagnosis of primary syphilis often must be made clinically.

Secondary syphilis presents several weeks to months after the chancre appears, and classically appears as a non-pruritic macular rash that can involve any part of the body, including the palms and soles of the feet. Other manifestations include condyloma lata, wart-like lesions on the genitals or anus, and leukoplakia-like plaques on the oral mucosa. Systemic signs and symptoms may include fatigue, myalgias, malaise, sore

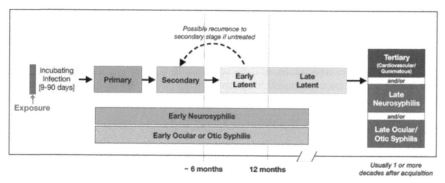

Fig. 1. The natural history of untreated syphilis. (Source: New York City Department of Health and Mental Hygiene, and the New York City STD Prevention Training Center. The Diagnosis and Management of Syphilis: An Update and Review. March 2019. A PDF version is available at www.nycptc.org. http://bit.ly/SyphilisMonograph2019PTC.)

throat, headaches, weight loss, patchy hair loss, fever, lymphadenopathy, pharyngitis, hepatosplenomegaly, and hepatitis. While secondary syphilis is a clinical diagnosis, this diagnosis can be supported by positive serology (see syphilis testing in the following sections).

During **latent syphilis**, *T pallidum* remains viable but asymptomatic. During the early latent stage (<1 year), the infection is still transmissible. Latent syphilis can only be diagnosed via serology. Important and relatively common syphilis complications that can occur at any stage are shown in **Box 3**.

Tertiary syphilis occurs years or decades after the initial infection in untreated cases. Manifestations include (a) skin/soft tissue: gummas, large soft sores on the skin or internal organs; (b) cardiovascular: aortic valve insufficiency, coronary artery obstruction, aortitis and associated aortic aneurysm and dissection; (c) neurologic: neurosyphilis, including tabes dorsalis (degeneration of dorsal columns), radicular pain and ataxia, gradual blindness, loss of reflexes, mood changes and psychiatric syndromes, paresis, seizures, and progressive dementia. These severe late complications are rarely seen as they are preventable with the detection and treatment of the disease in its initial stages. Additional syphilis complications that can occur at any stage are shown in **Box 3**.

Screening and testing for syphilis in EDs is recommended when testing for other STIs. Testing should also be strongly considered in pregnant ED patients, particularly in those with limited prenatal care access. Clinical decision support has been used to improve appropriate syphilis testing.[102] Universal ED syphilis screening, including

---

Box 3
Complications of syphilis

Severe complications of syphilis that can occur at any stage
- Ocular syphilis: Conjunctivitis, red eye, pain, anterior uveitis, interstitial keratitis, optic neuropathy, and retinal vasculitis. Can be vision threatening.
- Otic syphilis: Tinnitus, vertigo, and sensorineural hearing loss. Can be hearing threatening.
- Neurosyphilis: Headache and difficulty coordinating muscle movements, severe dementia, or stroke

patients without a suspected STI, has also been proposed[103] (See the following STI screening section).

The traditional syphilis testing algorithm **(Fig. 2)** starts with a nontreponemal serology test to detect antibodies to a cardiolipin antigen; examples include the rapid plasma reagin (RPR) and venereal disease research laboratory (VDRL). The RPR is more sensitive than the VDRL but both tests have lower sensitivity in early and late disease, and thus false negatives are possible. Additionally, false positives are possible and may occur due to a variety of causes, such as systemic lupus erythematosus, leprosy, brucellosis, atypical pneumonia, HIV, IV drug use, or pregnancy. As such, a positive RPR or VDRL must be followed by a syphilis-specific antibody serology, also called a direct treponemal test. Examples include the fluorescent treponemal antibody absorption or *T pallidum* particle agglutination test.

The reverse sequence algorithm is now increasingly used to reduce false negative syphilis screening and improve laboratory workflow. It begins with a *T pallidum* antibody test, also called a direct treponemal test, typically an enzyme immunoassay or chemiluminescence immunoassay. These tests are highly sensitive for syphilis antibodies, even in cases where nontreponemal test titers might be low or non-reactive. If this initial treponemal test is positive or equivocal, it is followed by a nontreponemal test (ie, RPR) for confirmation, which then reflexes to a titer. If there is a discrepancy between the 2, a different type of direct treponemal test (eg, *T pallidum* antibody, particle agglutination), may be used to confirm the diagnosis, which, if negative, suggests an initial false positive or early infection.

Notably, in both testing algorithms, there is a "window period" of 1 to 6 weeks between the infection and the appearance of detectable antibodies. Depending on the test, this window period may be between 1 and 6 weeks, but a chancre may appear as early as 10 days post-exposure. Thus, if there are signs of primary or secondary syphilis and/ or there is a high index of suspicion, the patient should be empirically treated.

Since treponemal test serologies remain positive after treatment, in order to determine whether a positive syphilis test represents a new or prior infection and to judge treatment effectiveness, it is necessary to interpret the change of nontreponemal (RPR or VDRL) titers. An increase in titer of ≥ 2 dilutions (eg, 1:1–1:4) represents re-infection or active infection, whereas declining titers suggest effective treatment or the absence of active disease. Titers can persist at low levels even after adequate therapy, known as the serofast state.

Parenteral benzathine penicillin G remains the mainstay of syphilis treatment (see **Table 2**). Doxycycline can be used for patients reporting penicillin allergy but is

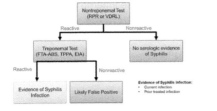

Traditional Algorithm

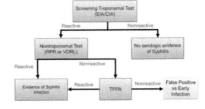

Reverse Sequence Algorithm

Fig. 2. Syphilis laboratory testing algorithms: traditional versus reverse algorithm. CIA, chemiluminescence immunoassay; EIA, enzyme immunoassay; FTA-ABS, fluorescent treponemal antibody absorption; RPR, rapid plasma reagin; TP-PA; *Treponema pallidum* particle agglutination; TPPA, *Treponema pallidum* antibody, particle agglutination; VDRL, venereal disease research laboratory.

considered less effective. Skin testing or direct oral challenge for penicillin allergy should be considered. If compliance or follow-up cannot be ensured, the CDC recommends patients be desensitized and treated with benzathine penicillin G. Due to the seriousness of congenital syphilis, pregnant women with syphilis require penicillin, and those with a proven penicillin allergy must be desensitized. For neurosyphilis, ocular syphilis, and otic syphilis, aqueous crystalline penicillin G administered via IV is also required and for proven penicillin allergy, desensitization is recommended. Inform patients, especially those in early stages of syphilis, of the possibility of a Jarisch-Herxheimer reaction (occurs in up to 30%–50% of patients)[104] of fever, headache, or myalgia that may occur within the first day of treatment. Symptoms may be managed with antipyretics.

Less Common Syndromes and Sexually Transmitted Pathogens

Acute human immunodeficiency virus infection

HIV remains a significant public health threat in the United States. While a thorough discussion of this disease is beyond the scope of this article, the authors wish to highlight acute HIV infection, a syndrome which is critical yet very challenging to recognize. In 2021, 36,136 people in the United States received a new HIV diagnosis.[105] MSM contact accounted for 67% of new cases, while heterosexual contact accounted for 22%.[105] ED visits for acute HIV infection represent an opportunity for very early HIV diagnosis. Broad ED opt-out HIV testing (screening) improves the ability to pick up early infection beyond that of clinician-initiated testing.[106,107] Emergency clinicians, therefore, stand to play a critical role in early HIV diagnosis, treatment, and interruption of further transmission (**Box 4**).

When acute HIV is suspected, immediate testing via HIV-1/HIV-2 antigen/antibody (Ag/Ab) test is indicated. If there is a possibility of very early HIV infection leading to a nonreactive initial Ag/Ab test, such as recent sexual exposure to HIV within the previous days to weeks, HIV ribonucleic acid (viral load) testing is recommended.[108] Nontargeted HIV screening and non-occupational post-exposure prophylaxis are discussed elsewhere. Early antiretroviral therapy initiation is strongly recommended during the acute phase of HIV infection for a number of reasons, including: to reduce the risk of transmission, lessen the severity of acute symptoms, lower the viral setpoint, reduce the size of the viral reservoir, suppress viral replication, and help preserve immune function.[109]

Epididymitis

Acute epididymitis is characterized by unilateral swelling, pain, and tenderness in the region of the epididymis, present for less than 6 weeks.[110] The inflammatory process

---

Box 4
Early human immunodeficiency virus infection symptoms[74]

- *Acute viral syndrome (2–6 weeks post-exposure):* fever (most common), fatigue/malaise, myalgias, lymphadenopathy, rash, oral ulcers, pharyngitis, diarrhea,

- Additional symptoms of early HIV infection: aseptic meningitis-headache, photophobia, meningismus

- Some may be asymptomatic

- **Laboratory findings**: leukopenia, lymphopenia, transaminitis, thrombocytopenia, and other transient and nonspecific laboratory findings are common.

Abbreviation: HIV, human immunodeficiency virus.

may progress to epididymo-orchitis. Sudden and severe pain suggests testicular torsion, a surgical emergency.[111] In men under age 35, GC and CT are the predominant causative organisms.[110,102] In men who engage in insertive anal sex,[110] enteric organisms such as *Escherichia coli* are common. Non-STI epididymitis, caused by *E coli* and other typical bacterial uropathogens, occurs in men older than 35 years, usually associated with partial bladder outlet obstruction from benign prostatic hyperplasia.[110–112] The diagnosis can be made clinically, followed by empiric treatment, provided there is no concern for testicular torsion or cancer. Urinalysis, urine culture, and a urine NAAT for GC/CT should be obtained in all suspected cases. Though not required for diagnosis, ultrasound may reveal hydrocele and epididymal enlargement or hyperemia, or may be normal.[111] Selection of presumptive therapy is based on risk for CT and GV versus enteric organisms, with sexually active patients receiving presumptive CT/GC treatment[110,111] (see **Table 2**.). Effective treatment may prevent infertility or chronic pain.

Proctitis and lymphogranuloma venereum[70]

Proctitis is inflammation of the lower rectum. Infectious etiologies are linked to oral-anal, digital-anal, or receptive anal sex. Symptoms include tenesmus, rectal pain, and discharge. Sexually transmitted etiologies include GC, CT (including lymphogranuloma venereum [LGV] serovars), and syphilis. In HIV patients, HSV, LGV, and Mgen are more prevalent. With acquired immunodeficiency syndrome or immunosuppression, CMV should also be considered. LGV is caused by CT serovars L1, L2, or L3, which can lead to severe inflammation and invasive infections. LGV is very uncommon in the United States, but outbreaks of LGV proctocolitis, predominantly affecting MSM, have occurred.[113] LGV can also be a cause of genital, anal, or perianal ulcers. Non-STI proctitis pathogens include *Campylobacter, Shigella, Entamoeba histolytica, Escherichia coli,* and *Salmonella.* Inflammatory bowel disease is an important noninfectious cause to consider.

Diagnosis can be aided by anoscopy, to assess for lesions and to collect diagnostic specimens. All patients should undergo testing for GC/CT and HSV with NAAT (via rectal swabs), syphilis, and HIV. A conclusive diagnosis of LGV requires LGV-specific PCR-based genotyping. Because these tests are not widely available, diagnosis relies on clinical suspicion, epidemiologic data, and a positive CT NAAT from a swab of the involved anatomic site. Treatment details are provided in **Table 2**. Those with severe infection (tenesmus, rectal ulcers) should be presumptively treated for LGV if specific testing is not available.[114]

Mycoplasma genitalium

Mgen is a sexually transmitted bacterium that affects the urogenital tract. It is increasingly recognized as a cause of urethritis and cervicitis, especially recurrent or persistent urethritis, and may also contribute to PID, preterm delivery, spontaneous abortion, and infertility.[44] Mgen can cause typical urethritis and cervicitis symptoms, such as dysuria or discharge, but is also frequently asymptomatic. The impact of asymptomatic infections is not well understood, and the bacterium's ability to develop antibiotic resistance contributes to limited treatment options.[115] Hence, the CDC only recommends testing for Mgen in cases of recurrent or persistent nongonococcal urethritis and cervicitis, or for sex partners of patients diagnosed with the bacteria. Mgen NAATs by urine or vaginal swab specimen are increasingly available for testing ED patients. Treatment is complicated by the need for prolonged treatment with multiple agents (see **Table 2**).[116–118]

Mpox

Mpox is an orthopoxvirus illness that had a recent outbreak that started in Spain and spread to Europe and North America in May 2022, increased in June to July 2022 during Pride events, and ended in May 2023, likely due to immunity, behavior change, and vaccinations.[85,119,120] Mpox is spread through direct contact with infectious skin or lesions and through mucosal contact, then presents with a prodrome of flulike symptoms followed by a rash of pruritic or painful blister lesions on the genital, perianal, and anorectal area or pharynx, lasting 2 to 4 weeks.[121,122] During the 2022 outbreak, atypical presentations with only skin or mucosal lesions and prodrome occurring after lesions have been common. Mpox continues to be a clinical concern as sporadic cases continue to occur across the United States.

NEWER SEXUALLY TRANSMITTED INFECTION DIAGNOSTIC STRATEGIES
Extragenital Sexually Transmitted Infection Testing for gonorrhea and chlamydia

EDs should have protocols for performing extragenital testing (EGT) for STIs, when indicated. This is also called triple-site testing, referring to genitourinary, pharyngeal, and rectal sampling. Studies show that STIs are missed when STI testing is limited to urine samples, a common practice in most EDs.[123–125] Further, extragenital sites may represent asymptomatic reservoirs for GC and CT.[44,123] The CDC now recommends that MSM should routinely be offered EGT when testing for a suspected STI. For heterosexual women, shared decision-making regarding EGT is recommended, based on the specific sexual history.[44] FDA-approved STI NAAT swabs for EGT are available from common suppliers of medical equipment already carried in many EDs, which should facilitate stocking these supplies.[126] Additionally, new POC tests are being developed for EGT.[127]

Patient-Collected Samples

Patient-collected samples can enhance the feasibility and accuracy of STI testing in women, especially in crowded EDs with limited examination space.[128] In circumstances where emergency clinicians do not plan to perform a pelvic examination as part of the workup, patient-collected vaginal swabs are preferable to urine samples because they are more sensitive for GC/CT.[48,51–54,129,130] Moreover, patient-collected samples are as effective as clinician-collected samples, are preferred by patients,[54,131] and[49,51–54] lead to a greater willingness for future testing.[49]

Point-of-Care Diagnostic Tests

ED STI testing continues to be primarily laboratory-based, with turn-around times that typically exceed the ED length of stay. POC tests are little used in the ED despite studies showing they can improve antibiotic stewardship.[132–135] There are FDA-approved POC tests for CT/GC (GeneXpert, Binx io); TV (Solana); syphilis (Syphilis Health Check, Dual Path Platform Test); and combination CT/GC/TV (Visby).[55,56] POC STI tests can reduce reliance on empiric treatment, [56,136,137,55,138,55,131] an approach that lacks accuracy for identifying infected patients.[139,140] POC testing also increases the opportunity to provide counseling, offer partner care, target HIV prevention, and minimize patients lost to follow-up of undertreated infections.[55,133,141] However, there are several barriers to POC test utilization in EDs, which are detailed in **Box 5**.

Sexually Transmitted Infection Screening in the Emergency Department

There have not yet been consensus recommendations regarding the role of EDs in communicable disease screening for asymptomatic patients. The notion that EDs should perform this public health function remains controversial and has yet to be widely adopted. Yet, screening is critical to STI identification and control, and is strongly embraced by the CDC. Ultimately, whether a particular ED embraces asymptomatic screening will depend on community disease prevalence, patient sociodemographics, and access to primary care and screening outside of the ED. For CT and GC,

---

Box 5
Barriers to extragenital testing and point-of-care test implementation

- Eligible patient population may be limited because certain POC tests are approved for females only.[142]
- Laboratories may require additional validation for FDA-approved EGT specimens from some anatomic sites
- Clinical workflow change
- Increased emergency clinician and nurse task burden
- Staff training with refreshers is required
- Billing for POC tests
- Costs of POC tests
- Linking POC test results to electronic health records

Abbreviations: EGT, extragenital testing; FDA, Food and Drug Administration; POC, point-of-care.

---

the US Preventive Services Task Force (USPSTF) recommends screening all sexually active women under age 25 and older groups at high risk.[143] The USPSTF recommends syphilis screening for those "at increased risk" for infection[144] (**Box 6**). A limitation of such targeted screening is that patients may not be asked about or disclose risk factors that would prompt screening. Additionally, with rising rates of congenital syphilis and declining access to US maternity care,[145] EDs should consider liberal syphilis testing in pregnant patients in all trimesters.[101]

Co-testing for STIs is a form of targeted screening strongly recommended by the CDC. Co-testing for both HIV and syphilis is recommended when testing for suspected CT/GC or TV.[146,147] Although HCV is more frequently transmitted through

---

Box 6
Factors associated with higher prevalence of syphilis according to US Preventive Services Task Force

- MSM
- HIV infection
- Men
- Young adults
- Incarceration
- Sex work
- Military service
- Methamphetamine use
- Another STI
- Condomless sex

Abbreviations: HIV, human immunodeficiency virus; MSM, men who have sex with men; STI, sexually transmitted infection.

Adapted from Luetkemeyer AF, Donnell D, Dombrowski JC, et al. Postexposure Doxycycline to Prevent Bacterial Sexually Transmitted Infections. N Engl J Med. 2023;388(14):1296-1306. https://doi.org/10.1056/NEJMoa2211934

---

blood and injection drug use, sexual transmission can occur. Thus, HCV testing can also be bundled with STI tests to achieve the CDC-recommended universal HCV screening (at least once per lifetime and more frequently depending on risk factors for all adults aged 18).[44]

NEWER APPROACHES TO SEXUALLY TRANSMITTED INFECTION TREATMENT
Notable Centers for Disease Control and Prevention 2021 Guidelines Updates[44]

Based on changing STIs and antibiotic resistance patterns, the CDC issued updated treatment guidelines in 2021, which are summarized in **Box 7**.

Expedited Partner Therapy

EPT refers to providing treatment to the sex partner(s) of patients treated for GC and CT without a clinical assessment of those partners.[149] EPT reduces the risk of persistent or

---

Box 7
Centers for Disease Control and Prevention 2021 guideline notable updates and rationale

- Testing:
  - **Extragenital testing** (pharyngeal and rectal) for CT/GC encouraged
    - Most cases of GC/CT in MSM would be missed with urine testing alone, one-third cases of CT/GC in heterosexual individuals would be missed with genitourinary testing alone.[148]
  - *Mycoplasma genitalium (Mgen)* NAAT testing recommended for persistent genital and urinary symptoms
- Treatment:
  - **Gonorrhea**: treat with ceftriaxone 500 mg (or if > 150 kg, 1 g)
    - Previous: dual therapy recommended with ceftriaxone 250 mg and azithromycin 1g
    - Increasing GC and enteric bacteria azithromycin resistance; higher ceftriaxone dose needed for pharyngeal GC
  - **Chlamydia**: doxycycline 100 mg bid x 7d regimen preferred to azithromycin, except in pregnancy
    - Previous: azithromycin 1 g was a recommended option
    - Doxycycline is non-inferior to azithromycin; conserves azithromycin
  - **Syphilis**: For reported penicillin allergy in pregnant patients, or those for whom compliance or follow-up cannot be ensured, desensitize and treat with benzathine penicillin G.
  - **Trichomonas**: metronidazole 500 mg bid x 7d is recommended for females
    - Previous: metronidazole 2g single dose was recommended for both females and males, now just for males
    - 7-day course more effective in females
  - **Pelvic inflammatory disease**: metronidazole 500 mg bid x 14d routinely should be included in regimen
    - Previous: addition of metronidazole was optional
    - Anaerobic organisms and co-occurrence of bacterial vaginosis are prevalent
  - *Mgen*: doxycycline 100 mg po bid x 7d, then moxifloxacin 460 mg bid x7 d; if known to be macrolide sensitive, azithromycin 1gm once, then 500 mg × 3d
- Prevention:
  - **EPT**: Consider this strategy when partners are unlikely or unable to seek treatment; use oral cefixime for GC treatment in EPT
  - **HIV prevention**: routine for eligibility for nPEP and PrEP recommended

Abbreviations: CT, chlamydia; EPT, expedited partner therapy; GC, gonorrhea; HIV, human immunodeficiency virus; MSM, men who have sex with men; NAAT, nucleic acid amplification test; nPEP, non-occupational post-exposure prophylaxis; PrEP, pre-exposure prophylaxis; STI, sexually transmitted infection.

recurrent CT/GC in index patients by 29%, with no reported adverse events.[150,151] As a harm-reduction approach, EPT is intended for circumstances where the partner will not get timely care otherwise. It remains preferable for the partner to undergo comprehensive STI testing and for GC to be treated with intramuscular ceftriaxone rather than oral cefixime that is used for EPT.

EPT is supported by the CDC and the American College of Emergency Physicians.[152] It is permissible or potentially allowable in every US state[153] and there have been no legal cases involving EPT.[154] Unfortunately, EPT remains underused because of a lack of awareness and difficulty prescribing through electronic health records, which require a pre-existing chart for electronic prescriptions.[155,156] Pharmacists may be unaware of EPT laws and regulations[157] that permit filling prescriptions without the partner's personally identifiable information.[153] Electronic prescribing can be facilitated by creating a generic profile called "expedited partner" to send nameless prescriptions for partners,[158] a practice recommended by national prescription guidelines.[159] Take-home medication packs for EPT are CDC-recommended and have been piloted.[160]

Doxycycline for Post-Exposure Prophylaxis

Doxy-PEP refers to the use of doxycycline for post-exposure prophylaxis to prevent the acquisition of bacterial STIs, particularly GC, CT, and syphilis. In 2 recent studies involving MSM and transgender women, 200 mg of doxycycline given within 72 hours of condomless sex, substantially reduced rates of GC, CT, and syphilis infection.[161,162] In November 2023, the CDC released preliminary guidance recommending consideration of doxy-PEP for MSM and transgender women with a history of at least 1 bacterial STI in the last 12 months and who are at ongoing risk for bacterial STIs. ED clinicians should familiarize themselves with doxy-PEP education and follow-up from their local institutions as the practice has already begun to be recommended by official guideline organizations and state and local departments of health.[163-165] Important caveats include the following: doxy-PEP has yet to be shown effective in real-world studies, there is no published experience with its use in the ED setting, and its potential to increase antibiotic resistance requires further study.

SUMMARY

EDs can play an important role in combating the STI and HIV epidemics and improving population health throughout the community in which they are located. This requires ongoing provider education, as well as investing in and developing newer systems and strategies for STI diagnosis and treatment. Important examples include

- Ensuring that emergency clinicians stay abreast of changing STI epidemiology, such as the re-emergence of syphilis and recognition of Mgen as a cause of persistent urethritis or cervicitis
- Following current CDC STI testing and treatment guidelines
- Rapid POC testing for more accurate STI diagnosis for a precision medicine approach to treatment
- EGT (pharyngeal and rectal) for STIs, especially in MSM
- Systems to provide treatment to partners of patients with STIs, such as EPT electronic prescribing
- Doxy-PEP is a novel post-exposure prophylaxis approach to reduce the risk of STI acquisition.

CLINICS CARE POINTS

- Emergency clinicians should be familiar with updated recommendations contained in the 2021 CDC STI treatment guidelines.
- For GC treatment, the standard dose of ceftriaxone has been increased, and for CT, doxycycline is the preferred agent, rather than azithromycin.
- Extragenital STI testing is recommended for many patients.
- Expedited partner therapy (EPT) should be considered to ensure all partners are treated.
- Emergency clinicians should be familiar with the evolving epidemiology of syphilis and understand the now widely used "reverse algorithm" approach to syphilis testing.
- Doxy-PEP, with shared decision making, is now recommended by public health officials to reduce the risk of STI acquisition in certain high risk patients.

DISCLOSURE

No disclosures for any author

REFERENCES

1. Preliminary 2021 STD surveillance data. 2022. Available at: https://www.cdc.gov/std/statistics/2021/default.htm. [Accessed 11 January 2023].
2. National Academies of Sciences, Engineering, and Medicine, Health and Medicine Division. Sexually transmitted infections: adopting a sexual health paradigm. National Academies Press; 2021. Available at: https://books.google.com/books/about/Sexually_Transmitted_Infections.html?hl=&id=2ldizgEACAAJ.
3. Trichomoniasis statistics. 2021. Available at: https://www.cdc.gov/std/trichomonas/stats.htm. [Accessed 5 November 2023].
4. Kreisel KM, Spicknall IH, Gargano JW, et al. Sexually transmitted infections among US Women and Men: prevalence and incidence estimates, 2018. Sex Transm Dis 2021;48(4):208–14.
5. Ollstein AM. STDs are surging. The funding to fight them is not. POLITICO. Available at: https://www.politico.com/news/2022/04/12/stds-funding-00024678. [Accessed 6 November 2022].
6. Nagendra G, Carnevale C, Neu N, et al. The potential impact and availability of sexual health services during the COVID-19 pandemic. Sex Transm Dis 2020;47(7):434–6.
7. Fang J, Silva RM, Tancredi DJ, et al. Examining associations in congenital syphilis infection and socioeconomic factors between California's small-to-medium and large metro counties. J Perinatol 2022;42(11):1434–9.
8. Schmidt R, Carson PJ, Jansen RJ. Resurgence of syphilis in the United States: an assessment of contributing factors. Infect Dis 2019;12. 1178633719883282.
9. Chesson HW, Spicknall IH, Bingham A, et al. The estimated direct lifetime medical costs of sexually transmitted infections acquired in the United States in 2018. Sex Transm Dis 2021;48(4):215–21.
10. National Institute of Allergy and Infectious Diseases. Sexually transmitted diseases. 2015. Available at: https://www.NIAID.nih.org.

11. Hosenfeld CB, Workowski KA, Berman S, et al. Repeat infection with Chlamydia and gonorrhea among females: a systematic review of the literature. Sex Transm Dis 2009;36(8):478–89.
12. Detailed STD facts - HIV/AIDS & STDs. 2022. Available at: https://www.cdc.gov/std/hiv/stdfact-std-hiv-detailed.htm. [Accessed 11 January 2023].
13. Cohen MS, Council OD, Chen JS. Sexually transmitted infections and HIV in the era of antiretroviral treatment and prevention: the biologic basis for epidemiologic synergy. J Int AIDS Soc 2019;22(Suppl 6):e25355.
14. Sexually transmitted infections workgroup. Available at: https://health.gov/healthypeople/about/workgroups/sexually-transmitted-infections-workgroup. [Accessed 11 January 2023].
15. Hogben M, Leichliter JS. Social determinants and sexually transmitted disease disparities. Sex Transm Dis 2008;35(12 Suppl):S13–8.
16. Copen CE, Haderxhanaj LT, Renfro KJ, et al. County-level chlamydia and gonorrhea rates by social vulnerability, United States, 2014-2018. Sex Transm Dis 2022;49(12):822–5.
17. Flagg EW, Meites E, Phillips C, et al. Prevalence of trichomonas vaginalis among civilian, noninstitutionalized male and female population aged 14 to 59 Years: United States, 2013 to 2016. Sex Transm Dis 2019;46(10):e93–6.
18. Dailey AF, Gant Z, Hu X, et al. Association between social vulnerability and rates of HIV diagnoses among black adults, by selected characteristics and region of residence—United .... and Mortality Weekly ..... 2022. Available at: https://www-ncbi-nlm-nih-gov.proxy.lib.umich.edu/pmc/articles/PMC8812837/.
19. Noah AJ, Yang TC, Wang WL. The black-white disparity in sexually transmitted diseases during pregnancy: how do racial segregation and income inequality matter? Sex Transm Dis 2018;45(5):301–6.
20. Stoltey JE, Li Y, Bernstein KT, et al. Ecological analysis examining the association between census tract-level incarceration and reported chlamydia incidence among female adolescents and young adults in San Francisco. Sex Transm Infect 2015;91(5):370–4.
21. Wiehe SE, Rosenman MB, Aalsma MC, et al. Epidemiology of sexually transmitted infections among offenders following arrest or incarceration. Am J Public Health 2015;105(12):e26–32.
22. Dauria EF, Elifson K, Arriola KJ, et al. Male incarceration rates and rates of sexually transmitted infections: results from a longitudinal analysis in a Southeastern US City. Sex Transm Dis 2015;42(6):324–8.
23. Thomas JC, Sampson LA. High rates of incarceration as a social force associated with community rates of sexually transmitted infection. J Infect Dis 2005;191(Suppl 1):S55–60.
24. Thomas JC, Levandowski BA, Isler MR, et al. Incarceration and sexually transmitted infections: a neighborhood perspective. J Urban Health 2008;85(1):90–9.
25. Pearson WS, Peterman TA, Gift TL. An increase in sexually transmitted infections seen in US emergency departments. Prev Med 2017;100:143–4.
26. Batteiger TA, Dixon BE, Wang J, et al. Where do people go for gonorrhea and chlamydia tests: a cross-sectional view of the Central Indiana Population, 2003–2014. Sex Transm Dis 2019;46(2):132.
27. Solnick RE, Rothenber C, Merchant RC, et al. 273 racial and gender disparities in the diagnosis and empiric treatment of sexually transmitted infections. Acad Emerg Med 2022;29(S1). https://doi.org/10.1111/acem.14511.

28. Jamison CD, Greenwood-Ericksen M, Richardson CR, et al. Association between chlamydia and routine place for healthcare in the United States: NHANES 1999-2016. PLoS One 2021;16(5):e0251113.

29. Gift TL, Cuffe KM, Leichliter JS. The impact of budget cuts on sexually transmitted disease programmatic activities in state and local health departments with staffing reductions in fiscal year 2012. Sex Transm Dis 2018;45(11):e87–9.

30. Ware CE, Ajabnoor Y, Mullins PM, et al. A retrospective cross-sectional study of patients treated in US EDs and ambulatory care clinics with sexually transmitted infections from 2001 to 2010. Am J Emerg Med 2016;34(9):1808–11.

31. Pearson WS, Tromble E, Jenkins WD, et al. Choosing the emergency department as an alternative for STD care: potential disparities in access. J Health Care Poor Underserved 2022;33(3):1163–8.

32. Bergquist EP, Trolard A, Zhao Y, et al. Single and repeated use of the emergency department for chlamydia and gonorrhea care. Sex Transm Dis 2020; 47(1):14–8.

33. Reno H, Park I, Workowski K, et al. A guide to taking a sexual history. Centers for Disease Prevention and Control. 2022. Available at: https://www.cdc.gov/std/treatment/SexualHistory.htm. [Accessed 28 August 2023].

34. GOALS Framework for sexual history taking in primary care. Available at: https://www.hivguidelines.org/guideline/goals-framework/. [Accessed 4 November 2023].

35. Ahmad FA, Jeffe DB, Plax K, et al. Computerized self-interviews improve chlamydia and gonorrhea testing among youth in the emergency department. Ann Emerg Med 2014;64(4):376–84.

36. Goyal MK, Shea JA, Hayes KL, et al. Development of a sexual health screening tool for adolescent emergency department patients. Acad Emerg Med 2016; 23(7):809–15.

37. Ahmad FA, Fischer K, Gu H, et al. Impact of risk-based sexually transmitted infection screening in the emergency department. Acad Emerg Med 2022. https://doi.org/10.1111/acem.14465.

38. Williams AM, Gift TL, O'Donnell LN, et al. Assessment of the cost-effectiveness of a brief video intervention for sexually transmitted disease prevention. Sex Transm Dis 2020;47(2):130–5.

39. Monti PM, Mastroleo NR, Barnett NP, et al. Brief motivational intervention to reduce alcohol and HIV/sexual risk behavior in emergency department patients: a randomized controlled trial. J Consult Clin Psychol 2016;84(7):580–91.

40. Miller MK, Champassak S, Goggin K, et al. Brief behavioral intervention to improve adolescent sexual health: a feasibility study in the emergency department. Pediatr Emerg Care 2016;32(1):17–9.

41. Peterman TA, Tian LH, Metcalf CA, et al. High incidence of new sexually transmitted infections in the year following a sexually transmitted infection: a case for rescreening. Ann Intern Med 2006;145(8):564–72.

42. Potterat JJ. Active detection of men with asymptomatic chlamydial or gonorrhoeal urethritis. Int J STD AIDS 2005;16(6):458.

43. Scholes D, Stergachis A, Heidrich FE, et al. Prevention of pelvic inflammatory disease by screening for cervical chlamydial infection. N Engl J Med 1996; 334(21):1362–6.

44. Workowski KA, Bachmann LH, Chan PA, et al. Sexually transmitted infections treatment guidelines, 2021. MMWR Recomm Rep 2021;70(4):1–187.

45. By P, Papp JR, Schachter J, et al. Recommendations for the laboratory-based detection of chlamydia trachomatis and Neisseria gonorrhoeae — 2014. 2014.

Available at: https://www.cdc.gov/mmwr/preview/mmwrhtml/rr6302a1.htm. [Accessed 10 December 2023].

46. Michel CEC, Sonnex C, Carne CA, et al. Chlamydia trachomatis load at matched anatomic sites: implications for screening strategies. J Clin Microbiol 2007; 45(5):1395–402.

47. Shafer MA, Moncada J, Boyer CB, et al. Comparing first-void urine specimens, self-collected vaginal swabs, and endocervical specimens to detect Chlamydia trachomatis and Neisseria gonorrhoeae by a nucleic acid amplification test. J Clin Microbiol 2003;41(9):4395–9.

48. Coorevits L, Traen A, Bingé L, et al. Identifying a consensus sample type to test for Chlamydia trachomatis, Neisseria gonorrhoeae, Mycoplasma genitalium, Trichomonas vaginalis and human papillomavirus. Clin Microbiol Infect 2018; 24(12):1328–32.

49. van der Helm JJ, Hoebe CJPA, van Rooijen MS, et al. High performance and acceptability of self-collected rectal swabs for diagnosis of Chlamydia trachomatis and Neisseria gonorrhoeae in men who have sex with men and women. Sex Transm Dis 2009;36(8):493.

50. Freeman AH, Bernstein KT, Kohn RP, et al. Evaluation of self-collected versus clinician-collected swabs for the detection of Chlamydia trachomatis and Neisseria gonorrhoeae pharyngeal infection among men who have sex with men. Sex Transm Dis 2011;38(11):1036–9. Available at: https://journals.lww.com/stdjournal/FullText/ 2011/11000/Evaluation_of_Self_Collected_Versus.9.aspx?casa_token=xWBMiia Wd_0AAAAA:V0rTbDwwUEYYZUHfuzo_-I0ZrGzgFK6to1T8cwlGQCK8l1K2aQyn i6Ar0dnx_OHI9h89DkZBsVPKtNGOQUzv57MmTCS8ieY.

51. Berwald N, Cheng S, Augenbraun M, et al. Self-administered vaginal swabs are a feasible alternative to physician-assisted cervical swabs for sexually transmitted infection screening in the emergency department. Acad Emerg Med 2009;16(4):360–3.

52. Lunny C, Taylor D, Hoang L, et al. Self-collected versus clinician-collected sampling for chlamydia and gonorrhea screening: a systemic review and meta-analysis. PLoS One 2015;10(7):e0132776.

53. Krause A, Miller JB, Samuel L, et al. Vaginal swabs are non-inferior to endocervical swabs for sexually transmitted infection testing in the emergency department. West J Emerg Med 2022;23(3):408–11.

54. Chinnock B, Yore M, Mason J, et al. Self-obtained vaginal swabs are not inferior to provider-performed endocervical sampling for emergency department diagnosis of Neisseria gonorrhoeae and Chlamydia trachomatis. Acad Emerg Med 2021;28(6):612–20.

55. Gaydos CA, Manabe YC, Melendez JH. A narrative review of where we are with point-of-care sexually transmitted infection testing in the United States. Sex Transm Dis 2021;48(8S):S71–7.

56. Dawkins M, Bishop L, Walker P, et al. Clinical integration of a highly accurate polymerase chain reaction point-of-care test can inform immediate treatment decisions for chlamydia, gonorrhea, and trichomonas. Sex Transm Dis 2022;49(4): 262–7.

57. Soa-Aids Amsterdam. CC BY-SA 3.0 File:SOA-Chlamydia-trachomatis-female.jpg. File:SOA-Chlamydia-trachomatis-female.jpg. Available at: https:// commons.wikimedia.org/w/index.php?curid=45718. [Accessed 2 December 2023].

58. Young A, Toncar A, Wray AA. Urethritis. StatPearls Publishing; 2022. Available at: https://www.ncbi.nlm.nih.gov/books/NBK537282/. [Accessed 7 November 2023].

59. Workowski K, Bachmann L, Chan P, et al. Sexually transmitted infections treatment guidelines, 2021. MMWR Recomm Rep 2021;70:1–187. Available at: https://www.cdc.gov/std/treatment-guidelines/STI-Guidelines-2021.pdf.

60. Ngan V, Vanousova D, Renaud N, et al. Gonorrhea. DermNet. 2005. Available at: https://dermnetnz.org/topics/gonorrhoea. [Accessed 9 November 2023].

61. Details - Public Health Image Library(PHIL) -11255. Available at: https://phil.cdc.gov/Details.aspx?pid=11255. [Accessed 4 December 2023].

62. Buder S, Schöfer H, Meyer T, et al. Bacterial sexually transmitted infections. J Dtsch Dermatol Ges 2019;17(3):287–315.

63. Pfennig CL. Sexually transmitted diseases in the emergency department. Emerg Med Clin North Am 2019;37(2):165–92.

64. Handsfield HH, Lipman TO, Harnisch JP, et al. Asymptomatic gonorrhea in men. Diagnosis, natural course, prevalence and significance. N Engl J Med 1974; 290(3):117–23.

65. Syphilis Images. DermNet. 2009. Available at: https://dermnetnz.org/topics/syphilis-images. [Accessed 9 November 2023].

66. Towns JM, Leslie DE, Denham I, et al. Painful and multiple anogenital lesions are common in men with Treponema pallidum PCR-positive primary syphilis without herpes simplex virus coinfection: a cross-sectional clinic-based study. Sex Transm Infect 2016;92(2):110–5.

67. Ghanem KG. REVIEW: neurosyphilis: a historical perspective and review. CNS Neurosci Ther 2010;16(5):e157–68.

68. CDC. STI treatment guidelines. Centers for Disease Control and Prevention; 2022. Available at: https://www.cdc.gov/std/treatment-guidelines/default.htm. [Accessed 18 October 2022].

69. Details - Public Health Image Library (PHIL) 18038. Available at: https://phil.cdc.gov/Details.aspx?pid=18038. [Accessed 2 July 2023].

70. Lymphogranuloma Venereum (LGV). 2021. Available at: https://www.cdc.gov/std/treatment-guidelines/lgv.htm. [Accessed 23 June 2023].

71. Details - Public Health Image Library (PHIL)- 6514. Available at: https://phil.cdc.gov/Details.aspx?pid=6514. [Accessed 4 December 2023].

72. Martin DH. Mycoplasma genitalium infection in males and females. In: Marrazzo J, Bloom A, editors. UpToDate. UpToDate; 2021. Available at: https://www.uptodate.com/contents/mycoplasma-genitalium-infection-in-males-and-females?search=mycoplasma%20genitalium%20infection&source=search_result&selectedTitle=1~31&usage_type=default&display_rank=1.

73. Tallon B. Pruritic papular eruption of HIV. DermNet. 2021. Available at: https://dermnetnz.org/topics/pruritic-papular-eruption-of-hiv. [Accessed 9 November 2023].

74. Knight CL. Physical examination in Human Immunodeficiency Virus disease. Med Clin North Am 2022;106(3):527–36.

75. Details 15822 - Public Health Image Library (PHIL). Available at: https://phil.cdc.gov/Details.aspx?pid=15822. [Accessed 1 July 2023].

76. Twede JV. MedPix Topic - case 16 (27th Annual Uniformed Services Dermatology Seminar, 2003) VERRUCIFORM XANTHOMA. 2005. Available at: https://medpix.nlm.nih.gov/topic?id=0c0602d0-f9e2-4261-bd40-9a2fa8b2fef9. [Accessed 2 July 2023].

77. STD facts - human papillomavirus (HPV). 2022. Available at: https://www.cdc.gov/std/hpv/stdfact-hpv.htm. [Accessed 23 June 2023].
78. Soheili M, Keyvani H, Soheili M, et al. Human papilloma virus: a review study of epidemiology, carcinogenesis, diagnostic methods, and treatment of all HPV-related cancers. Med J Islam Repub Iran 2021;35:65.
79. Manini I, Montomoli E. Epidemiology and prevention of human papillomavirus. Ann Ig 2018;30(4 Supple 1):28–32.
80. Details - Public Health Image Library (PHIL)- 2860. Available at: https://phil.cdc.gov/Details.aspx?pid=2860. [Accessed 4 December 2023].
81. Seeff LB. Natural history of hepatitis C. Hepatology 1997;26(3 Suppl 1):21S–8S.
82. Feld JJ. Clinical manifestations, diagnosis, and treatment of acute hepatitis C virus infection in adults. In: Di Bisceglie AM, Bloom A, editors. UpToDate. UpToDate; 2022. https://www.uptodate.com/contents/clinical-manifestations-diagnosis-and-treatment-of-acute-hepatitis-c-virus-infection-in-adults?search=acute%20infection%20hepatitis%20c%20symptoms&source=search_result&selectedTitle=1~91&usage_type=default&display_rank=1.
83. Chopra S. Clinical manifestations and natural history of chronic hepatitis C virus infection. In: Di Bisceglie AM, Bloom A, editors. UpToDate. UpToDate; 2023. Available at: https://www.uptodate.com/contents/clinical-manifestations-and-natural-history-of-chronic-hepatitis-c-virus-infection?search=hepatitis%20c%20symptoms&source=search_result&selectedTitle=1~150&usage_type=default&display_rank=1.
84. Gilbourne, Marika (Nottingham University), Oakley A, Coulson I. Mpox (monkeypox). DermNet. 2023. Available at: https://dermnetnz.org/topics/mpox. [Accessed 9 November 2023].
85. Chauhan RP, Fogel R, Limson J. Overview of diagnostic methods, disease prevalence and transmission of Mpox (Formerly Monkeypox) in humans and animal reservoirs. Microorganisms 2023;11(5). https://doi.org/10.3390/microorganisms11051186.
86. Center for Devices, Radiological Health. Monkeypox (mpox) and Medical Devices. U.S. Food and Drug Administration; 2023. Available at: https://www.fda.gov/medical-devices/emergency-situations-medical-devices/monkeypox-mpox-and-medical-devices. [Accessed 29 June 2023].
87. Suñer C, Ubals M, Tarín-Vicente EJ, et al. Viral dynamics in patients with monkeypox infection: a prospective cohort study in Spain. Lancet Infect Dis 2023;23(4):445–53.
88. CDC. Guidelines for collecting and handling specimens for mpox testing. Centers for Disease Control and Prevention; 2023. Available at: https://www.cdc.gov/poxvirus/mpox/clinicians/prep-collection-specimens.html. [Accessed 29 June 2023].
89. Schumann JA, Plasner S. Trichomoniasis. In: StatPearls. StatPearls Publishing; 2022. Available at: https://www.ncbi.nlm.nih.gov/pubmed/30521247.
90. Details - Public Health Image Library (PHIL) 16402. Available at: https://phil.cdc.gov/Details.aspx?pid=16402. [Accessed 2 July 2023].
91. Association of Public Health Laboratories. Advances in laboratory detection of Trichomonas Vaginalis (updated). 2016. Available at: https://www.aphl.org/aboutAPHL/publications/Documents/ID_2016November-Laboratory-Detection-of-Trichomonas-update.pdf.
92. Ravel J, Moreno I, Simón C. Bacterial vaginosis and its association with infertility, endometritis, and pelvic inflammatory disease. Am J Obstet Gynecol 2021;224(3):251–7.

93. Villanueva DDH, Staton JP, Gupte AA. A report of haemophilus influenzae bacteremia with acute pelvic inflammatory disease. Cureus 2022;14(9):e28970.

94. Portman MD. Re: pelvic inflammatory disease. BMJ 2023;346(f3189). Available at: https://www.bmj.com/content/346/bmj.f3189/rr/657322. [Accessed 10 December 2023].

95. Schoeman SA, Stewart CMW, Booth RA, et al. Assessment of best single sample for finding chlamydia in women with and without symptoms: a diagnostic test study. BMJ 2012;345:e8013.

96. Schachter J, Chernesky MA, Willis DE, et al. Vaginal swabs are the specimens of choice when screening for Chlamydia trachomatis and Neisseria gonorrhoeae: results from a multicenter evaluation of the APTIMA assays for both infections. Sex Transm Dis 2005;32(12):725–8.

97. Suzich JB, Cliffe AR. Strength in diversity: understanding the pathways to herpes simplex virus reactivation. Virology 2018;522:81–91.

98. McQuillan G, Kruszon-Moran D, Flagg EW, et al. Prevalence of herpes simplex virus type 1 and type 2 in persons aged 14-49: United States, 2015-2016. NCHS Data Brief 2018;(304):1–8. Available at: https://www.ncbi.nlm.nih.gov/pubmed/29442994.

99. Herpes - STI treatment guidelines. 2022. Available at: https://www.cdc.gov/std/treatment-guidelines/herpes.htm. [Accessed 21 July 2023].

100. The diagnosis, management and prevention of syphilis: an update and review. New York City Department of Health and Mental Hygiene Burea of Sexually Transmitted Infections and the New York City STD Prevention Training Center. 2019. Available at: https://www.nycptc.org/x/Syphilis_Monograph_2019_NYC_PTC_NYC_DOHMH.pdf. [Accessed 10 November 2023].

101. McDonald R. Vital signs: missed opportunities for preventing congenital syphilis — United States, 2022. MMWR Morb Mortal Wkly Rep 2023;72. https://doi.org/10.15585/mmwr.mm7246e1.

102. Ford JS, Chechi T, Otmar M, et al. ED syphilis and gonorrhea/chlamydia cotesting practices before and after the implementation of an electronic health record-based alert. Emerg Med J 2021. https://doi.org/10.1136/emermed-2020-210331.

103. Stanford KA, Hazra A, Friedman E, et al. Opt-Out, routine emergency department syphilis screening as a novel intervention in at-risk populations. Sex Transm Dis 2021;48(5):347–52.

104. Hook EW 3rd. Syphilis. Lancet. 2017;389(10078):1550–7.

105. HIV Basic statistics. 2023. Available at: https://www.cdc.gov/hiv/basics/statistics.html. [Accessed 8 November 2023].

106. White DAE, Warren OU, Scribner AN, et al. Missed opportunities for earlier HIV diagnosis in an emergency department despite an HIV screening program. AIDS Patient Care STDS 2009;23(4):245–50.

107. Missed opportunities for earlier diagnosis of HIV infection — South Carolina, 1997–2005. 2006. Available at: https://www.cdc.gov/mmwr/preview/mmwrhtml/mm5547a2.htm. [Accessed 3 January 2023].

108. HIV - STI treatment guidelines. 2021. Available at: https://www.cdc.gov/std/treatment-guidelines/hiv.htm. [Accessed 8 November 2023].

109. CDC. STI treatment guidelines. 2022. Available at: https://www.cdc.gov/std/treatment-guidelines/default.htm. [Accessed 18 October 2022].

110. Eyre RC. Acute scrotal pain in adults. In: O'Leary MP, Law K, editors. UpToDate. UpToDate; 2023. Available at: https://www.uptodate.com/contents/acute-

scrotal-pain-in-adults?search=epididymitis%20&source=search_result&selected
Title=1~84&usage_type=default&display_rank=1.

111. Epididymitis. 2021. Available at: https://www.cdc.gov/std/treatment-guidelines/
epididymitis.htm. [Accessed 21 June 2023].

112. Ludwig M. Diagnosis and therapy of acute prostatitis, epididymitis and orchitis.
Andrologia 2008;40(2):76–80.

113. de Voux A, Kent JB, Macomber K, et al. Notes from the field: cluster of lymphogranuloma venereum cases among men who have sex with men - Michigan,
August 2015-April 2016. MMWR Morb Mortal Wkly Rep 2016;65(34):920–1.

114. Proctitis, proctocolitis, and enteritis. 2021. Available at: https://www.cdc.gov/
std/treatment-guidelines/proctitis.htm. [Accessed 27 July 2023].

115. DiMarco DE, Urban MA, McGowan JP, et al. Mycoplasma genitalium management in adults. Johns Hopkins University; 2022. Available at: https://www.ncbi.
nlm.nih.gov/books/NBK583532/. [Accessed 30 January 2024].

116. Gossé M, Nordbø SA, Pukstad B. Evaluation of treatment with two weeks of
doxycycline on macrolide-resistant strains of Mycoplasma genitalium: a retrospective observational study. BMC Infect Dis 2021;21(1):1225.

117. Lau A, Bradshaw CS, Lewis D, et al. The efficacy of azithromycin for the treatment of genital Mycoplasma genitalium: a systematic review and meta-analysis.
Clin Infect Dis 2015;61(9):1389–99.

118. Li Y, Le WJ, Li S, et al. Meta-analysis of the efficacy of moxifloxacin in treating
Mycoplasma genitalium infection. Int J STD AIDS 2017;28(11):1106–14.

119. WHO declares end of mpox emergency, calls for sustained efforts for long-term
management of the disease. Pan American Health Organization; 2023. Available at: https://www.paho.org/en/news/11-5-2023-who-declares-end-mpox-
emergency-calls-sustained-efforts-long-term-management-disease#:
~:text=May%2011%2C%202023%2D%20The%20Emergency,General%
20accepted%20the%20Committee's%20advice. [Accessed 8 November 2023].

120. Kirby T. What happened to the mpox pandemic? 2023. https://doi.org/10.1016/
S0140-6736(23)01956-6.

121. Clinical Recognition. Centers of Disease Control and Prevention. 2023. Available
at: https://www.cdc.gov/poxvirus/mpox/clinicians/clinical-recognition.html. [Ac-
cessed 1 July 2023].

122. Mpox (monkeypox). World Health Organization; 2023. Available at: https://www.
who.int/news-room/fact-sheets/detail/monkeypox. [Accessed 8 November
2023].

123. Rawre J, Agrawal S, Dhawan B. Sexually transmitted infections: need for extragenital screening. Indian J Med Microbiol 2018;36(1):1–7.

124. Assaf RD, Cunningham NJ, Adamson PC, et al. High proportions of rectal and
pharyngeal chlamydia and gonorrhoea cases among cisgender men are
missed using current CDC screening recommendations. Sex Transm Infect
2022;98(8):586–91.

125. Jann JT, Cunningham NJ, Assaf RD, et al. Evidence supporting the standardisa-
tion of extragenital gonorrhoea and chlamydia screenings for women. Sex
Transm Infect 2021;97(8):601–6.

126. Aptima® Multitest Swab. Hologic Women's Health. 2020. Available at: https://
hologicwomenshealth.com/products/aptimamultitestswab/. [Accessed 1 July
2023].

127. Adamson PC, Klausner JD. Diagnostic tests for detecting Chlamydia trachomatis and Neisseria gonorrhoeae in rectal and pharyngeal specimens. J Clin Microbiol 2022;60(4). e0021121.

128. Locklear M. Emergency department crowding hits crisis levels, risking patient safety. YaleNews 2022. Available at: https://news.yale.edu/2022/09/30/emergency-department-crowding-hits-crisis-levels-risking-patient-safety. [Accessed 27 June 2023].

129. Gaydos CA, Quinn TC, Willis D, et al. Performance of the APTIMA Combo 2 assay for detection of Chlamydia trachomatis and Neisseria gonorrhoeae in female urine and endocervical swab specimens. J Clin Microbiol 2003;41(1):304–9.

130. Aaron KJ, Griner S, Footman A, et al. Vaginal swab vs urine for detection of Chlamydia trachomatis, Neisseria gonorrhoeae, and Trichomonas vaginalis: a meta-analysis. Ann Fam Med 2023;21(2):172–9.

131. Hsieh YH, Lewis MK, Viertel VG, et al. Performance evaluation and acceptability of point-of-care Trichomonas vaginalis testing in adult female emergency department patients. Int J STD AIDS 2020;31(14):1364–72.

132. Lehto E, Anderson B, Reed J, et al. Impact of rapid testing for gonorrhea and chlamydia in an urban pediatric emergency department. J Adolesc Health 2022. https://doi.org/10.1016/j.jadohealth.2022.01.219.

133. Gaydos CA, Ako MC, Lewis M, et al. Use of a rapid diagnostic for Chlamydia trachomatis and Neisseria gonorrhoeae for women in the emergency department can improve clinical management: report of a randomized clinical trial. Ann Emerg Med 2019;74(1):36–44.

134. Rapid testing for Chlamydia and gonorrhea in emergency departments. 2017. Available at: http://chlamydiacoalition.org/rapid-testing-for-chlamydia-and-gonorrhea-in-emergency-departments/. [Accessed 7 August 2022].

135. May L, Ware CE, Jordan JA, et al. A randomized controlled trial comparing the treatment of patients tested for chlamydia and gonorrhea after a rapid polymerase chain reaction test versus standard of care testing. Sex Transm Dis 2016;43(5):290.

136. Blachford A. The rising importance of urgent care in the fight against the STI epidemic. J Urgent Care Med 2022. Available at: https://www.jucm.com/the-rising-importance-of-urgent-care-in-the-fight-against-the-sti-epidemic/. [Accessed 28 June 2023].

137. Caruso G, Giammanco A, Virruso R, et al. Current and future trends in the laboratory diagnosis of sexually transmitted infections. Int J Environ Res Public Health 2021;18(3). https://doi.org/10.3390/ijerph18031038.

138. Adamson PC, Loeffelholz MJ, Klausner JD. Point-of-care testing for sexually transmitted infections: a review of recent developments. Arch Pathol Lab Med 2020;144(11):1344–51.

139. Breslin K, Tuchman L, Hayes KL, et al. Sensitivity and specificity of empiric treatment for sexually transmitted infections in a pediatric emergency department. J Pediatr 2017;189:48–53.

140. Solnick R, Patel R, Chang E, et al. 211 gender differences in empiric treatment in US emergency departments for chlamydia and gonorrhea: a systematic review and meta-analysis. Ann Emerg Med 2023;82(4):S96.

141. Fisk KM, Derouin A, Holm G, et al. Getting it right: the impact of point-of-care testing for gonorrhea and chlamydia in the urgent care setting. J Nurse Pract 2020;16(5):388–93.

142. Sexual Health Test — POC rapid PCR device. Visby medical. Available at: https://www.visbymedical.com/sexual-health-test/. [Accessed 1 July 2023].

143. Cantor A, Dana T, Griffin JC, et al. Screening for chlamydial and gonococcal infections: updated evidence report and systematic review for the US Preventive Services Task Force. JAMA 2021;326(10):957–66.

144. US Preventive Services Task Force, Mangione CM, Barry MJ, et al. Screening for syphilis infection in nonpregnant adolescents and adults: US Preventive Services Task Force Reaffirmation Recommendation Statement. JAMA 2022; 328(12):1243–9.

145. Kozhimannil KB. Declining access to US maternity care is a systemic injustice. BMJ 2023;382:2038.

146. Getting tested. 2023. Available at: https://www.cdc.gov/hiv/basics/hiv-testing/getting-tested.html. [Accessed 10 November 2023].

147. Chlamydial infections. 2022. Available at: https://www.cdc.gov/std/treatment-guidelines/chlamydia.htm. [Accessed 10 November 2023].

148. Bamberger DM, Graham G, Dennis L, et al. Extragenital gonorrhea and chlamydia among men and women according to type of sexual exposure. Sex Transm Dis 2019;46(5):329–34.

149. Expedited partner therapy. 2022. Available at: https://www.cdc.gov/std/ept/default.htm. [Accessed 13 January 2023].

150. Trelle S, Shang A, Nartey L, et al. Improved effectiveness of partner notification for patients with sexually transmitted infections: systematic review. BMJ 2007; 334(7589):354.

151. Ferreira A, Young T, Mathews C, et al. Strategies for partner notification for sexually transmitted infections, including HIV. Cochrane Database Syst Rev 2013;(10):CD002843.

152. American College of Emergency Physicians (ACEP). Expedited partner therapy for selected sexually transmitted infections. Policy Statements. 2022. Available at: https://www.acep.org/patient-care/policy-statements/expedited-partner-therapy-for-selected-sexually-transmitted-infections/. [Accessed 12 January 2023].

153. Legal Status of expedited partner therapy. 2021. Available at: https://www.cdc.gov/std/ept/legal/default.htm. [Accessed 8 November 2022].

154. Arizona State University, Centers for Disease Control and Prevention. Legal/policy toolkit for adoption and implementation of expedited partner therapy. 2011. Available at: https://www.cdc.gov/std/ept/legal/ept-toolkit-complete.pdf.

155. Solnick RE, Cortes R, Chang E, et al. A national study of expedited partner therapy use in emergency departments: a survey of medical director knowledge, attitudes and practices. medRxiv 2023. https://doi.org/10.1101/2023.04.01.23287999.

156. McCool-Myers M, Goedken P, Henn MC, et al. Who is practicing expedited partner therapy and why? Insights from providers working in specialties with high volumes of sexually transmitted infections. Sex Transm Dis 2021;48(7):474–80.

157. Mmeje OO, Qin JZ, Wetmore MK, et al. Breakdown in the expedited partner therapy treatment cascade: from reproductive healthcare provider to the pharmacist. Am J Obstet Gynecol 2020. https://doi.org/10.1016/j.ajog.2020.02.038.

158. Minnesota Department of Health. Expedited Partner Treatment (EPT) toolkit for implementation in clinical settings: guidance from the Minnesota. Department of Health; 2023. Available at: https://www.health.state.mn.us/diseases/stds/hcp/ept/eptimptoolkit.pdf.

159. National Council for Prescription Drug Programs. SCRIPT implementation recommendations. National Council for Prescription Drug Programs, Inc.; 2023.

Available at: https://www.ncpdp.org/NCPDP/media/pdf/SCRIPT-Implementation-Recommendations.pdf.

160. Ager EE, Sturdavant W, Curry Z, et al. Mixed-methods evaluation of an expedited partner therapy take-home medication program: pilot emergency department intervention to improve sexual health equity. West J Emerg Med 2023; 24(5):993–1004.

161. Luetkemeyer AF, Donnell D, Dombrowski JC, et al. Postexposure doxycycline to prevent bacterial sexually transmitted infections. N Engl J Med 2023;388(14): 1296–306.

162. Molina JM. ANRS 174 DOXYVAC: an open-label randomized trial to prevent STIs in MSM on PrEP. Presented at: CROI; March 4, 2023; Seattle. Available at: https://www.croiconference.org/abstract/anrs-174-doxyvac-an-open-label-randomized-trial-to-prevent-stis-in-msm-on-prep/. [Accessed 30 June 2023].

163. Doxycycline post-exposure prophylaxis to prevent bacterial sexually transmitted infections. Available at: https://www.hivguidelines.org/guideline/sti-doxy-pep/. [Accessed 30 January 2024].

164. California Department of Health. Doxycycline post-exposure prophylaxis (doxy-PEP) for the prevention of bacterial sexually transmitted infections (STIs). 2023. Available at: https://www.cdph.ca.gov/Programs/CID/DCDC/CDPH%20Document%20Library/CDPH-Doxy-PEP-Recommendations-for-Prevention-of-STIs.pdf.

165. Quinn C, Pathela P, NYC Department of Health. Postexposure doxycycline to prevent bacterial sexually transmitted infections. N Engl J Med 2023;388(14): 1296–306.

Communicable Disease Screening and Human Immunodeficiency Virus Prevention in the Emergency Department

Douglas A.E. White, MD[a],*, Rachel E. Solnick, MD, MSc[b]

KEYWORDS

- Emergency department • Screening • HIV • Hepatitis C virus • Syphilis
- Pre-exposure prophylaxis • PrEP

KEY POINTS

- Emergency departments (EDs) can play a critical role in the screening, treatment, and prevention of communicable diseases like HIV, HCV, and syphilis.
- National guidelines recommend routine screening for HIV and HCV at least once per lifetime and syphilis screening annually or more frequently for at-risk individuals.
- Successful integration of communicable disease screening into ED operations requires simple consent processes, leveraging the electronic health record, utilizing standard testing procedures, full-time patient navigators, and multidisciplinary collaboration.
- Rapid ED initiation of same-day antiretroviral HIV treatment can improve HIV-related health outcomes.
- Emergency department communicable disease screening programs can be leveraged to provide HIV prevention service delivery and referral.

INTRODUCTION

Emergency department (ED) screening for communicable infectious diseases such as acquired immunodeficiency syndrome, hepatitis, and syphilis reaches patient populations who do not routinely access screening and prevention services elsewhere, many of whom have high rates of infection. In this article, we review the state of the art in ED communicable disease screening, treatment, and linkage to care.

---

[a] Department of Emergency Medicine, Alameda Health System, Wilma Chan Highland Hospital, 1411 East 31st Street, Oakland, CA 94602, USA; [b] Icahn School of Medicine at Mount Sinai Hospital, 555 West 57th Street 5-25, New York, NY 10019, USA
* Corresponding author.
E-mail address: dwhite@alamedahealthsystem.org

Emerg Med Clin N Am 42 (2024) 369–389
https://doi.org/10.1016/j.emc.2024.02.007
0733-8627/24/© 2024 Elsevier Inc. All rights reserved.

emed.theclinics.com

National Guidelines in Support of Communicable Infectious Disease Screening

National guidelines for human immunodeficiency virus (HIV), hepatitis C virus (HCV), and syphilis screening from the Centers for Disease Control and Prevention (CDC), US Preventive Services Task Force (USPSTF), and the American College of Emergency Physicians (ACEP) are shown in **Table 1**.[1–5] The CDC and USPSTF recommend screening adult patients for HIV and HCV infection at least once per lifetime, with more frequent screening targeting patients with ongoing risk for acquiring disease, as well as targeted syphilis screening for at-risk individuals and pregnant patients.[1–4] Updated in April 2023, the ACEP policy on "Bloodborne Pathogens in Emergency Medicine" endorses these CDC and USPSTF screening recommendations for HIV and HCV infections if mechanisms are in place to link patients screening positive to treatment.[5] The ACEP policy further supports the ED initiation of rapid start antiretroviral treatment (ART) for patients diagnosed with HIV and recommends an expansion of HIV prevention services, including providing HIV pre-exposure prophylaxis (PrEP) to patients at risk for HIV. At this time, national guidelines support syphilis screening for pregnant women and for patients at increased risk and have not yet endorsed routine, screening for all patients. Some states, however, are recommending routine syphilis screening in combination with HIV and HCV screening.[6]

Rationale for Locating Infectious Disease Screening in the Emergency Department

Over the past 20 years, the ED has emerged as an important venue for the screening and prevention initiatives recommended by the CDC and USPSTF. With over 130 million ED visits each year and a continuously replenished population of patients, many of whom are medically underserved, experiencing poverty, and have substance use disorders (SUDs), US EDs are strategically positioned to identify and treat people communicable infectious diseases.[7,8] EDs have developed innovative screening and testing programs for HIV, HCV, and syphilis.[9–12] Programs have demonstrated the ability to identify new cases of infections, link patients to care, and integrate procedures into standard ED operations. More recently, reports have demonstrated the feasibility and clinical effectiveness of integrating HIV prevention services into existing screening programs.[13]

Human Immunodeficiency Virus Screening Inception, Expansion, and Impact

In 2006, the CDC expanded its recommendations to support universal HIV screening in acute care settings to promote earlier disease identification, reduce stigma, and improve testing uptake nationally.[1] Since that time, the US has seen a steady increase in the implementation of ED-based HIV screening programs.[14–16] Experts believe that ED-based HIV screening has been an important factor contributing to improvements in HIV diagnosis, linkage to care, treatment, and viral suppression.

Human Immunodeficiency Virus Screening as a Foundation for Expanded Screening for Other Infections

The impact that ED-based HIV screening has made toward ending the HIV epidemic both exemplifies why ED screening should be embraced and provides a basis for implementing broader screening. Over the past decade, programs have found that having the infrastructure in place and experience with HIV screening provides a convenient foundation to expand screening, particularly for HCV and, to a lesser extent, syphilis.

Although navigating through outpatient linkage and treatment is indeed more complex when screening for a variety of diseases instead of just one, it can be readily accomplished. There are multiple examples of HCV screening being successfully

Table 1
Recommendations for human immunodeficiency virus, hepatitis c virus, and syphilis screening

Test	Organization	Target Population for Screening	Restrictions for Screening	Frequency of Screening	Consent
HIV screening	• CDC[a]	• 13–64 y of age • All patients seeking STI treatment • All pregnant women	• All health care settings with a prevalence of undiagnosed HIV infection >0.1%	• At least once in lifetime • At least once per year if ongoing HIV risk • Pregnant women: Consider repeat screening in third trimester, especially if at increased risk	• Voluntary, opt-out
	• USPSTF[b]	• 15–65 y of age • Younger adolescents and older adults if at increased risk • All pregnant women	• None specified	• At least once in lifetime • Repeat screening "reasonable" if ongoing risk, no recommendation on frequency • Pregnant women: Each pregnancy	• Voluntary, opt-out
	• ACEP[c]	• ≥13 y of age • Pregnant women	• Screening encouraged	• None specified	• Voluntary, opt-out
HCV screening	• CDC[d]	• ≥18 y of age • Pregnant women	• All health care settings with a prevalence of chronic HCV infection of >0.1%	• Once in lifetime • Periodic screening for persons with ongoing risk factors • Pregnant women: Each pregnancy	• None specified
	• USPSTF[e]	• 18–79 y of age • <18 and >79 y of age if at high risk	• None specified	• Once in lifetime • Periodic screening for persons with ongoing risk factors	• Voluntary
	• ACEP[c]	• All adults • High-risk patient populations • No age ranges specified	• Screening encourage when feasible	• Once in lifetime • Routine screening for high-risk patient populations	• Not specified

(continued on next page)

Table 1
(continued)

Test	Organization	Target Population for Screening	Restrictions for Screening	Frequency of Screening	Consent
Syphilis screening	• CDC[f]	• Nonpregnant persons at increased risk • All pregnant women • No age restrictions	• At increased risk (nonpregnant persons)	• Annually or more frequently depending on risk • Pregnant women: First prenatal visit and retest at 28 wk and at time of delivery if at increased risk	• Not specified
	• USPSTF[g,h]	• Nonpregnant persons at increased risk • All pregnant women • No age restrictions	• At increased risk (nonpregnant persons)	• Annually or more frequently depending on risk • Pregnant women: Early as possible when present for prenatal care and at time of delivery if no prenatal care	• Not specified
	• ACEP	—	—	—	—

Abbreviations: ACEP, American College of Emergency Physicians; CDC, Centers for Disease Control and Prevention; STI, sexually transmitted infection; USPSTF, United States Preventative Services Task Force.

[a] Reference: Revised Recommendations for HIV Testing of Adults, Adolescents, and Pregnant Women in Health Care Settings. MMWR, September 22, 2006 / 55(RR14);1-17.
[b] Reference: Screening for HIV Infection US Preventive Services Task Force Recommendation Statement JAMA. https://doi.org/10.1001/jama.2019.6587.
[c] Reference: https://www.acep.org/patient-care/policy-statements/bloodborne-pathogens-in-emergency-medicine. Date accessed: 9/25/23.
[d] Reference: CDC Recommendations for Hepatitis C Screening Among Adults — United States, 2020 MMWR / April 10, 2020 / Vol. 69 / No. 2.
[e] Reference: Screening for Hepatitis C Virus Infection in Adolescents and Adults US Preventive Services Task Force Recommendation Statement JAMA. https://doi.org/10.1001/jama.2020.1123.
[f] Reference: https://www.cdc.gov/std/treatment-guidelines/screening-recommendations.htm. Date accessed: 9/25/23.
[g] Reference: Screening for Syphilis Infection in Nonpregnant Adolescents and Adults. US Preventive Services Task Force Reaffirmation Recommendation Statement JAMA. 2022;328(12):1243-1249. https://doi.org/10.1001/jama.2022.15322.
[h] Reference: Screening for Syphilis in Pregnant Women. US Preventive Services Task Force Reaffirmation Recommendation Statement JAMA. 2018;320(9):911-917. https://doi.org/10.1001/jama.2018.11785.

added to established HIV screening programs, mirroring the procedures already in place, like notification and test ordering.[17] Expanding triage-based screening protocols and electronic health record (EHR)-driven algorithms have also been reported.[18] In a project conducted at the University of Chicago, syphilis testing was bundled with their existing HIV screening prompt, a simple enhancement with minimal additional end-user effort, which increased the number monthly syphilis tests by almost 1000.[10]

In addition to identifying individuals living with HIV and linking them to care and ART treatment, an HIV screening program is an essential foundation for newer programs that seek to identify ED patients at increased risk for HIV acquisition—but who have screened negative—and link them to HIV PrEP services.

ESSENTIAL ELEMENTS OF SUCCESSFUL EMERGENCY DEPARTMENT COMMUNICABLE DISEASE SCREENING

Informed by a large body of implementation science research, best practice for ED infectious disease screening are shown in **Box 1**. Here we discuss what we believe are the essential elements of a successful screening program that is integrated into the ED setting.

Multidisciplinary Collaboration

Successful screening programs rely on multidisciplinary collaboration, requiring clinical and administrative support from ED staff, infectious disease and HIV specialists, inpatient hospitalists, laboratory directors, community referral partners, disease surveillance officers from local health jurisdictions, community outreach workers, and hospital administrators. Despite the importance of collaboration, many programs rely on a single champion, often an ED or infectious disease physician, who assumes responsibility for program implementation, clinical oversight, and assessment of outcomes for quality improvement.

Consent

Separate written informed consent is not required for infectious disease screening, including for HIV. It is recommended (and in most cases legislated) that screening be voluntary and free from coercion.[5] Patients should be given the opportunity to decline screening, ask questions, and be provided information. EDs vary in where consent for infectious disease screening occurs, whether integrated into the general consent for medical care, triage registration, IV/phlebotomy processes, or during assessments by emergency providers.[19] Many EDs notify patients of screening policies through signage in the waiting room and patient care areas and provide more detailed testing information through brochures, handouts, and discharge printouts. *Opt-out consent* for screening (whereby patients are notified that screening is routinely performed and are given the opportunity to decline) is recommended by the CDC and others as a strategy to minimize stigma and improve testing rates and is the standard of care for ED-based screening programs.[1,5,19]

Electronic Health Record Strategies

EHR technology has greatly improved ED infectious disease screening, allowing consistent integration of appropriate screening into ED operations, as compared to simply relying on clinical staff.[20–24] The EHR can be used to determine whether a patient is eligible for screening. For example, patients can be flagged electronically as eligible for HIV screening based on custom criteria, including age (such as between the ages of 13–64 years), not previously identified as living with HIV (via laboratory

Box 1
Best practice recommendations for integrating HIV, HCV, and/or syphilis screening into emergency department processes

- The screening program is led by an ED clinical champion with collaboration from infectious disease specialists, HIV specialists, laboratory managers, community partners, clinical pharmacists, hospital administration, and local health jurisdictions.
- Integrate consent for screening into the general consent for hospital care or triage processes.
- Employ verbal, opt-out consent practices.
- Notify patients of the screening policy through signage in the waiting room, triage, and patient care areas.
- Screen patients who are otherwise having blood drawn and laboratory tests performed.
  - Takes advantage of existing ED processes, results in minimal to no interruptions of clinical care, and has a negligible impact on throughput.
- Leverage the EHR to facilitate screening:
  - Program the EHR to identify and/or flag eligible patients.
  - Utilize an EHR best practice advisory dialog box to prompt the offer/order of screening tests for eligible patients.
  - Develop comprehensive order sets inclusive of HIV, HCV, and syphilis screening.
  - Configure EHR algorithms, which automatically add screening tests to any laboratory order initiated by clinicians.
- Use a fourth-generation HIV antibody/antigen test for HIV screening.
  - Allows for the early detection of HIV infection, including acutely infected patients.
- Consider the reverse sequence algorithm for syphilis screening.
  - Ideal for laboratories that perform large volume syphilis testing because the algorithm uses automated treponemal testing for the initial screening.
- Perform screening tests "STAT."
  - Allows for same-day disclosure and counseling of patients with reactive test results, treatment initiation (when appropriate, feasible, and clinically indicated) and referral. Barriers to outpatient follow-up can be addressed.
- Employ automatic, reflex confirmatory testing for all reactive screening tests to determine who is truly infected and who requires linkage to care and treatment.
  - For example, reactive anti-HCV antibody tests reflex to HCV nucleic acid testing to determine who has chronic HCV infection.
  - Reactive HIV antigen/antibody tests reflex to HIV-1/HIV-2 antibody differentiation immunoassays and HIV nucleic acid tests to identify who is confirmed HIV (acute or chronic) and who is HIV negative (false-positive screening test).
- Fund dedicated ED-based navigators to assist with disclosure and linkage to care.
  - Disclosure and linkage to care can be time-consuming and often require intensive case management to address patient barriers and assist with navigation to outpatient care resources. This often requires complex care referrals for interventions unrelated to the infectious disease identified, such as housing assistance, behavioral health, and substance use management.
- Consider developing policies that enable the rapid initiation of ART for patients testing HIV positive.
  - Rapid antiretroviral therapy is well accepted by ED patients, reported to be "empowering," and maybe a powerful motivator for linkage.
- Develop a network of partnering clinics to provide rapid follow-up and treatment.

These strategies for integrating HIV, HCV, and/or Syphilis Screening into ED processes are based on personal experience, webinars, review of the published literature, and interviews with key ED personnel across the US. *Abbreviations:* ED, emergency department; HCV, hepatitis C virus.

query for reactive HIV tests and/or detectable HIV viral loads or through a keyword query of information documented in the past medical field, including "HIV"), and not recently tested (via laboratory query of HIV test within the previous 12 months). Eligibility can be tailored to the infection (HCV and syphilis), patient population needs (lifetime screen vs annual screen), and institutional limitations (laboratory capacity, funding). Once identified as eligible, the EHR can be programmed in various ways to facilitate screening. In some cases, a best practice advisory dialog box may appear as a clinical reminder to staff to offer opt-out testing and to place the screening test order. Some EHR algorithms automatically add an order for screening tests whenever other blood tests are ordered as a part of an eligible patient's clinical care. The simplest way to leverage the EHR to support broad screening, requiring minimal information technology assistance, is to include testing for HIV, HCV, and/or syphilis in commonly used order sets, such as those initiated for chest and abdominal pain. Additionally, instead of "a la carte" ordering of tests for specific sexually transmitted infections (STIs), an STI order panel should be used as a low-barrier strategy to target high-risk populations for appropriate, broad infectious disease screening (**Table 2**).

Choosing the Correct Screening Test

For HIV screening, using a laboratory-based, fourth-generation antibody/antigen assays is ideal because large numbers of tests can be processed efficiently and with reasonable turn-around times. This technology is highly sensitive and specific and identifies early HIV infection, including patients who are acutely seroconverting.[25]

Additionally, phlebotomy and laboratory systems should be designed to perform automatic, reflex confirmatory testing for all reactive ED-based screening tests. For HIV, HCV, and syphilis, additional tests (beyond the initial screening test) are required to correctly classify a patient as positive and to guide treatment and urgency of follow-up care. For example, all reactive anti-HCV antibody screening tests should reflex to HCV nucleic acid testing to determine which patients have chronic HCV infection. All reactive HIV antigen/antibody tests should reflex to HIV-1/HIV-2 antibody differentiation immunoassays and HIV nucleic acid tests to identify who is confirmed HIV positive and who is HIV negative (false-positive screening test). For syphilis, reverse screening algorithms, which begin with treponemal antibody testing and

Table 2	
Order panel for sexually transmitted infections	
Screening Test	**Automated Reflex Confirmatory Testing**
Gonorrhea/chlamydia	—
Trichomoniasis test	—
Syphilis (reverse sequence algorithm)	RPR and RPR titer
HIV antigen/antibody	HIV-1/HIV-2 antibody differentiation assay and HIV quantitative viral load
HCV antibody	HCV viral load and genotype
Hepatitis B Virus serologies (surface antibody, surface antigen, and core antibody)	—
Pregnancy	—
CBC	—
Metabolic panel	—
Exact orders may vary based on local laboratory preferences	

Abbreviation: HCV, hepatitis C virus.

reflex to nontreponemal testing (such as an rapid plasma reagin [RPR]) for reactive samples, are increasingly being used by high-volume laboratories because treponemal antibody testing can be automated with rapid turn-around times[26] and minimized technician time.[27]

Navigators

Many emergency physicians are reticent to support screening for diseases like HIV, often expressing concerns that systems are not in place to ensure disclosure and follow-up.[28] ED-based navigators, working in parallel with clinical staff, not only address this common barrier to implementation but have proven vital to the success and sustainability of screening programs. Often designated as community outreach workers, navigators can be trained to assist in all aspects of a screening program, serving as test result counselors, disease educators, case managers, social workers, insurance specialists, linkage specialists, and data managers. They address individual patient barriers and care needs and serve as a safety net for all patients screening positive.

Linkage Pathways

Appropriate systems for follow-up and treatment must be in place for patients screening newly positive for HIV, HCV, or syphilis, as well as for those previously infected but out of care and in need of treatment.[29] This essential yet logistically challenging element of successful screening programs is discussed in the next section. In brief, ED navigators are important facilitators of linkage and work closely with referral partners. Practice agreements between ED and clinic navigators are necessary to allow the free flow of patient information and assessment of follow-up metrics. Scheduled meetings between navigators to discuss cases, address barriers, and identify foci for improvement are recommended.

LINKAGE TO CARE FOR INFECTIONS IDENTIFIED THROUGH SCREENING

Successful linkage to care and treatment of ED patients identified with HIV, HCV, and/ or syphilis is challenging.[30] Screening programs must ensure support from institutional and community partners and local health jurisdictions to guarantee rapid, barrier-free access to outpatient services, as well as outreach for patients who cannot be reached and are lost to follow-up. The complexity and scope of a referral system will be driven by the types of ED screening, disease prevalence, insurance status, existing infrastructure, clinic capacity, and types of social determinants of health (SDOH) faced by patients requiring linkage.

EDs with the best outcomes employ a dedicated team of navigators responsible for supporting patients and collaborating with clinic networks to ensure timely follow-up and treatment. Success requires simultaneously addressing patients' SDOH, often through coordination between social services, street medicine teams, local health jurisdictions, and substance use and mental health specialists. A successful linkage to the care cascade also begins with timely result disclosure. Performing screening tests "STAT," if possible, allows for same-day result disclosure, counseling, and linkage planning. Navigators and ED clinicians can initiate treatment if appropriate, address barriers to outpatient follow-up, and confirm best contact information.

Immediate Emergency Department Treatment for Patients Screening Positive

Rapid antiretroviral treatment

EDs should consider developing protocols for same-day rapid initiation of ART for eligible patients who screen positive for HIV.[31,32] Rapid ART, defined as the initiation of ART within 7 days or as soon as possible for those newly diagnosed with HIV, has been shown to improve linkage to care and retention in care, reduce time to viral suppression, decrease viral transmission, and improve morbidity and mortality.[33–37] The results of a recently published study demonstrated that the initiation of ED rapid ART is feasible, well accepted, safe, and may be an important facilitator of linkage to care.[32] Organizations such as the Alameda Health System and East Bay Getting to Zero provide algorithms to assist in same-day ED Rapid ART, as summarized in **Box 2**.

Syphilis and hepatitis C virus

Similarly, the results of syphilis screening tests should be processed immediately by on-site laboratories so that treatment decisions can be made while patients are still in the ED, minimizing the need for syphilis callbacks and appointment scheduling for treatment. In addition, with the expansion of coverage for HCV antiviral treatment and the removal of prior authorizations in many states, coupled with the advent of rapid HCV RNA tests, ED providers may soon begin exploring the initiation of ED-based HCV antiviral therapy. Similar to ART and HIV, starting anti-HCV treatment of ED patients testing positive may facilitate follow-up in the outpatient setting.

Linkage to care in patients with substance use disorders

Patients with SUDs have increased rates of coinfections with HIV, HCV, and syphilis.[38] Linking ED patients with SUD to outpatient treatment of HIV, HCV, and syphilis is particularly challenging and often unsuccessful. One fortunate consequence of the national response to the opioid and substance use epidemic has been the development of ED Bridge Programs, which provide treatment of patients with SUD after they are

---

Box 2
ED-initiated rapid HIV antiretroviral treatment (rapid ART)[31,37]

- Disclose HIV result and offer treatment
- Laboratories
  - CBC, HIV viral load (RNA/ NAAT), HIV genotype, CD4 count, CMP, and pregnancy
  - Hepatitis B testing
  - Additional labs can be obtained at follow-up appointments, including comprehensive STI testing (including syphilis), hepatitis A and C, lipids, and tuberculosis screening.
- Screening questions to determine if it is safe to start rapid ART (*ineligible* if any of the following)
  - Previous ART
  - Symptoms of current opportunistic infections
    - Headache, visual change, diplopia, weakness, gait instability, confusion, seizure: cryptococcal meningitis, toxoplasmosis, tuberculosis meningitis, and cytomegalovirus retinitis.
    - Cough/shortness of breath greater than 1 week, respiration greater than 30: PCP pneumonia, pulmonary tuberculosis
    - Weight loss past month: *Mycobacterium avium* complex
  - Renal disease (estimated glomerular filtration rate [eGFR] <30 mL/min)
- Prescription for either (check with local institution):
  - *Biktarvy:* (BIC/FTC/TAF) 1 tab PO daily, 30 d supply,
    OR
  - If pregnant or potentially pregnant: *Tivicay:* Dolutegravir 50 mg 1 tab PO daily AND *Truvada:* (TDF/FTC) 1 tab PO daily, 30 day supply OR *Descovy* (TAF/FTC) 1 tab PO daily
- Warm hand-off to community providers via EHR messaging and phone contacts.
- HIV team intake within 2 days

discharged from the ED or hospital.[39–41] These programs take a harm reduction approach with flexible drop-in hours and are often staffed by a multidisciplinary team of pharmacists, social workers, navigators, and addiction specialists who provide stigma-free, nonjudgmental services.[39,41] As these low-barrier SUD clinics expand throughout the country, the need to integrate services beyond SUD to include treatment of coexisting infections like HIV, HCV, and syphilis—to colocalize SUD and infection disease treatment—has been identified as a promising innovation that deserves to be studied.[42–45] For example, the feasibility and cost-effectiveness of adding a part-time HIV or infectious disease specialist to the staff at a substance use clinic to manage coinfected patients, oversee prevention efforts, and provide guidance to addiction specialists should be explored.

Linkage to human immunodeficiency virus prevention and pre-exposure prophylaxis services in the emergency department
Recent CDC guidance on HIV prevention has broadened the groups that should be informed about HIV PrEP to all sexually active adults and adolescents.[46] ED clinicians may use the ED visit as an opportunity to provide education that patients may not receive elsewhere, educate patients from high prevalence groups or areas, and especially those with indications, should be prescribed PrEP. Indications for PrEP include shared IV injection equipment, condomless sex with partner(s) of unknown HIV status, STI in a man who has sex with men, or gonorrhea or syphilis in any sexually active person. With this expansion of the target education group, more eligible individuals may be identified through the ED and warrant linkage for continued PrEP services, as discussed later.

HUMAN IMMUNODEFICIENCY VIRUS PREVENTION AND PRE-EXPOSURE PROPHYLAXIS SERVICES IN THE EMERGENCY DEPARTMENT

Pharmacologic HIV prevention strategies include PrEP for at-risk patients and post-exposure prophylaxis (PEP) for those who have had a recent potential exposure. Recognizing the ongoing threat of HIV transmission and the development of new Food and Drug Administration-approved medications for PrEP, the CDC in 2021[46] and the USPSTF in 2023[47] issued reports in support of PrEP in persons at increased risk due to sexual activity or injection drug use. With the federal recognition of net benefit in the expansion of PrEP, and the relative underutilization of nonoccupational post-exposure prophylaxis (nPEP),[48] the ED can play a key role in expanding both of these opportunities with the linkage network and systems in place for follow-up care.

Rationale for Locating Human Immunodeficiency Virus Prevention/Pre-exposure Prophylaxis Services in the Emergency Department

EDs are well positioned to provide HIV prevention services, including PrEP, for patients who screen HIV negative. PrEP for patients at high risk of HIV acquisition is safe and well tolerated and significantly reduces the risk of acquiring HIV through sex by 99% and through injection drug use by 74%.[49–51] Despite being promoted as a key component in the National HIV/AIDS Strategy and the Ending the HIV Epidemic, however, PrEP uptake has been slow, and major disparities in PrEP use among racial, ethnic, gender, and economic lines exist.[52–55] Importantly, patients with opioid and stimulant use have alarmingly low rates of PrEP use, with recent estimates being less than 1 per 1000 individuals with SUD.[56]

Awareness of PrEP poses a major challenge for PrEP initiation. Data from the CDC found that only 32% of heterosexual adults who were at an increased risk for HIV were aware of PrEP,[55] and women and heterosexual men have low-PrEP uptake.[57] Those with increased behavioral HIV risk factors, and lower income,[58] had lower awareness of PrEP.[59]

HIV has a disparate impact on marginalized populations, such as racial/ethnic and sexual and gender minorities. Despite a high incidence of HIV infection in minority communities, PrEP use is lower and faces major implementation challenges.[54,60] Overlapping structural factors and social vulnerabilities such as low-income, intergenerational poverty, insecure housing and employment, incarceration, and stigma contribute both to higher HIV incidence and lower PrEP access and use.[61] Lower use of PrEP may also be to blame for a widening racial gap in HIV incidence that has been observed since oral PrEP was approved.[62]

EDs are critical access points for individuals at an increased risk for HIV. A recent review estimated up to a third of ED patients may be PrEP-eligible.[13] Black patients, a focus population for the Ending the HIV Epidemic, are overrepresented in national ED visits, constituting 22% of visits.[7] Moreover, certain groups (non-White, public insurance) that have a higher risk for STIs[63] — a known risk factor for HIV acquisition,[64-67] are also more likely to use the ED for care than an outpatient clinic.[68] Less than half of ED PrEP-eligible patients had prior knowledge of PrEP, and only a few that were interested in PrEP were ever prescribed it.[13]

Strategies and Recommendations for Implementing Emergency Department Human Immunodeficiency Virus Prevention/Pre-exposure Prophylaxis Services

Despite a growing body of implementation science research, best practice for implementing ED HIV prevention/PrEP services are still being evaluated. Strategies and recommendations for integrating HIV prevention/PrEP services into the ED setting are outlined in **Box 3** and discussed later. Many of the principles we recommend for successful communicable disease screening are applicable to a successful HIV prevention/PrEP services program. These include multidisciplinary collaborations and a reliance on dedicated navigators.

Building human immunodeficiency virus prevention/pre-exposure prophylaxis services on existing emergency department human immunodeficiency virus screening programs

Most ED HIV prevention programs are nested within a pre-existing HIV screening program; patients who screen HIV negative serve as the primary target population for prevention.[69-74] Recently, several US EDs have trialed HIV prevention programs as an expansion of their HIV screening programs. These programs have adopted a variety of screening criteria for PrEP eligibility and various models for real-time integration of HIV prevention education, counseling, and referral to outpatient comprehensive prevention services.[13,71,75] Several models have been described, ranging from interviewing patients who screen HIV negative using structured risk assessments based on CDC criteria to smart EHR algorithms that use natural language processing and/or laboratory data, to identify risk cohorts eligible for HIV prevention services.[69,76]

How to identify emergency department patients that might benefit from human immunodeficiency virus prevention/pre-exposure prophylaxis services

ED patients who screen HIV negative are not necessarily at an increased risk for acquiring HIV compared to ED patients who are not screened.[69] This means that an additional assessment of an individual's risk for acquiring HIV, beyond simply screening HIV negative, is a critical step in any ED prevention program. Determining the individual patient's risk of acquiring HIV infection is important to inform their need for and scope of HIV prevention services provided by a navigator. Estimating risk for acquiring HIV infection is typically based on responses to standard behavioral

Box 3
Best practice recommendations for integrating HIV prevention services/PrEP into emergency department processes

- The HIV prevention services program is led by an ED clinical champion in collaboration with infectious disease specialists, HIV specialists, laboratory managers, community partners, clinical pharmacists, hospital administration, and local health jurisdictions.
- Fund dedicated ED-based prevention navigators.
  - Completing risk assessments, providing ED-based prevention counseling, and linking eligible and interested patients to outpatient comprehensive prevention services, including PrEP, can be time-consuming and often require intensive case management and attention to social determinants of health. Referrals for interventions unrelated to, but important to, the success of HIV prevention, including housing assistance, behavioral health, and substance use management, are often required.
- ED HIV prevention services interventions may include basic HIV education, undetectable = untransmissible messaging, risk reduction counseling, instruction on proper condom use, PEP/PrEP education, substance use counseling and referral, and information on safe injection practices.
- HIV prevention services programs are usually integrated as an adjunct service within an existing HIV screening program and predicated on a framework that patients who screen HIV negative serve as the primary target population for HIV prevention.
- Characterizing risk for acquiring HIV infection is often based on responses to a standard behavioral risk assessment administered by a navigator, using questions adapted from CDC recommendations for PrEP.
  - Patients may be reluctant to disclose stigmatizing risk behaviors that may limit the efficacy of structured risk assessments.
  - Replacing traditional risk assessments with open-ended questions that emphasize an individual's sexual health goals and concerns may provide more accurate information about a patient's actual behavior, risk, and readiness for PrEP.
- Leverage the EHR to identify patients at an increased risk for HIV acquisition using automation.
  - Program the EHR to identify and/or flag eligible patients with objective risk criteria, such as injection drug use or recent positive STI tests.
  - Configure EHR algorithms that automatically add screening tests to any laboratory order initiated by clinicians.
- Consider developing policies that enable the rapid initiation of PrEP.
  - Rapid antiretroviral therapy is well accepted by ED patients newly diagnosed with HIV infection, reported to be "empowering," and may be a powerful motivator for linkage.
  - The same benefits may be seen with same-day PrEP initiation, although prospective effectiveness evaluations are needed.
- Develop a network of partnering clinics to provide rapid follow-up and treatment for comprehensive prevention treatment services.
  - Direct appointment scheduling and same-day appointments may improve outpatient follow-up.
- Colocalize outpatient comprehensive prevention services, including PrEP, with the receipt of care for other diseases associated with HIV acquisition, such as STIs and substance use disorders.

These strategies for integrating HIV Prevention/PrEP Services into ED processes are based on personal experience, webinars, review of the published literature, and interviews with key ED personnel across the United States. *Abbreviations:* ED, emergency department; EHR, electronic health record; PEP, postexposure prophylaxis; PrEP, pre-exposure prophylaxis; STI, sexually transmitted infection.

risk assessment, using structured questions adapted from CDC recommendations for PrEP eligibility.[77] Patients, however, may be reluctant to disclose stigmatizing risk behaviors, which can hamper risk assessments. Replacing traditional risk assessments with open-ended questions that emphasize an individual's sexual health goals and concerns may provide more accurate information about a patient's true behavior, risk, and readiness for PrEP.[78] Leveraging the EHR to automatically identify patients who may be at an increased risk using natural language processing to identify risk (eg, "injection drug use") and objective outcomes associated with HIV exposures (eg, positive STI test) may be efficient and less stigmatizing.

Linking patients to human immunodeficiency virus prevention/pre-exposure prophylaxis services
Many of the same strategies employed to facilitate linkage to care and treatment of patients identified with HIV, HCV, and syphilis also apply to patients referred to outpatient HIV prevention services. Follow-up from the ED for outpatient HIV prevention/PrEP services tends to be low, and there are limited reports on HIV prevention effectiveness, including the receipt of and adherence to PrEP for ED patients.[72,74,79]

Although initiating *same-day ED PrEP* reduces barriers to access, may increase patient uptake, and is supported by CDC guidelines, it remains largely unexplored by the ED.[77,80] Ongoing clinical trials are evaluating same-day PrEP utilizing ED-based starter packs, and published abstracts have found the feasibility of an ED-based PrEP immediate access program in which patients were discharged with a PrEP prescription, where 20% of patients accepted these additional services.[81] EDs with existing teams of navigators adept at outpatient warm-handoffs may consider developing their own same-day PrEP protocols based on CDC guidance.[77] Approaches may vary based on local needs, policies, and resources; important considerations are listed in **Box 4**. Same-day ED-PrEP implementation challenges include a lack of knowledge and familiarity with PrEP among ED providers, lack of laboratory data necessary before starting PrEP, lack of reliable, established referral networks for patient follow-up, and concerns about prescription coverage and out-of-pocket costs to patients. Prospective feasibility studies are needed that include patients who are at risk for HIV acquisition through needle sharing as well as sexual exposure and that assess PrEP adherence and long-term outcomes.

Low-barrier follow-up
Experience has shown that minimizing barriers to follow-up for outpatient HIV prevention and PrEP initiation will be critical to the success of any future ED HIV prevention programs. For example, direct appointment scheduling has been shown to improve outpatient follow-up for ED patients requiring primary care.[71] Mahal and colleagues described a protocol where ED navigators scheduled a same-day appointment with hospital-affiliated PrEP providers, with good results.[71]

Colocalization prevention/pre-exposure prophylaxis treatment
Another tool to improve linkage to PrEP services may be to colocalize HIV prevention services and PrEP treatment, with care for other diseases associated with HIV acquisition, such as STIs and SUDs.

Human Immunodeficiency Virus Nonoccupational Post-exposure Prophylaxis

Nonoccupational post-exposure prophylaxis is an essential intervention strategy to prevent the transmission of HIV following potential exposure.[83,84] When individuals present to the ED after recent condomless sex, sharing needles, or experiencing sexual assault, nPEP should be considered. HIV seroconversion is a low but nonzero risk after

---

Box 4
ED-initiated same-day HIV pre-exposure prophylaxis[46,82]

- Patient identification and eligibility:
  - Behavioral risk factors:
    - Sexually active AND either: inconsistent condom use, gonorrhea, chlamydia, or syphilis in the past 6 months
    - People with injection drug use and shared equipment
  - Clinical exclusion:
    - HIV positive, Acute HBV, Renal insufficiency (contraindicated if eGFR <60 mL/min for Truvada, or eGFR <30 mL/min for Descovy), caution osteoporosis or fragility fractures for Truvada
  - Screening eligibility questions:
    - No signs/symptoms of acute HIV if exposure within past 4 weeks (ie, fever with sore throat, rash, swollen lymph nodes, or headache)
    - No potential HIV exposure within 72 hours, consider nPEP instead
    - Reliable contact phone number for follow-up
- Laboratory tests:
  - HIV RNA, fourth-generation HIV antigen/antibody, HBV (surface antibody, core antibody, antigen), HCV antibody w/reflex, STI tests (gonorrhea/chlamydia throat/rectal/vaginal/urine as applicable) syphilis, trichomoniasis test for females, complete metabolic panel, and pregnancy test
- Potential options for ED same-day PrEP prescription:
  - *Truvada:* TDF/FTC 1 tab PO daily × 30 days
    - Alternative for patients with renal or bone dysfunction (exclusion—individuals at risk from vaginal sex or injection drug use):
      - *Descovy:* FTC/TAF 1 tab PO daily × 30 days
- Linkage to care:
  - Health care access—if available, an HIV navigator to assist with medication payment and 30 day follow-up PrEP appointment
  - Follow-up appointment within 30 days and then every 3 months.

---

sexual assault. For consensual sex, the HIV risk per act of vaginal intercourse is 0.08% and receptive anal intercourse is 1.38%, according to the CDC.[84] Nonoccupational postexposure prophylaxis is recommended due to substantial risk when a source is known to have HIV and the exposure is of the following anatomic areas: vagina, penis, rectum, eye, mouth, or other mucous membrane with the following fluids: blood, semen, vaginal secretions, and rectal secretions. Receptive (anal and vaginal) sex is higher risk than insertive (anal or vaginal) sex. If the source is of unknown HIV status, the clinician may offer nPEP on a case-by-case basis. Exposure to urine, nasal secretions, saliva, sweat, or tears is negligible risk for HIV acquisition. Nonoccupational postexposure prophylaxis involves a combination of antiretroviral medications, which should be initiated as soon as possible, ideally within 72 hours of exposure. ED clinicians play a crucial role in this time-sensitive intervention by assessing risk, counseling, and initiating nPEP. EDs should have a referral process to facilitate follow-up care and monitoring. In cases of sexual assault, the cost of PEP medications and care may qualify for reimbursement.[85] Despite the importance of nPEP, a recent study of ED clinicians found that 89% of respondents thought it was their responsibility to provide PEP, but only 40% felt they could confidently prescribe it, and only 25% had prescribed it in the last year.[86] While local protocols may vary, national guidelines for PEP are shown in **Box 5**. Individuals treated with nPEP, if at ongoing risk of HIV exposure, may consider transitioning to daily PrEP after completing PEP and testing negative for HIV.

Box 5
HIV nonoccupational post-exposure nonoccupational prophylaxis within 72 hours of exposure[82,83,87]

- Assess risk of HIV from exposure
- Screen for acute HIV infection: flu/mono-like symptoms, if so, add HIV viral load
- Laboratory tests:
  - HIV RNA, fourth-generation HIV antigen/antibody, HBV (surface antibody, core antibody, antigen), HCV antibody w/reflex, STI tests (gonorrhea/chlamydia throat/rectal/vaginal/urine as applicable) syphilis, trichomoniasis for females, complete metabolic panel, and pregnancy test
- Possible regimens (check with local formulary/infectious disease consultation):
  - *Truvada*[a]: TDF/FTC 1 tab PO once daily OR *Descovy*[a]: FTC/TAF 1 tab PO once daily AND
    Tivicay: dolutegravir 50 mg 1 tab PO daily OR *Isentress*[b]: raltegravir 400 mg 1 tab PO twice a day for 28 days
    - Alternate: *Biktarvy:* BIC/FTC/TAF 1 tab PO once daily for 28 days
- Follow-up:
  - Scheduled for HIV Ag/Ab retest 4 to 6 weeks after nPEP and 3 months
  - Assess and if appropriate, offer PrEP after 28 days of PEP

[a]Truvada: eGFR must be over ≥60 mL/min, Descovy: eGFR must be over ≥30 mL/min [b]If first trimester pregnancy or high pregnancy potential: Truvada AND Tivicay OR Isentress. Some institutions substitute dolutegravir for raltegravir. However, more recent guidance has found that exposure to dolutegravir has not been associated with an increased risk of congenital abnormalities.[88]

SUMMARY

EDs play a key role in ending epidemics of communicable infectious diseases, including HIV, HCV, and syphilis, through the integration of routine and targeted screening, rapid diagnosis, treatment, and outpatient linkage to long-term care. Wide scale adoption of these programs is achievable through EHR automation, clinical navigators, and collaborations with community treatment partners.

CLINICS CARE POINTS

- EDs can play a critical role in the screening, treatment, and prevention of communicable diseases like HIV, HCV, and syphilis, particularly for medically underserved populations who may not otherwise have health care access.
- National guidelines recommend routine screening for HIV and HCV at least once per lifetime and syphilis screening annually or more frequently for at-risk individuals, including pregnant women.
- EHRs have significantly improved the screening process, allowing for efficient integration of screening into ED operations and identification of eligible patients for testing.
- Successful ED communicable disease screening programs require multidisciplinary collaboration, consent processes, test selection, navigators to facilitate patient education, linkage to care, and follow-up processes.
- Rapid ART in the ED for patients testing positive for HIV can improve HIV health outcomes.
- Initiation of HIV PrEP and HIV nPEP is a developing field for EDs that holds promise to increase HIV prevention through ED-based education, immediate prescriptions, and referral.

DISCLOSURE

Dr White is supported by funding through Gilead Sciences, FOCUS; the California Department of Public Health, Office of AIDS (#23-10041); and the California Department of Public Health #22-11182). Dr Solnick has no financial disclosures. Dr White receives a non-research grant from Gilead Sciences, FOCUS. The Gilead FOCUS program is a public health initiative that supports HIV, hepatitis C virus, and hepatitis B virus screening, prevention, and linkage to a first appointment. This work was prepared by the authors in a personal capacity. The opinions expressed in this article are those of the authors and do not necessarily reflect the views of their affiliated institutions, employers, or funding agencies. Dr Solnick has no disclosures.

REFERENCES

1. Branson BM, Handsfield HH, Lampe MA, et al. Revised recommendations for HIV testing of adults, adolescents, and pregnant women in health-care settings. MMWR Recomm Rep (Morb Mortal Wkly Rep) 2006;55(RR-14):1–17 [quiz: CE1–4]. Available at: https://www.ncbi.nlm.nih.gov/pubmed/16988643.
2. US Preventive Services Task Force, Owens DK, Davidson KW, et al. Screening for HIV infection. JAMA 2019;321(23):2326.
3. Schillie S, Wester C, Osborne M, et al. CDC recommendations for hepatitis C screening among adults — United States, 2020. MMWR Recomm Rep (Morb Mortal Wkly Rep) 2020;69(2):1–17.
4. US Preventive Services Task Force, Mangione CM, Barry MJ, et al. Screening for Syphilis Infection in Nonpregnant Adolescents and Adults: US Preventive Services Task Force Reaffirmation Recommendation Statement. JAMA 2022;328(12):1243–9.
5. Bloodborne Pathogens in Emergency Medicine. Available at: https://www.acep.org/patient-care/policy-statements/bloodborne-pathogens-in-emergency-medicine. [Accessed 1 February 2024].
6. California Department of Public Health. Opt-Out ED HIV, HCV, and Syphilis Screening. 2022. Available at: https://www.cdph.ca.gov/Programs/CID/DCDC/CDPH%20Document%20Library/DCL-Opt-Out-ED-HIV-HCV-and-Syphilis-Screening.pdf. (Accessed 3 January 2024).
7. Cairns C. and Kang K., National Hospital Ambulatory Medical Care Survey: 2020 Emergency Department Summary Tables. National Center for Health Statistics. Available at: chrome-extension://efaidnbmnnnibpcajpcglclefindmkaj/https://www.cdc.gov/nchs/data/nhamcs/web_tables/2020-nhamcs-ed-web-tables-508.pdf. (Accessed 1 February 2024).
8. Cohen RA, Martinez ME, Cha AE, Terlizzi EP. Health insurance coverage: Early release of estimates from the National Health Interview Survey, January–June 2021. National Center for Health Statistics 2021.
9. Galbraith JW, Willig JH, Rodgers JB, et al. Evolution and Escalation of an Emergency Department Routine, Opt-out HIV Screening and Linkage-to-Care Program. Public Health Rep 2016;131(Suppl 1):96–106.
10. Stanford KA, Hazra A, Schneider J. Routine opt-out syphilis screening in the emergency department: A public health imperative. Acad Emerg Med 2020;27(5):437–8.
11. Ford J, Chechi T, Toosi K, et al. Universal screening for hepatitis C virus in the ED using a best practice advisory. West J Emerg Med 2021;22(3). https://doi.org/10.5811/westjem.2021.1.49667.

12. Galbraith JW, Anderson ES, Hsieh YH, et al. High prevalence of hepatitis C infection among adult patients at four urban emergency departments - Birmingham, Oakland, Baltimore, and Boston, 2015-2017. MMWR Morb Mortal Wkly Rep 2020;69(19):569–74.

13. Gormley MA, Nagy TR, Moschella P, et al. HIV Preexposure Prophylaxis in the Emergency Department: A Systematic Review. Ann Emerg Med 2022. https://doi.org/10.1016/j.annemergmed.2022.07.015.

14. Hoover KW, Huang YLA, Tanner ML, et al. HIV Testing Trends at Visits to Physician Offices, Community Health Centers, and Emergency Departments - United States, 2009-2017. MMWR Morb Mortal Wkly Rep 2020;69(25):776–80.

15. Hsieh YH, Wilbur L, Rothman RE. HIV testing in U.S. emergency departments: at the crossroads. Acad Emerg Med 2012;19(8):975–7.

16. Haukoos JS. The impact of nontargeted HIV screening in emergency departments and the ongoing need for targeted strategies. Arch Intern Med 2012;172(1):20.

17. Galbraith JW, Franco RA, Donnelly JP, et al. Unrecognized chronic hepatitis C virus infection among baby boomers in the emergency department. Hepatology 2015;61(3):776–82.

18. Galbraith JW, Anderson ES, Hsieh Y, et al. High Prevalence of Hepatitis C Infection Among Adult Patients at Four Urban Emergency Departments —. MMWR Morb Mortal Wkly Rep 2015–2017;69(2020):569–74.

19. Centers for Disease Control, State HIV Testing Laws: Consent and Counseling Requirements, Available at: https://www.cdc.gov/hiv/policies/law/states/testing.html (Accessed 2 February 2024).

20. White DAE, Todorovic T, Petti ML, et al. A comparative effectiveness study of two nontargeted HIV and hepatitis C virus screening algorithms in an urban emergency department. Ann Emerg Med 2018;72(4):438–48.

21. Larios Venegas A, Melbourne HM, Castillo IA, et al. Enhancing the routine screening infrastructure to address a syphilis epidemic in Miami-Dade County. Sex Transm Dis 2020;47(5S):S61–5.

22. Ford JS, Chechi T, Otmar M, et al. ED syphilis and gonorrhea/chlamydia cotesting practices before and after the implementation of an electronic health record-based alert. Emerg Med J 2021. https://doi.org/10.1136/emermed-2020-210331.

23. Stanford KA, Hazra A, Friedman E, et al. Opt-out, routine emergency department syphilis screening as a novel intervention in at-risk populations. Sex Transm Dis 2021;48(5):347–52.

24. Haas O, Maier A, Rothgang E. Machine learning-based HIV risk estimation using incidence rate ratios. Front Reprod Health 2021;3. https://doi.org/10.3389/frph.2021.756405.

25. Bernard MB, Centers for Disease Control and Prevention (U.S.), S. Michele O, et al. Laboratory Testing for the Diagnosis of HIV Infection : Updated Recommendations 2. Centers for Disease Control and Prevention 2014. https://doi.org/10.15620/cdc.23447.

26. Ortiz DA, Shukla MR, Loeffelholz MJ. The traditional or reverse algorithm for diagnosis of syphilis: Pros and cons. Clin Infect Dis 2020;71(Supplement_1):S43–51.

27. Satyaputra F, Hendry S, Braddick M, et al. The Laboratory Diagnosis of Syphilis. J Clin Microbiol 2021;59(10):e0010021.

28. Arbelaez C, Wright EA, Losina E, et al. Emergency provider attitudes and barriers to universal HIV testing in the emergency department. J Emerg Med 2012;42(1):7–14.

29. Weber W, Heins A, Jardine L, et al. Principles of Screening for Disease and Health Risk Factors in the Emergency Department. Ann Emerg Med 2022. https://doi.org/10.1016/j.annemergmed.2022.06.015.

30. Houri I, Horowitz N, Katchman H, et al. Emergency department targeted screening for hepatitis C does not improve linkage to care. World J Gastroenterol 2020;26(32):4878–88.

31. East Bay Getting to Zero, HIV Access, Alameda Health System. HIV Rapid ART: Emergency Department Algorithm, Available at: https://www.ebgtz.org/wp-content/uploads/2020/12/AHS-ED-Rapid-ART-algorithm-v.3.19.21.pdf. (Accessed: 11 November 2023).

32. White DAE, Jewett M, Burns M, et al. Implementing a rapid antiretroviral therapy program using starter packs for emergency department patients diagnosed with HIV infection. Open Forum Infect Dis 2023;10(7). https://doi.org/10.1093/ofid/ofad292.

33. McNulty M, Schmitt J, Friedman E, et al. Implementing Rapid Initiation of Antiretroviral Therapy for Acute HIV Infection Within a Routine Testing and Linkage to Care Program in Chicago. J Int Assoc Provid AIDS Care 2020;19. 2325958220939754.

34. Michienzi SM, Barrios M, Badowski ME. Evidence Regarding Rapid Initiation of Antiretroviral Therapy in Patients Living with HIV. Curr Infect Dis Rep 2021;23(5):7.

35. Nosyk B, Audoin B, Beyrer C, et al. Examining the evidence on the causal effect of HAART on transmission of HIV using the Bradford Hill criteria. AIDS 2013;27(7):1159–65.

36. Cohen MS, Chen YQ, McCauley M, et al. Prevention of HIV-1 infection with early antiretroviral therapy. N Engl J Med 2011;365(6):493–505.

37. Rapid ART. East Bay Getting to Zero. Available at: https://www.ebgtz.org/rapid/. [Accessed 27 November 2023].

38. Serota DP, Barocas JA, Springer SA. Infectious complications of addiction: A call for a new subspecialty within infectious diseases. Clin Infect Dis 2020;70(5):968–72.

39. Snyder H, Kalmin MM, Moulin A, et al. Rapid adoption of low-threshold buprenorphine treatment at California emergency departments participating in the CA bridge program. Ann Emerg Med 2021;78(6):759–72.

40. Taylor JL, Wakeman SE, Walley AY, et al. Substance use disorder bridge clinics: models, evidence, and future directions. Addict Sci Clin Pract 2023;18(1). https://doi.org/10.1186/s13722-023-00365-2.

41. CA bridge program. DHCS Opioid Response. Published April 10, 2019. Available at: https://californiamat.org/matproject/california-bridge-program/. [Accessed 1 February 2024].

42. Harvey L, Taylor JL, Assoumou SA, et al. Sexually transmitted and blood-borne infections among patients presenting to a low-barrier substance use disorder medication clinic. J Addict Med 2021;15(6):461–7.

43. Gryczynski J, Nordeck CD, Mitchell SG, et al. Pilot studies examining feasibility of substance use disorder screening and treatment linkage at urban sexually transmitted disease clinics. J Addict Med 2017;11(5):350–6.

44. Yu J, Appel P, Rogers M, et al. Integrating intervention for substance use disorder in a healthcare setting: practice and outcomes in New York City STD clinics. Am J Drug Alcohol Abuse 2016;42(1):32–8.

45. Serota DP, Bartholomew TS, Tookes HE. Evaluating differences in opioid and stimulant use-associated infectious disease hospitalizations in Florida, 2016–2017. Clin Infect Dis 2021;73(7):e1649–57.

46. Centers for Disease Control and Prevention, Preexposure Prophylaxis for the Prevention of HIV Infection in the United States – 2021 Update Clinical Practice Guideline, Available at: https://www.cdc.gov/hiv/pdf/risk/prep/cdc-hiv-prep-guidelines-2021.pdf, 2021. (Accessed 11 Novemebr 2023).

47. Final Recommendation Statement. Prevention of Acquisition of HIV: Preexposure Prophylaxis. 2023. Available at: https://www.uspreventiveservicestaskforce.org/uspstf/document/RecommendationStatementFinal/prevention-of-human-immuno deficiency-virus-hiv-infection-pre-exposure-prophylaxis. [Accessed 2 February 2024].

48. Wang Z, Zou H. P566 The uptake of non-occupational HIV postexposure prophylaxis among MSM: a systematic review and meta-analysis. Sex Transm Infect 2019;95(Suppl 1):A255.

49. Grant RM, Lama JR, Anderson PL, et al. Preexposure chemoprophylaxis for HIV prevention in men who have sex with men. N Engl J Med 2010;363(27):2587–99.

50. Choopanya K, Martin M, Suntharasamai P, et al. Antiretroviral prophylaxis for HIV infection in injecting drug users in Bangkok, Thailand (the Bangkok Tenofovir Study): a randomised, double-blind, placebo-controlled phase 3 trial. Lancet 2013;381(9883):2083–90.

51. Baeten JM, Donnell D, Ndase P, et al. Antiretroviral prophylaxis for HIV prevention in heterosexual men and women. N Engl J Med 2012;367(5):399–410.

52. Shull JA, Attys JM, Amutah-Onukagha NN, et al. Utilizing emergency departments for pre-exposure prophylaxis (PrEP). J Am Coll Emerg Physicians Open 2020;1(6):1427–35.

53. The White House, National HIV/AIDS Strategy for the United States 2022-2025, Available at: https://files.hiv.gov/s3fs-public/NHAS-2022-2025.pdf, 2021. (Accessed 2 October 2023).

54. Huang YLA, Zhu W, Smith DK, et al. HIV Preexposure Prophylaxis, by Race and Ethnicity - United States, 2014-2016. MMWR Morb Mortal Wkly Rep 2018;67(41):1147–50.

55. Baugher AR, Trujillo L, Kanny D, et al. Racial, Ethnic, and Gender Disparities in Awareness of Preexposure Prophylaxis Among HIV-Negative Heterosexually Active Adults at Increased Risk for HIV Infection - 23 Urban Areas, United States, 2019. MMWR Morb Mortal Wkly Rep 2021;70(47):1635–9.

56. Streed CG Jr, Morgan JR, Gai MJ, et al. Prevalence of HIV preexposure prophylaxis prescribing among persons with commercial insurance and likely injection drug use. JAMA Netw Open 2022;5(7):e2221346.

57. Siegler AJ, Mouhanna F, Giler RM, et al. The prevalence of pre-exposure prophylaxis use and the pre-exposure prophylaxis–to-need ratio in the fourth quarter of 2017, United States. Ann Epidemiol 2018;28(12):841–9.

58. Namara D, Xie H, Miller D, et al. Awareness and uptake of pre-exposure prophylaxis for HIV among low-income, HIV-negative heterosexuals in San Francisco. Int J STD AIDS 2021;32(8):704–9.

59. Keddem S, Dichter ME, Hamilton AB, et al. Awareness of HIV Preexposure Prophylaxis Among People at Risk for HIV: Results From the 2017-2019 National Survey of Family Growth. Sex Transm Dis 2021;48(12):967–72.

60. Schneider JA, Bouris A, Smith DK. Race and the Public Health Impact Potential of Pre-Exposure Prophylaxis in the United States. J Acquir Immune Defic Syndr 2015;70(1):e30–2.

61. Millett GA, Peterson JL, Flores SA, et al. Comparisons of disparities and risks of HIV infection in black and other men who have sex with men in Canada, UK, and USA: a meta-analysis. Lancet 2012;380(9839):341–8.

62. CDC. HIV in the United States by Race/Ethnicity: HIV Diagnoses. Centers for Disease Control and Prevention. 2023. Available at: https://www.cdc.gov/hiv/group/racialethnic/other-races/diagnoses.html. [Accessed 1 July 2023].

63. Ware CE, Ajabnoor Y, Mullins PM, et al. A retrospective cross-sectional study of patients treated in US EDs and ambulatory care clinics with sexually transmitted infections from 2001 to 2010. Am J Emerg Med 2016;34(9):1808–11.

64. Wasserheit JN. Epidemiologies! Synergy: Interrelationships between Human Immunodeficiency Virus Infection and Other Sexually Transmitted Diseases. Sex Transm Dis 1992;19(2):61–77. Available at: http://www.jstor.org/stable/44964413.

65. Fleming DT, Wasserheit JN. From epidemiological synergy to public health policy and practice: the contribution of other sexually transmitted diseases to sexual transmission of HIV infection. Sex Transm Infect 1999;75(1):3–17.

66. Bernstein KT, Marcus JL, Nieri G, et al. Rectal gonorrhea and chlamydia reinfection is associated with increased risk of HIV seroconversion. J Acquir Immune Defic Syndr 2010;53(4):537–43.

67. Katz DA, Dombrowski JC, Bell TR, et al. HIV Incidence Among Men Who Have Sex With Men After Diagnosis With Sexually Transmitted Infections. Sex Transm Dis 2016;43(4):249–54.

68. Jamison CD, Greenwood-Ericksen M, Richardson CR, et al. Association between Chlamydia and routine place for healthcare in the United States: NHANES 1999-2016. PLoS One 2021;16(5):e0251113.

69. Haukoos JS, White DAE, Rowan SE, et al. HIV Risk and Pre-Exposure Prophylaxis Eligibility Among Emergency Department Patients. AIDS Patient Care STDS 2021;35(6):211–9.

70. Kulie P, Castel AD, Zheng Z, et al. Targeted screening for HIV pre-exposure prophylaxis eligibility in two emergency departments in Washington, DC. AIDS Patient Care STDS 2020;34(12):516–22.

71. Mahal J, Deccy S, Seu R. Linking emergency department patients at risk for human immunodeficiency virus to pre-exposure prophylaxis. Am J Emerg Med 2022;54:87–90.

72. Ridgway JP, Almirol EA, Bender A, et al. Which Patients in the Emergency Department Should Receive Preexposure Prophylaxis? Implementation of a Predictive Analytics Approach. AIDS Patient Care STDS 2018;32(5):202–7.

73. Faryar KA, Ancona RM, Braun RS, et al. Estimated proportion of an urban academic emergency department patient population eligible for HIV preexposure prophylaxis. Am J Emerg Med 2021;48:198–202.

74. Zhao Z, Jones J, Arrington-Sanders R, et al. Emergency Department-Based Human Immunodeficiency Virus Preexposure Prophylaxis Referral Program-Using Emergency Departments as a Portal for Preexposure Prophylaxis Services. Sex Transm Dis 2021;48(8):e102–4.

75. Jackson KJ, Chitle P, McCoy SI, et al. A Systematic Review of HIV Pre-exposure Prophylaxis (PrEP) Implementation in U.S. Emergency Departments: Patient Screening, Prescribing, and Linkage to Care. J Community Health 2023. https://doi.org/10.1007/s10900-023-01320-7.

76. Carlisle NA, Booth JS, Rodgers JB, et al. Utilizing laboratory results to identify emergency department patients with indications for HIV pre-exposure prophylaxis. AIDS Patient Care STDS 2022;36(8):285–90.

77. Centers for Disease Control and Prevention. US Public Health Service. Preexposure prophylaxis for the prevention of HIV infection in the United States—2021 Update: a clinical practice guideline. Published 2021. https://www.cdc.gov/hiv/pdf/risk/prep/cdc-hiv-prep-guidelines-2021.pdf. [Accessed 1 January 2023].

78. Golub SA. PrEP stigma: Implicit and explicit drivers of disparity. Curr HIV AIDS Rep 2018;15(2):190–7.
79. Stanford KA, Almirol E, Eller D, et al. Routine, opt-out, emergency department syphilis testing increases HIV PrEP uptake. Sex Transm Dis 2023. https://doi.org/10.1097/OLQ.0000000000001774.
80. Kamis KF, Marx GE, Scott KA, et al. Same-day HIV pre-exposure prophylaxis (PrEP) initiation during drop-in sexually transmitted diseases clinic appointments is a highly acceptable, feasible, and safe model that engages individuals at risk for HIV into PrEP care. Open Forum Infect Dis 2019;6(7):ofz310.
81. Dashler G, Rudolph D, Cho MH, et al. 322 A Novel, Emergency Department Based Human Immunodeficiency Virus Preexposure Prophylaxis Program. Academic Emergency Medicine SAEM23 Abstracts 2023. https://doi.org/10.1111/acem.14718.
82. AETC Pacific AIDS Education and Training Center. Clinical Essentials: HIV testing, Rapid ART, PEP, PrEP. Published May 2023. Available at: https://www.ebgtz.org/wp-content/uploads/2023/08/HIV-testing-PEP-PrEP-rapid-ART-2-pager-v.2023.pdf. [Accessed 2 February 2024].
83. AIDS Education and Training Center Program. nPEP Non-Occupational Post-Exposure HIV prevention. Published November 2021. Available at: https://aidsetc.org/sites/default/files/resources_files/AETC-nPEP-guide-111721.pdf. [Accessed 1 February 2024].
84. Workowski K, Bachmann L, Chan P, et al. Sexually Transmitted Infections Treatment Guidelines, 2021. Morbidity and Mortality Weekly Report (MMWR) Recomm Rep 2021;70:2021. Available at: https://www.cdc.gov/std/treatment-guidelines/STI-Guidelines-2021.pdf.
85. Paying for PEP. Published July 13, 2022. Available at: https://www.cdc.gov/hiv/basics/pep/paying-for-pep.html. [Accessed 2 July 2023].
86. O'Connell KA, Kisteneff AV, Gill SS, et al. HIV post-exposure prophylaxis in the emergency department: An updated assessment and opportunities for HIV prevention identified. Am J Emerg Med 2021;46:323–8.
87. nPEP Quick Guide for Providers. Available at: https://aidsetc.org/resource/npep-quick-guide-providers. [Accessed 2 July 2023].
88. Recommendations for the Use of Antiretroviral Drugs During Pregnancy and Interventions to Reduce Perinatal HIV Transmission in the United States. Integrase Inhibitors. Available at: https://clinicalinfo.hiv.gov/en/guidelines/perinatal/safety-toxicity-arv-agents-integrase-inhibitors-dolutegravir-tivicay. (Accessed 2 February 2024).

The Intersection of Substance Use Disorders and Infectious Diseases in the Emergency Department

Erik S. Anderson, MD[a,b,*], Bradley W. Frazee, MD[a]

KEYWORDS

- Social determinants of health • Infectious diseases • Substance use
- Human immunodeficiency syndrome • Hepatitis C virus

KEY POINTS

- Infectious diseases and substance use commonly intersect and are deeply influenced by social determinants of health.
- Emergency medicine has developed a deeper understanding of how these conditions overlap, as well as how they can be treated more comprehensively.
- Emergency departments can implement strategies to treat and refer patients with co-occuring substance use disorders and infectious diseases.
- Substance use navigators and low-threshold clinics offer important opportunities for emergency departments to integrate substance use and infectious disease services.
- Harm reduction services have robust evidence and can be integrated into emergency department substance use programs.

INTRODUCTION

Encounters with alcohol and other substance use disorders (SUDs) are increasingly common in emergency departments (EDs). Approximately 1 in 11 ED visits and 1 in 9 hospitalizations are related to SUDs, with increases seen over the last decade.[1] Additionally, mortality rates continue to rise, with more than 100,000 deaths attributed to drug overdoses in 2021 and nearly 100,000 deaths attributed to excessive alcohol use per year.[2,3] It is now well recognized that integrating SUD treatment into emergency medicine practice has important population health benefits; perhaps most importantly, EDs can be a point of entry for treatment initiation for SUDs for patients otherwise unconnected to the health care system.[4,5]

[a] Department of Emergency Medicine, Alameda Health System, Wilma Chan Highland Hospital, 1411 East 31st Street, Oakland, CA 94602, USA; [b] Division of Addiction Medicine, Highland Hospital, Alameda Health System, 1411 East 31st Street, Oakland, CA 94602, USA
* Corresponding author.
E-mail address: esoremanderson@gmail.com

Emerg Med Clin N Am 42 (2024) 391–413
https://doi.org/10.1016/j.emc.2024.02.004
0733-8627/24/© 2024 Elsevier Inc. All rights reserved.

emed.theclinics.com

A significant contributor to SUD-related mortality are co-occurring infectious diseases, which range from acute conditions, such as necrotizing soft tissue infections (NSTIs), to more chronic diseases including human immunodeficiency virus (HIV) and hepatitis C virus (HCV).[6] Approaching this intersection of SUD and infectious diseases requires a framework that addresses both conditions in parallel, while also integrating social factors that further affect morbidity and mortality.

In this article, we use a lens of common SUDs and practices, including *opioid use disorder (OUD), alcohol use disorder (AUD), stimulant use disorders (StUD), and injection drug use (IDU)*, to frame the diagnosis and treatment of co-occurring infectious diseases. We hope to provide emergency clinicians with a deeper understanding of these complex and intersecting conditions, and introduce cutting-edge approaches for screening, diagnosis, and linkage to care from the ED.

SUBSTANCE USE DISORDER TREATMENT IN THE EMERGENCY DEPARTMENT: A NEW PARADIGM

The treatment of SUDs is an increasingly important part of emergency medicine clinical practice. The most common substances that impact clinical care in the ED include opioids, alcohol, and stimulants. **Table 1** shows medications and other effective treatments that can be deployed in the ED for each of these SUDs. Many EDs have become central to population health approaches and treatment initiation for OUD.[5] This is, in large part, because EDs are the only part of the United States health care system open to anyone, any day, and any time. A landmark study by D'Onofrio and colleagues at Yale found that ED patients started on buprenorphine had 78% engagement in addiction treatment after ED discharge compared with 37% who had a brief intervention and referral to treatment; this study set the stage for widespread implementation of OUD treatment in EDs across the country.[5,7,8] For the treatment of AUD, the Food and Drug Administration (FDA) has approved several medications, and EDs are beginning to use these in treatment protocols with positive results.[9,10] StUD, including methamphetamine and cocaine use disorder, is increasingly prevalent in United States EDs; while there are no FDA-approved pharmacotherapies for StUD, some EDs have developed dedicated treatment pathways for ED patients who use stimulants, which include evidence-based pharmacotherapy.[4,11–13]

Even as SUD treatment in the ED is increasingly recognized as essential, it does constitute an undeniable paradigm shift for emergency medicine that some clinicians may be reluctant to embrace. While this shift to ED-based SUD treatment is important in its own right, leveraging it to improve the diagnosis and management of co-occurring infectious diseases represent an opportunity to further improve population health outcomes in the communities in which EDs are located.

OPIOID USE DISORDER

Emergency medicine is on the front lines of the opioid epidemic. OUD-related acute care encounters have skyrocketed in the last decade, with more than 1 million ED visits in 2021.[14] Alongside this epidemic, there has been a rise in infectious disease complications from OUD, including HIV, HCV, skin and soft tissue infections (SSTIs), bacterial endocarditis, and osteomyelitis.[6] Treatment outcomes for these infections are tied not only to early recognition and management of the infection itself, but also to how well OUD can be managed. Fortunately, OUD has very effective medical therapy in the form of buprenorphine and methadone. The number needed to treat, with either medication, to prevent return to illicit opioid use, is 2, with a 50% reduction in all-cause mortality.[15–18]

Table 1
Approved and commonly used pharmacotherapy for addiction treatment

Substance Use Disorder	Approved Medications[a]	Off-Label Medications with Varying Levels of Evidence	Comments
Opioids	Buprenorphine Methadone Extended-release naltrexone	—	NNT 2 to prevent illicit opioid use; 50% reduction in all-cause mortality. Buprenorphine most commonly implemented in EDs
Alcohol	Naltrexone (oral or extended-release) Disulfiram Acamprosate	Gabapentin Topiramate Baclofen	Naltrexone NNT 12 to prevent return to heavy drinking. Gabapentin NNT as low as 8 for alcohol abstinence in some studies; gabapentin can also be used for alcohol withdrawal as monotherapy or as an adjunct
Methamphetamines	—	Bupropion Mirtazapine Extended-release naltrexone	Mixed evidence, most often used by addiction specialists
Cocaine	—	Disulfiram	Mixed evidence, most often used by addiction specialists

[a] Food and Drug Administration-approved medications. ED, emergency department; NNT, number needed to treat.

Opioid Use Disorder and Blood-Borne Viral Infections: Human Immunodeficiency Virus, Hepatitis C Virus, and Hepatitis B Virus

Global strategic goals for HIV are known as 90-90-90, and aim to have 90% of all people living with HIV to know their status, 90% of those who know their status receive treatment, and 90% of those on treatment that achieve viral suppression.[18] Largely driven by injection opioid use, OUD is estimated to account for approximately 1 in 10 new cases of HIV.[19] Notable outbreaks of HIV have occurred among networks of people who inject drugs, most notably in Scott County, Indiana, and northeastern Massachusetts.[20,21] It is also clear that successful HIV treatment among patients who also have OUD is closely correlated with successful SUD treatment. Multiple studies have found that providing medications for OUD (MOUD) leads to higher rates of viral suppression and increased retention in HIV care.[22,23]

People with OUD also have significantly higher rates of HCV, again largely driven by IDU. Some studies have found up to an over 40% prevalence of HCV among patients who inject drugs.[24] People who inject drugs are estimated to account for 80% of new HCV infections worldwide and 60% of current infections.[25] With the advent of curative direct-acting antiviral treatments for HCV, developing successful HCV screening strategies has become critical. Focusing screening and treatment efforts on people who inject drugs is one of the highest priority strategies to eliminate HCV.[26] As an example of the potential impact for this population, modeling has shown that in a community of people who inject drugs with a chronic HCV prevalence of 25%, treating 40 per 1000 patients with chronic HCV annually could reduce the prevalence of HCV approximately 90% within 15 years.[27] This suggests that efforts to identify patients with HCV in the ED and link them to care are likely to be much more impactful when paired with ED-based substance use treatment and linkage to care.

Hepatitis B virus is also closely tied to OUD and IDU. Effective implementation of HBV vaccination over the previous several decades initially led to a decrease in the prevalence of HBV across the United States; however, the opioid epidemic and IDU have been linked to a surge in cases of HBV.[28] The Center for Disease Control recommends that all patients with OUD be offered HBV screening wherever they interact with the health care system.[29] In one study among people experiencing homelessness in Los Angeles, California, the prevalence of HBV was 7 to 10 times higher than the general population in the United States with OUD and IDU each as independent predictors of infection.[30]

ED-based programs for treatment and linkage to care for various SUDs will tend to support ED-based screening efforts for blood-borne viral infections, and vice versa. In our institution, screening for blood-borne viral infections occurs alongside substance use treatment, with linkage to a low-threshold clinic that is capable of treating HIV, HCV, as well as any SUD. There are significant advantages to co-located SUD and infectious disease treatment in the same clinic, which will be discussed later in this article, and models for parallel linkage from the ED for linkage are relatively novel and deserve ongoing formal study. One simple strategy to help pair SUD treatment and infectious disease screening is through electronic health record ordersets, and an example of the orderset from our institution can be found in **Table 2**. See also the article in this issue, "Communicable Disease Screening in the Emergency Department."

METHAMPHETAMINE AND COCAINE USE DISORDERS

Methamphetamine and other amphetamine-related substances are the second most commonly used illicit substances in the world, trailing only cannabis.[31] Methamphetamines, cocaine, and other psychostimulants including 3,4-methylenedioxymethamphetamine (also known as "ecstasy") contribute to nearly half of all overdose deaths in the United States; additionally, EDs and hospitals have seen a significant increase in visits, particularly on the West Coast, over the past decade.[1,32,33] While there are no medications for methamphetamine and cocaine use disorders approved by the FDA, there are several promising behavioral and pharmacologic treatments utilized by Addition Medicine clinicians.[11,12,34]

The top 3 reasons for ED visits related to stimulant use are related to psychiatric emergencies but are closely followed by sepsis and SSTIs.[1] In addition, people who use methamphetamine have high rates of sexually transmitted infections, including gonorrhea, chlamydia, and syphilis, as well as HIV and HCV.[35–40] Rates of bacterial sexually transmitted infections (STIs) have been found to be up to 3 times higher

Table 2
Order panel for blood-borne viral and sexually transmitted infections for patients with substance use disorders

Screening Test	Automated Reflex Confirmatory Testing
HIV antigen/antibody	HIV-1/HIV-2 antibody differentiation assay and HIV quantitative viral load
Hepatitis C virus antibody	HCV viral load and genotype
Hepatitis B virus serologies (surface antibody, surface antigen, and core antibody)	—
Treponemal antibody (Reverse sequence algorithm)	RPR and RPR titer
Gonorrhea and chlamydia	—
CBC and metabolic panel with liver function testing	—
Consult SUD treatment	—

Exact orders may vary based on local laboratory preferences.
Abbreviation: RPR, rapid plasma reagin.

among patients with methamphetamine use disorder. Patients who use methamphetamine represent 1 in 3 new HIV seroconversions among sexual and gender minorities and have a 5 to 10 times higher rate of chronic HCV infection compared to patients who do not use methamphetamines.[39,40] There are also some data to suggest that chronic pulmonary damage related to inhalational use of cocaine can lead to higher rates of pulmonary tuberculosis (TB).[41] Lastly, some communities who use drugs to enhance sexual experiences, also know as "chemsex," will use stimulants with or without other substance including alcohol or newer psychoactive drugs such as gamma-hydroxybutyric acid, gamma-butyrolactone, and mephedrone. This population is particularly at high risk for STI acquisition and transmission.[42]

Stimulant Use and Syphilis

Rates of syphilis had reached a low point in the year 2000, with sporadic cases largely isolated to communities of men who have sex with men (MSM); however, from 2000 to 2013, there was an increase in syphilis rates among MSM, followed by a rise in cases among heterosexual men and women.[43,44] Along with these trends has come an alarming rise in congenital syphilis in the United States, with a 460% increase from 2012 to 2019.[45,46]

The increase in syphilis incidence in the last decade is, in part, connected to increases in methamphetamine use, heroin use, IDU, and to sex with people who inject drugs.[44,47] The Center for Disease Control found that nearly 10% of patients with primary and secondary syphilis reported methamphetamine use, compared to 1% who reported heroin use, supporting other data that show a strong link between stimulant use and sex.[44] Methamphetamine use is also associated with high-risk sexual behaviors, including having multiple sexual partners, infrequent condom usage, and sex work.[48] While the link between rising stimulant use and syphilis transmission has caught the recent attention of public health officials, a similar phenomenon occurred with rising cocaine usage and risky sexual behaviors in the 1980s and 1990s.[49] In a recent study of birthing parents in California, rates of congenital syphilis were highest among people using methamphetamines and those experiencing homelessness, and increasing access to prenatal care improved outcomes for patients regardless of their substance use or housing status.[46]

There have also been several reports describing successful integration of SUD services into STI clinics, as well as programs that integrate STI screening and treatment into low-threshold SUD clinics.[50–52] Emergency physicians who are interested in developing programs for either substance use or STI screening, should consider pathways to integrate screening and treatment processes.

INJECTION DRUG USE

There are between 1.8 and 7.2 million people who inject drugs in the United States, according to a 2023 estimate.[53] Drugs can be injected at almost any anatomic location, and IDU encompasses intravenous, intramuscular, and subcutaneous injecting with needles. Traditionally, heroin has been the main drug that was injected, but injection of stimulants and other drugs has increased in recent years.[53] There are also significant regional differences; for example, approximately 50% of overdose deaths in the Northeast and Midwest involved IDU, as compared to 30% to 40% in the West and Southern United States, where smoking and intranasal routes of substance use are more common.[53] Rates of IDU and acute care visits for bacterial infections are directly linked, with highest rates of hospitalization in those demographic groups that also have the highest rates of IDU.[54,55]

Injection Drug Use and Skin and Soft Tissue Infections

SSTIs encompass cellulitis, abscesses, and NSTIs. These infections are common in people who inject drugs. While largely the result of nonsterile injection itself, there are some data to suggest that methamphetamines produce a particular impairment of the local immune response.[56] IDU can introduce bacteria into the dermis, subdermal tissues, and muscle, as well as the blood stream, from a number of sources, including skin flora, contaminated supplies, or other impurities in the drug itself. Tar heroin was known for its many impurities and bacterial contaminants, including spore-forming clostridial species, like *Clostridium perfringens* and *Clostridium botulinum*. However, as patterns of substance use have changed and fentanyl has begun to supplant heroin in the drug market, it is less common to see bacterial contamination in the drugs themselves. Rather, high rates of SSTIs are increasingly related to injection practices and high-frequency use patterns.[57,58] Additionally, the introduction of specific adulterants into the drug market, most notably xylazine, has contributed to an increase of severe SSTIs among people who inject drugs.[59]

Table 3 shows the typical microbiology of SSTIs and their management. Most IDU-related NSTIs are purulent (abscesses with or without associated purulent cellulitis). Older studies reported that methicillin-resistant *Staphylococcus aureus* (MRSA) infections were more common among patients who use methamphetamines, though more recent data have called this into question.[56,57] An ED study conducted in Colorado in 2007 to 2012 found slightly lower rates of MRSA, but more streptococcal and anaerobic bacteria in IDU-related as compared to non-IDU-related cutaneous abscesses.[56] Polymicrobial abscesses are also common.[58] The etiologic pathogen responsible for nonpurulent cellulitis—lacking a culturable focus—among people who inject drugs is unclear. While beta-hemolytic streptococci predominate in typical cases of nonpurulent cellulitis, some experts caution that MRSA should be considered a potential pathogen in people who inject drugs, and covered empirically in this population, especially if the patient is febrile.[60] The bacteriology of NSTIs, which may be monomicrobial (type 2) or polymicrobial (type 1), includes *Streptococcus* species, *Staphylococcus* species

Table 3
Microbiology and clinical considerations for skin and soft tissue infections and invasive bacterial infections in patients who use injection drugs

Infection	Microbiology	Diagnostic Considerations	Management
Abscess and purulent cellulitis	S aureus (incl. MRSA) most common; streptococcal species; abscesses may be polymicrobial and include oral-type anaerobic bacteria	Consider culture of pus for recurrent abscesses or those warranting admission	For abscess, incision and drainage is mandatory. Cover MRSA with trimethoprim/ sulfamethoxazole, doxycycline, linezolid, or vancomycin
Nonpurulent cellulitis	Beta-hemolytic streptococci; proportion due to S aureus unclear in IDU population	Strongly consider blood cultures prior to empiric therapy in PWID and febrile cellulitis	Provide streptococcal and MSSA coverage with cephalexin, dicloxacillin, and cefazolin. In febrile cases, consider MRSA coverage with linezolid, vancomycin
NSTI	Often polymicrobial; staphylococcal species, streptococcal species, anaerobes incl. clostridial species	Contrast CT scan is the recommended initial imaging modality. Obtain emergent surgical consultation for exploration	Emergent surgical debridement required. Typical recommended broad antimicrobial regimen: Pip/tazo or amp/sulbactam plus vancomycin plus clindamycin; may substitute linezolid for vancomycin plus clindamycin
Pyogenic spinal infections	S aureus (incl MRSA) most common; streptococcal species; gram-negative bacteria, incl. P aeruginosa; Candida spp rarely implicated	Contrast MRI of the entire spine is the recommended initial imaging modality. C-reactive protein and erythrocyte sedimentation rate almost always elevated. Obtain blood cultures prior to empiric therapy	Cover common gram-positive (incl. MRSA) and gram-negative pathogens. Typical recommended regimen: vancomycin plus cefixime

(continued on next page)

		Diagnostic	
Table 3 **(continued)**			
Infection	**Microbiology**	**Considerations**	**Management**
IE	S aureus most common; high rates of polymicrobial infections. Fungal infections rare but increasing	Three sets of blood cultures and formal echocardiography recommended when suspected. Infectious disease, cardiology consultation recommended; cardiothoracic surgery consultation, depending on echocardiography results	Vancomycin. Adjust regimen to isolate species and susceptibility as soon as possible. Surgery often indicated; eg, acute valvular heart failure and perivalvular extension

(including MRSA), and anaerobes—both so-called oral anaerobes and *Clostridium* species. Gram-negative bacteria are less commonly implicated. NSTIs that are related to injection of tar heroin are distinguished by the predominance of the spore-forming anaerobic species, *C perfringens* and *Clostridium sordelli*.[60] Purulent SSTIs that require hospitalization should undergo wound/pus culture. Blood cultures should be strongly considered in people who inject drugs who are febrile with an SSTI.

Diagnosis of cutaneous abscesses is often straightforward and can be aided by the use of point-of-care ultrasound.[61] A thorough search for a pus pocket is recommended before concluding that a cutaneous infection is nonpurulent. Identifying an NSTI is notoriously challenging.[62] Since IDU is a leading risk factor for this life-threatening form of SSTI, occult NSTI should be considered in all IDU-related SSTIs and whenever a person who injects drugs presents with musculoskeletal pain or swelling. While laboratory findings such as extreme leukocytosis and hyponatremia may offer a clue to the diagnosis, immediate computed tomographic scanning or surgical exploration are required to evaluate suspected NSTI.[63]

Cutaneous abscesses should be drained in the ED, with the addition of adjunctive antibiotics as needed. Whether to alter empiric antimicrobial selection based on drug use behavior is not clear, with limited prospective data that predate the emergence of community-associated MRSA. Experts generally maintain that MRSA and streptococcal gram-positive coverage is adequate, even for IDU-related abscesses, where anaerobic bacteria are frequently isolated.[59,64] While immediate surgical debridement is the cornerstone of NSTI treatment, broad empiric antimicrobial treatment should provide excellent, streptococcal, MRSA and anaerobic coverage, and should include either clindamycin or linezolid (see **Table 3**).

Using an SUD lens, emergency providers can view many of these infections as preventable. Initiating SUD treatment in the ED, with successful linkage and long-term treatment, may lead to a reduction in IDU-associated SSTIs.[65] Since particular injection practices and used or shared equipment are linked to SSTI incidence, incorporating a harm reduction approach, such as providing clean needles, should be a routine component of comprehensive treatment of SSTIs in people who inject drugs[66] (see "Harm Reduction" section).

Injection Drug Use and Osteomyelitis, Spinal Epidural Abscess, and Paraspinous Abscess

The frequent bacteremia associated with IDU and SSTIs can lead to a variety of hematogenous orthopedic infections, including osteomyelitis and septic arthritis. We focus here on pyogenic spinal infections, a group of often overlapping infections, which include spinal osteomyelitis, paraspinous abscess (eg, psoas abscess), and spinal epidural abscess.[67] While rare in the overall ED patient population, IDU is a leading risk factor for these infections, accounting for up to 60% of spinal epidural abscess cases, with rates increasing in parallel with the opioid epidemic and IDU.[68] The presentation is typically subtle and nonspecific, so initial misdiagnosis occurs in roughly 50% of cases.[69,70] Diagnostic delay is associated with often irreversible neurologic deficits. Compared to non-IDU-related cases, pyogenic spinal infections in PWID have longer hospitalizations, higher surgery rates, and higher monetary costs.[71]

Microbiology of the various subtypes of pyogenic spinal infections is similar[67,68] (see **Table 3**). *S aureus* is by far the most common pathogen, with MRSA accounting for roughly one-third of *S aureus* isolates. Coagulase-negative *Staphylococcus* and other skin commensals can cause infection following a spinal procedure. Gram-negative bacteria account for roughly 5-20% of cases, with *Pseudomonas aeruginosa* associated in particular with IDU.[69] *Candida* vertebral osteomyelitis can occur in PWID, as well as in immunocompromised patients.[72]

Back or neck pain is the most common—and sometimes only—presenting symptom. About one-half of patients are febrile. Neurologic signs or symptoms, including radiculopathy or bowel and bladder dysfunction, are present in about one-third of those with a spinal epidural abscess.[69] This lack of specific findings underscores the importance of recognizing IDU as a major red flag in patients with back pain.[72] Inflammatory markers, particularly erythrocyte sedimentation rate and C-reactive protein, are elevated in 80% to 100% of cases.[69,73] Gadolinium-enhanced MRI is the imaging study of choice. Because about 20% of infections involve multiple spinal regions, and may skip regions, imaging of the entire spine has been recommended to evaluate suspected pyogenic spinal infection.[67] Up to 60% of patients are bacteremic, not infrequently from associated endocarditis, so blood cultures prior to empiric antibiotics are mandatory, and knowing the blood isolate susceptibilities may obviate the need for an invasive biopsy for culture.

Patients with neurologic findings and spinal epidural abscess on MRI require immediate neurosurgical consultation for decompressive surgery; timely surgery (typically defined as within 24 hours) has been associated with better neurologic outcome.[69] Empiric antibiotics should cover MRSA and gram-negative bacteria, including *P aeruginosa* in the case of IDU-related infections[69] (see **Table 3**). Standard therapy entails a 6 week course of parenteral antibiotics, which can be challenging in people who inject drugs. Treatment failure is reduced when co-occurring substance use is treated aggressively by a multidisciplinary team that includes addiction medicine specialists[74,75] (see later discussion).

Injection Drug Use and Infectious Endocarditis

Infectious endocarditis (IE) is a notorious complication of IDU, which results from frequent bacteremia and occult valve damage caused by injected material. In parallel with the opioid epidemic, hospitalization for IDU-related IE doubled from 2008 to 2014, with the proportion of cases linked to IDU exceeding 50% in some hard-hit communities.[76] Development of injection-related endocardial damage, which disproportionately affects the right side of the heart, is poorly understood, but IE tends to be a mark of advanced IDU.[77] The source of bacteria may be from skin flora, cutaneous abscess, or material used in injection practices, like cottons, cookers, syringes, and water used to dilute drugs. The microbiology of IDU-related IE does not differ meaningfully from other forms of IE in developed nations, where *S aureus* has emerged as the most common pathogen, with MRSA accounting for almost 15% of cases.[78]

IE presents in myriad ways, from subacute febrile illness with nonspecific symptoms like headache and myalgias, to acute heart failure, to altered mental status or focal neurologic deficits from central nervous system septic emboli. The presentation in people who inject drugs is distinguished by a higher proportion of tricuspid vegetations and septic pulmonary emboli, which can easily be mistaken for simple pneumonia.[77] Fever is present during the ED visit in about 80% of cases. While a murmur is heard during hospitalization in 68% of IE cases, it is rarely picked up in the ED. Peripheral embolic and vascular stigmata of IE (splinter hemorrhages, Janeway lesions, and Osler's nodes) together are detected in only about 15% of contemporary case series.[78,79] With such varied and nonspecific symptoms and often subtle signs, diagnosis of IE depends on having a very low threshold for initiating diagnostic testing in any PWID with a febrile illness.

The critical diagnostic first steps are to obtain 3 sets of blood cultures and order comprehensive echocardiography. A nondiagnostic transthoracic echocardiogram should be followed by a transesophageal study, which is significantly more sensitive for vegetations and cardiac complications of IE. A person who injects drugs with a fever and suspected IE should be admitted to the hospital. There is limited guidance on empiric antibiotic therapy since isolate-targeted therapy is critical, but until MRSA has been excluded, vancomycin is considered the essential, and likely sufficient, empiric agent in suspected IDU-related IE. Confirmed IE generally requires 4 to 6 weeks of antimicrobial therapy. Transition to oral therapy in selected patients is increasingly accepted for both left-sided and right-sided infections and has been validated in populations of patients who inject drugs.[80,81] Emergency providers must be aware of the indications for emergent surgical treatment, as modern IE therapy entails cardiothoracic surgery in about half of cases.[82]

Treatment of invasive staphylococcal infections like IE and pyogenic spinal infections typically involves long hospitalizations, followed by a period of close outpatient care. In people who inject drugs, the SUD and often other social barriers conspire to complicate clinical care, resulting in poor outcomes. In-hospital mortality for patients with IDU-related IE is as high as 8%, with up to a 34% mortality 1 year after initial hospitalization.[83–85] It is therefore critical that these patients receive treatment for their underlying SUD during hospitalization. The importance of a multidisciplinary "endocarditis team," composed of infectious disease, cardiology and cardiothoracic surgery specialists, has been promoted in current IE guidelines; in the case of IDU-related IE, the addition of an addiction medicine specialist is crucial.[86] Unsurprisingly, patients with IDU-related IE and other invasive staphylococcal infections who undergo simultaneous treatment of OUD have improved outcomes compared to patients not treated for their underlying SUD.[74] Hospital-based collaborations between infectious disease experts and addiction medicine specialists are cost-effective and have been shown to reduce readmissions, self-directed discharges, and all-cause mortality, largely driven by fewer overdoses and improved infection outcomes.[87,88]

ALCOHOL USE DISORDER

AUD is a significant public health issue across the world and has increased in prevalence in recent years.[89] Alcohol-related deaths account for approximately 1 in 10 deaths in the United States and cost the health care system upward of US$40 billion annually.[90,91] ED patients with AUD have a 6.5 times higher all-cause mortality rate than demographically similar peers.[92] Unfortunately, despite this burden of disease, and the availability of effective treatments, the vast majority of patients with AUD remain untreated. Additionally, the overlap between AUD and infectious disease complications is often underrecognized by clinicians.[93] Recognizing and treating AUD with evidence-based treatments, especially when it intersects with infectious diseases, can improve outcomes[90,94] (see **Table 1**).

Alcohol Use Disorder and Community-Acquired Pneumonia and Tuberculosis

Patients with AUD have higher rates of lower respiratory infections compared to patients without AUD.[95] In a meta-analysis, AUD was found to be a risk factor for acquisition of community-acquired pneumonia (CAP), and there appears to be a dose response; patients with higher amounts of alcohol intake had higher rates of CAP.[95] A recent study of patients with CAP requiring hospitalization found that while the microbiology of CAP is similar between those with and without AUD, clinical outcomes were worse in the AUD group, with higher rates of ventilator use, mortality, and hospital length of stay and costs.[96,97] While the exact mechanism for this relationship is unclear, it is likely that AUD causes an underlying immunocompromised state, as well as possibly higher rates of aspiration from impaired gag reflex during alcohol intoxication.[98] Additionally, the clinical course can be more complicated for patients with AUD hospitalized with CAP because of associated comorbidities and the development of alcohol withdrawal during hospitalization.[96]

Alcohol use has long been associated with higher rates of incident TB infection, as well as reactivation of disease and treatment failure.[99] This is thought to be due to a complex array of factors, including impaired immune responses, social barriers to healthcare services and the long course of treatment required for TB. TB is closely tied to social deprivation; specifically, marginalized and congregate housing situations, like shelters and incarceration – all of which are also associated with AUD and other substance use. This confluence of social determinants of health (SDOH), AUD, and active TB infection are more prevalent globally, with an estimated 10% of all TB infections attributable to alcohol worldwide.[100] Unfortunately, there are no studies that examine the impact of AUD treatment on TB treatment outcomes. However, with AUD treatment rates ranging from only 5% to 15%, there is certainly room to improve care for this population.[101,102]

Emergency clinicians have an opportunity to improve care for patients with AUD and CAP or TB infections. Practical strategies at the bedside include screening for and recognizing concurrent AUD in patients with suspected lower respiratory infections, having a lower threshold to admit patients with CAP and AUD to the hospital, and screening for TB in this population. Additionally, it is imperative not only to recognize alcohol withdrawal in ED patients but also to implement early withdrawal protocols including prophylaxis. There are several scoring systems that can be used to predict alcohol withdrawal, and these systems can help cue early treatment of patients who are at higher risk when admitted for any reason.[103] ED visits and hospitalizations in this population should be viewed as an opportunity to initiate AUD treatment, and there is an increasing interest and evidence regarding AUD treatment of ED and hospitalized patients.[10,104] Formal addiction medicine consult teams represent an important new paradigm for providing state-of-the-art AUD treatment of hospitalized patients. Having these services improves rates of AUD treatment and leads to shorter hospital length of stay and higher rates of linkage to care and treatment engagement after hospital discharge.[87,88,105]

NEW PARADIGMS: EMERGENCY DEPARTMENT SUBSTANCE USE NAVIGATORS AND LOW-THRESHOLD CLINICS

Successful integration of substance use and infectious disease management in the ED is dependent not only on recognizing the clinical overlap between these disease types, but also on embracing novel systems of care that "de-silo" clinical services that traditionally have been distinct. In the past, infectious disease management and substance use management operated independently, but there has been a growing recognition in recent years that providing these services alongside one another from start to finish is much more patient-centered and potentially more effective.[106,107]

In our institution, we have integrated SUD and communicable disease screening and initial treatment in the ED with a simplified linkage pathway that funnels patients to a single low-threshold co-located SUD and infectious disease clinic. The foundation of this program is a group of dedicated substance use navigators.[4] Navigators may have lived experience with substance use, though this is not a requirement. Some have training as community health workers or licensed substance use counselors. Their main role is to develop relationships with patients, help develop personalized treatment plans, provide bedside brief interventions, navigate barriers to SUD services in the community, and accompany patients across traditionally siloed aspects of the health care system. Navigators maintain a formal clinical footprint in the ED and hospital wards as well as in the dual SUD and infectious disease clinic. This program is predicated on a whole-person care framework, using a harm reduction lens and personalized treatment plans. Navigators, as well as substance use and infectious disease specialists in the clinic, seek to "meet patients where they are." In this way, SDOH and substance use are addressed and integrated into infection-related treatment.

This approach of co-locating treatment of SUD and infectious diseases has been formally evaluated at other centers, and there is increasing evidence that this novel paradigm is effective and improves outcomes for patients.[52,106,107] Implementing these programs in the ED can be complex, however, requiring a multidisciplinary approach, with emergency physicians, addiction medicine specialists, and infectious disease specialists collaborating together. (Various implementation strategies and best practices are discussed further in the "Communicable Disease Screening in the Emergency Department" article, in this volume.) Technical assistance is available through CA Bridge, a large organization that supports EDs that seek to implement SUD and infectious disease programs across the country.[108] As the number of programs and their experience grows, the approach to integrating emergency care, SUD treatment, and infectious disease treatment will naturally evolve. Meanwhile, more research is needed to establish and disseminate best practices.[109]

HARM REDUCTION

Harm reduction is an approach to treatment that engages directly with people who use drugs and alcohol and aims to reduce deaths and infectious disease transmission.[110] The notion of harm reduction, which does not expect abstinence as a treatment goal, has a robust literature base supporting it.[111–123] **Box 1** discusses common harm reduction interventions and supplies. While most harm reduction programs are community-based, there are increasing efforts to integrate harm reduction services into hospital-based care. A first step for many institutions may be the adoption of destigmatizing language and policies. Using "patient with opioid use disorder" as opposed to "addict" or "drug user," for example, is a simple way clinicians can model destigmatizing language for their departments. Such "person first" language can help reframe substance use as a disease rather than a character flaw.

Box 1
Common harm reduction supplies, interventions, and strategies

Supplies	Notes
Naloxone	Overdose education and naloxone distribution can be targeted toward patients, community members, or the family of patients. The FDA recently approved naloxone to be available over the counter. Naloxone distribution is widely viewed as a life-saving intervention and has been adopted across a wide variety of community and hospital-based care settings.
Fentanyl test strips	Fentanyl tests strips can be distributed to patients to test their own drugs for the presence of fentanyl. Various types are available, and test characteristics may limit their utility in some instances. Many harm reduction experts advise using test strips along with "test doses"—that is, using a small amount of a drug initially—to mitigate the harms of unintentional fentanyl use.
Clean syringes and sharps disposal	Offering clean syringes and sharps disposal has been shown to decrease the transmission of HIV and hepatitis C virus. Most syringe service programs are based in the community, though there are some examples of programs in hospital-based and ED settings.
Safe smoking supplies	Rubber smoking kits and clean supplies to prepare drugs for smoking can prevent transmission of blood-borne viral infections and decrease the risks of inhalational injuries from drugs.
Safe injection kits	Safe injection kits, distinct from clean syringes, will offer clean supplies used in preparation for injecting drugs; these supplies may include alcohol swabs, cookers, cotton balls, and tourniquets. These supplies can prevent blood-borne viral infections from shared equipment, SSTIs, or the injection of impurities from the drugs themselves.
Condoms and safer sex kits	Condoms and safer sex kits can be distributed alongside other harm reduction supplies; these may be particularly useful in certain communities, especially in those where drugs are used to enhance sexual experiences.
Personal hygiene supplies	Personal hygiene kits can include soap, deodorant, hand sanitizer, tampons, or toothbrushes. These kits can help to prevent a variety of infectious diseases.

| Educational materials on safer use of drugs and alcohol | There are a variety of handouts that can be distributed to patients to help provide tips for the safer use of drugs and alcohol. These may include patient-oriented advice including: do not use drugs alone, use test doses prior to a full dose, keep naloxone nearby with a trusted friend or family member, use in safe place, alternate hard alcohol with water or beer, do not use while driving, and avoid mixing drugs together. |

Harm reduction toolkits are available through the Substance Abuse and Mental Health Services Administration at samhsa.gov/find-help/harmreduction; we highly recommend partnering with local community-based harm reduction organizations.

Syringe service programs (SSPs), which distribute clean needles, syringes, and other sterile equipment to people who use drugs, represent another well-known, evidence-based harm reduction strategy. These programs are cost-effective and have been shown to reduce SSTI incidence, rates of HIV seroconversion and HCV transmission, while increasing rates of entrance into substance use treatment.[113–122] In fact, people who engage with SSPs are 5 times more likely to start substance use treatment and 3 times more likely to stop using drugs compared to people who do not access SSPs.[115] When SSPs and MOUD services are offered together—which can occur during an ED visit or hospitalization—HIV and HCV transmission is reduced by two-thirds.[122] The Centers for Disease Control and Prevention explicitly supports SSPs and provides a technical support package with strategies for effective implementation.[124]

In our institution, we have a formal partnership with one of the longest running harm reduction organizations on the United States West Coast, called the HIV Education and Prevention Project of Alameda County (HEPPAC). HEPPAC is contracted to provide on-site substance use navigation and harm reduction counseling for patients with SUDs in the ED and throughout the hospital, as well as supply harm reduction kits that

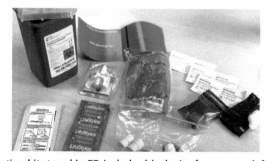

Fig. 1. Harm reduction kit stored in ED includes (clockwise from *upper left*): sharps container, naloxone spray, syringes, alcohol pads, rubber pipes, clean cottons, tourniquet and one-use cooker, condoms, and fentanyl test strips. Kits furnished courtesy of HEPPAC. Photo is of Medicine Kits and medicines. Kits furnished courtesy of HIV Education and Prevention Project of Alameda County (HEPPAC). Instagram HEPPAC_OAKLAND (@heppac_oakland) •Instagram photos and videos [https://www.instagram.com/heppac_oakland/] & Facebook HIV Education and Prevention Project of Alameda County Facebook [https://www.facebook.com/IHEARTHEPPAC/].

contain clean syringes and sharps containers.[125] Our ED itself is a certified SSP, which can provide safe injection supplies and other harm reduction tools, like rubber pipes for smoking, wound care supplies, fentanyl test strips, naloxone, and condoms (**Fig. 1**). Certain harm reduction supplies and intranasal naloxone can also be obtained for free in our ED lobby from a large electronic dispenser, similar to a soft drink vending machine.[126] While harm reduction has traditionally focused on people who inject drugs, our hospital has also adopted evidence-based harm reduction approaches for AUD, including when patients are hospitalized for infections or other conditions. Harm reduction in the contest of AUD may not directly reduce the transmission of infectious diseases but can reduce alcohol intake with attendant improvement in overall health.[123]

SUMMARY

Patients with concurrent SUD and infectious diseases frequently present to EDs. These patients require an approach to care that simultaneously and effectively treats both conditions. Such an approach constitutes a potential paradigm shift for emergency care. Yet experience and evidence are growing, which shows that integrating SUD treatment with infectious disease treatment, while using a harm reduction approach and addressing other SDOH, can mitigate infectious disease transmission, reduce disease burden, and improve the overall health of the community that an ED serves.

CLINICS CARE POINTS

- Infectious disease complications of IDU, related to underlying opioid and SUD, include blood-borne viral infections, superficial and NSTIs, and invasive orthopedic infections and IE.
- Stimulant use disorder is closely linked to rising rates of sexually transmitted infections, particularly syphilis.
- AUD can lead to pneumonia and TB, and significantly worsens the prognosis of these infections.
- Effective SUD treatment stands to both prevent and improve treatment of many types of severe infection.
- Many novel approaches to combined SUD and infectious disease treatment are being developed by emergency medicine researchers and piloted in the ED.
- Evidence-based, and highly cost-effective, harm reduction strategies can be deployed directly from the ED.
- Availability of SUD and communicable disease navigators, and low-barrier outpatient clinics that can manage both SUD and infectious diseases, are critical to the success of these cutting-edge programs.

DISCLOSURE

The authors have no conflicts of interest to disclose.

REFERENCES

1. Suen LW, Makam AN, Snyder HR, et al. National Prevalence of Alcohol and Other Substance Use Disorders Among Emergency Department Visits and Hospitalizations: NHAMCS 2014-2018. J Gen Intern Med 2022;37(10):2420–8.

2. Dyer O. A record 100 000 people in the US died from overdoses in 12 months of the pandemic, says CDC. BMJ 2021;375:2865–6.
3. Esser MB, Sherk A, Liu Y, et al. Deaths and years of potential life lost from excessive alcohol use – United States, 2011-2015. MMWR Morb Mortal Wkly Rep 2020;69:1428–33.
4. Anderson ES, Rusoja E, Luftig J, et al. Effectiveness of Substance Use Navigation for Emergency Department Patients With Substance Use Disorders: An Implementation Study. Ann Emerg Med 2023;81(3):297–308.
5. Snyder H, Kalmin MM, Moulin A, et al. Rapid Adoption of Low-Threshold Buprenorphine Treatment at California Emergency Departments Participating in the CA Bridge Program. Ann Emerg Med 2021;78(6):759–72.
6. Serota DP, Barocas JA, Springer SA. Infectious Complications of Addiction: A Call for a New Subspecialty Within Infectious Diseases. Clin Infect Dis 2020; 70(5):968–72.
7. D'Onofrio G, O'Connor PG, Pantalon MV, et al. Emergency department-initiated buprenorphine/naloxone treatment for opioid dependence: a randomized clinical trial. JAMA 2015;313(16):1636–44.
8. D'Onofrio G, Edelman EJ, Hawk KF, et al. Implementation Facilitation to Promote Emergency Department-Initiated Buprenorphine for Opioid Use Disorder. JAMA Netw Open 2023;6(4):e235439.
9. Murphy CE 4th, Coralic Z, Wang RC, et al. Extended-Release Naltrexone and Case Management for Treatment of Alcohol Use Disorder in the Emergency Department. Ann Emerg Med 2023;81(4):440–9.
10. Anderson ES, Chamberlin M, Zuluaga M, et al. Implementation of Oral and Extended-Release Naltrexone for the Treatment of Emergency Department Patients With Moderate to Severe Alcohol Use Disorder: Feasibility and Initial Outcomes. Ann Emerg Med 2021;78(6):752–8.
11. Coffin PO, Santos GM, Hern J, et al. Effects of Mirtazapine for Methamphetamine Use Disorder Among Cisgender Men and Transgender Women Who Have Sex With Men: A Placebo-Controlled Randomized Clinical Trial. JAMA Psychiatr 2020;77(3):246–55.
12. Trivedi MH, Walker R, Ling W, et al. Bupropion and Naltrexone in Methamphetamine Use Disorder. N Engl J Med 2021;384(2):140–53.
13. Simpson SA, Wolf C, Loh RM, et al. Evaluation of the BEAT Meth Intervention for Emergency Department Patients with Methamphetamine Psychosis. J Addict Med 2023;17(1):67–73.
14. Substance Abuse and Mental Health Services Administration. (2022). Drug Abuse Warning Network: Findings from Drug-Related Emergency Department Visits, 2021 (HHS Publication No. PEP22-07-03-002). Rockville, MD: Center for Behavioral Health Statistics and Quality, Substance Abuse and Mental Health Services Administration, Available at: https://www.samhsa.gov/data/. Accessed December 18, 2024.
15. Heikkinen M, Taipale H, Tanskanen A, et al. Real-world effectiveness of pharmacological treatments of opioid use disorder in a national cohort. Addiction 2022; 117(6):1683–91.
16. Larochelle MR, Bernson D, Land T, et al. Medication for Opioid Use Disorder After Nonfatal Opioid Overdose and Association With Mortality: A Cohort Study. Ann Intern Med 2018;169(3):137–45.
17. Santo T Jr, Clark B, Hickman M, et al. Association of Opioid Agonist Treatment With All-Cause Mortality and Specific Causes of Death Among People With Opioid Dependence: A Systematic Review and Meta-analysis. JAMA Psychiatr

2021;78(9):979–93 [published correction appears in JAMA Psychiatry. 2021 Sep 1;78(9):1044] [published correction appears in JAMA Psychiatry. 2022 May 1;79(5):516] [published correction appears in JAMA Psychiatry. 2023 Sep 1;80(9):972].

18. UNAIDS (2017). Ending AIDS Progress towards the 90-90-90 targets.
19. UNAIDS, Global AIDS update: confronting inequalities, Available at: https://www.unaids.org/sites/default/files/media_asset/2021-global-aids-update_en.pdf. Accessed December 18, 2024.
20. Peters PJ, Pontones P, Hoover KW, et al. Indiana HIV Outbreak Investigation Team HIV infec-tion linked to injection use of oxymorphone in Indiana, 2014–2015. N Engl J Med 2016;375:229–39.
21. Randall LM, Dasgupta S, Day J, et al. An outbreak of HIV infection among people who inject drugs in northeastern Massachusetts: findings and lessons learned from a medical record review. BMC Publ Health 2022;22:257.
22. Springer SA, Di Paola A, Azar MM, et al. Extended-Release Naltrexone Improves Viral Suppression Among Incarcerated Persons Living With HIV With Opioid Use Disorders Transitioning to the Community: Results of a Double-Blind, Placebo-Controlled Randomized Trial. J Acquir Immune Defic Syndr 2018;78(1):43–53.
23. Springer SA, Qiu J, Saber-Tehrani AS, et al. Retention on buprenorphine is associated with high levels of maximal viral suppression among HIV-infected opioid dependent released prisoners. PLoS One 2012;7(5):e38335.
24. Degenhardt L, Peacock A, Colledge S, et al. Global prevalence of injecting drug use and sociodemographic characteristics and prevalence of HIV, HBV, and HCV in people who inject drugs: a multistage systematic review. Lancet Global Health 2017;5(12). e1192–e1207.
25. Grebely J, Larney S, Peacock A, et al. Global, regional, and country-level estimates of hepatitis C infection among people who have recently injected drugs. Addiction 2019;114(1):150–66.
26. Day E, Hellard M, Treloar C, et al. Hepatitis C elimination among people who inject drugs: Challenges and recommendations for action within a health systems framework. Liver Int 2019;39(1):20–30.
27. Martin NK, Vickerman P, Grebely J, et al. Hepatitis C virus treatment for prevention among people who inject drugs: Modeling treatment scale-up in the age of direct-acting antivirals. Hepatology 2013;58(5):1598–609.
28. Johansson ED, Nunez M. Acute Hepatitis B Surge: Opioid Epidemic Implication and Management Challenges. Open Forum Infect Dis 2020;7(6):ofaa190.
29. Center for Disease Control. Viral Hepatitis. Available at: https://www.cdc.gov/hepatitis/hbv/testingchronic.htm. [Accessed 23 August 2023].
30. Khouzam Nour MD, Gelberg Lillian MD, MSPH, et al. Opiate Dependence: A Risk Factor for Hepatitis B Virus Exposure in Homeless Adults. Fam Community Health 2020;43(2):161–9.
31. United Nations Office on Drugs and Crime. Drug Statistics and Trends. Available at: https://www.unodc.org/documents/wdr/WDR_2010/2.0_Drug_statistics_and_Trends.pdf. [Accessed 23 August 2023].
32. Winkelman TNA, Admon LK, Jennings L, et al. Evaluation of Amphetamine-Related Hospitalizations and Associated Clinical Outcomes and Costs in the United States. JAMA Netw Open 2018;1(6):e183758.
33. Kariisa M, Seth P, Scholl L, et al. Drug Overdose Deaths Involving Cocaine and Psychostimulants with Abuse Potential among Racial and Ethnic Groups –

United States, 2004-2019. Drug Alcohol Depend 2021;227. https://doi.org/10.1016/j.drugalcdep.2021.109001.

34. Ronsley C, Nolan S, Knight R, et al. Treatment of stimulant use disorder: A systematic review of reviews. PLoS One 2020;15(6):e0234809.

35. Colfax GN, Mansergh G, Guzman R, et al. Drug use and sexual risk behavior among gay and bisexual men who attend circuit parties: a venue-based comparison. J Acquir Immune Defic Syndr 2001 Dec 1;28(4):373–9.

36. Shannon K, Strathdee S, Shoveller J, et al. Crystal methamphetamine use among female street-based sex workers: Moving beyond individual-focused interventions. Drug Alcohol Depend 2011;113(1):76–81.

37. Hart TA, Noor SW, Tavangar F, et al. Crystal methamphetamine use and bacterial sexually transmitted infections (STIs) among gay, bisexual and other sexual minority men in Canada. Drug Alcohol Depend 2023;242:109718.

38. Colfax G, Shoptaw S. The methamphetamine epidemic: implications for HIV prevention and treatment. Curr HIV AIDS Rep 2005;2(4):194–9.

39. Grov C, Westmoreland D, Morrison C, et al. The Crisis We Are Not Talking About: One-in-Three Annual HIV Seroconversions Among Sexual and Gender Minorities Were Persistent Methamphetamine Users. J Acquir Immune Defic Syndr 2020;85(3):272–9.

40. Riley DE, Liu L, Cohen B, et al. Characteristics and impact of methamphetamine use in patients with chronic hepatitis C. J Addict Med 2014;8(1):25–32.

41. Story A, Bothamley G, Hayward A. Crack cocaine and infectious tuberculosis. Emerg Infect Dis 2008 Sep;14(9):1466–9.

42. Hegazi A, Lee M, Whittaker W, et al. Chemsex and the city: sexualised substance use in gay bisexual and other men who have sex with men attending sexual health clinics. Int J STD AIDS 2017;28(4):362–6.

43. de Voux A, Kidd S, Grey JA, et al. State-Specific Rates of Primary and Secondary Syphilis Among Men Who Have Sex with Men - United States, 2015. MMWR Morb Mortal Wkly Rep 2017;66(13):349–54.

44. Kidd SE, Grey JA, Torrone EA, et al. Increased Methamphetamine, Injection Drug, and Heroin Use Among Women and Heterosexual Men with Primary and Secondary Syphilis - United States, 2013-2017. MMWR Morb Mortal Wkly Rep 2019;68(6):144–8.

45. Centers for Disease Control and Prevention. Sexually transmitted disease Surveillance 2019. US Department of Health and Human Services; 2019.

46. Plotzker RE, Burghardt NO, Murphy RD, et al. Congenital syphilis prevention in the context of methamphetamine use and homelessness. Am J Addict 2022;31(3):210–8.

47. Reno H, Fox B, Highfill C, et al. The Emerging Intersection Between Injection Drug Use and Early Syphilis in Nonurban Areas of Missouri, 2012-2018. J Infect Dis 2020;222(Suppl 5):S465–70.

48. Harvey L, Taylor JL, Assoumou SA, et al. Sexually Transmitted and Blood-borne Infections Among Patients Presenting to a Low-barrier Substance Use Disorder Medication Clinic. J Addict Med 2021;15(6):461–7.

49. Hibbs JR, Gunn RA. Public health intervention in a cocaine-related syphilis outbreak. Am J Public Health 1991;81(10):1259–62.

50. Gryczynski J, Nordeck CD, Mitchell SG, et al. Pilot studies examining feasibility of substance use disorder (SUD) screening and treatment linkage at urban sexually transmitted disease (STD) clinics. J Addict Med 2017;11:350–6.

51. Yu J, Appel P, Rogers M, et al. Integrating intervention for substance use disorder in a healthcare setting: practice and outcomes in New York City STD clinics. Am J Drug Alcohol Abuse 2016;42(1):32–8.

52. Falade-Nwulia O, Agee T, Kelly SM, et al. Implementing a peer-supported, integrated strategy for substance use disorder care in an outpatient infectious disease clinic is associated with improved patient outcomes [published online ahead of print, 2023 Sep 21]. Int J Drug Policy 2023;121:104191.

53. Bradley H, Hall EW, Asher A, et al. Estimated Number of People Who Inject Drugs in the United States. Clin Infect Dis 2023;76(1):96–102.

54. McCarthy NL, Baggs J, See I, et al. Bacterial Infections Associated With Substance Use Disorders, Large Cohort of United States Hospitals, 2012-2017. Clin Infect Dis 2020;71(7):e37–44.

55. Serota DP, Bartholomew TS, Tookes HE. Evaluating Differences in Opioid and Stimulant Use-associated Infectious Disease Hospitalizations in Florida, 2016-2017 [published correction appears in Clin Infect Dis. 2021 May 4;72(9):1686]. Clin Infect Dis 2021;73(7):e1649–57.

56. Jenkins TC, Knepper BC, Moore SJ, et al. Microbiology and initial antibiotic therapy for injection drug users and non-injection drug users with cutaneous abscesses in the era of community-associated methicillin-resistant Staphylococcus aureus. Acad Emerg Med 2015;22(8):993–7.

57. Moran GJ, Krishnadasan A, Gorwitz RJ, et al. Methicillin-resistant S. aureus infections among patients in the emergency department. N Engl J Med 2006; 355(7):666–74.

58. Saldana CS, Vyas DA, Wurcel AG. Soft Tissue, Bone, and Joint Infections in People Who Inject Drugs. Infect Dis Clin North Am 2020;34(3):495–509.

59. Malayala SV, Papudesi BN, Bobb R, et al. Xylazine-Induced Skin Ulcers in a Person Who Injects Drugs in Philadelphia, Pennsylvania, USA. Cureus 2022;14(8): e28160.

60. Chambers HF. Skin and Soft Tissue Infections in Persons Who Inject Drugs. Infect Dis Clin North Am 2021;35(1):169–81.

61. Gonzales y Tucker RD, Frazee B. View from the front lines: an emergency medicine perspective on clostridial infections in injection drug users. Anaerobe 2014;30:108–15.

62. Barbic D, Chenkin J, Cho DD, et al. In patients presenting to the emergency department with skin and soft tissue infections what is the diagnostic accuracy of point-of-care ultrasonography for the diagnosis of abscess compared to the current standard of care? A systematic review and meta-analysis. BMJ Open 2017;7(1):e013688 [published correction appears in BMJ Open. 2017 Sep 14; 7(9):e013688corr1].

63. Goh T, Goh LG, Ang CH, et al. Early diagnosis of necrotizing fasciitis. Br J Surg 2014;101(1):e119–25.

64. Fernando SM, Tran A, Cheng W, et al. Necrotizing Soft Tissue Infection: Diagnostic Accuracy of Physical Examination, Imaging, and LRINEC Score: A Systematic Review and Meta-Analysis. Ann Surg 2019;269(1):58–65.

65. Stevens DL, Bisno AL, Chambers HF, et al. Practice guidelines for the diagnosis and management of skin and soft tissue infections: 2014 update by the Infectious Diseases Society of America. Clin Infect Dis 2014;59(2):e10–52 [published correction appears in Clin Infect Dis. 2015 May 1;60(9):1448. Dosage error in article text].

66. Dunleavy K, Munro A, Roy K, et al. Association between harm reduction intervention uptake and skin and soft tissue infections among people who inject drugs. Drug Alcohol Depend 2017;174:91–7.

67. Dahlman D, Håkansson A, Kral AH, et al. Behavioral characteristics and injection practices associated with skin and soft tissue infections among people who inject drugs: A community-based observational study. Subst Abus 2017; 38(1):105–12.

68. Shroyer S, Boys G, April MD, et al. Imaging characteristics and CT sensitivity for pyogenic spinal infections. Am J Emerg Med 2022;58:148–53.

69. Sharfman ZT, Gelfand Y, Shah P, et al. Spinal Epidural Abscess: A Review of Presentation, Management, and Medicolegal Implications. Asian Spine J 2020;14(5):742–59.

70. Darouiche RO. Spinal epidural abscess. N Engl J Med 2006;355(19):2012–20.

71. Ananda RA, Attwood LO, Lancaster R, et al. Clinical and financial burden of spinal infections in people who inject drugs. Intern Med J 2022;52(10):1741–8.

72. Richaud C, De Lastours V, Panhard X, et al. Candida vertebral osteomyelitis (CVO) 28 cases from a 10-year retrospective study in France. Medicine (Baltim) 2017;96(31):e7525 [published correction appears in Medicine (Baltimore). 2017 Nov;96(47):e8910].

73. Davis DP, Salazar A, Chan TC, et al. Prospective evaluation of a clinical decision guideline to diagnose spinal epidural abscess in patients who present to the emergency department with spine pain. J Neurosurg Spine 2011;14(6):765–70.

74. Kimmel SD, Walley AY, Li Y, et al. Association of Treatment With Medications for Opioid Use Disorder With Mortality After Hospitalization for Injection Drug Use-Associated Infective Endocarditis. JAMA Netw Open 2020;3(10):e2016228.

75. Appa A, Adamo M, Le S, et al. Patient-Directed Discharges Among Persons Who Use Drugs Hospitalized with Invasive Staphylococcus aureus Infections: Opportunities for Improvement. Am J Med 2022;135(1):91–6.

76. Hartman L, Barnes E, Bachmann L, et al. Opiate Injection-associated Infective Endocarditis in the Southeastern United States. Am J Med Sci 2016;352(6): 603–8.

77. Mathew J, Addai T, Anand A, et al. Clinical features, site of involvement, bacteriologic findings, and outcome of infective endocarditis in intravenous drug users. Arch Intern Med 1995;155(15):1641–8.

78. Slipczuk L, Codolosa JN, Davila CD, et al. Infective endocarditis epidemiology over five decades: a systematic review. PLoS One 2013;8(12):e82665 [published correction appears in PLoS One. 2014;9(10):e111564].

79. Delgado V, Ajmone Marsan N, de Waha S, et al. 2023 ESC Guidelines for the management of endocarditis. Eur Heart J 2023;44(39):3948–4042 [published correction appears in Eur Heart J. 2023 Sep 20;:] [published correction appears in Eur Heart J. 2024 Jan 1;45(1):56].

80. Marks LR, Liang SY, Muthulingam D, et al. Evaluation of Partial Oral Antibiotic Treatment for Persons Who Inject Drugs and Are Hospitalized With Invasive Infections. Clin Infect Dis 2020;71(10):e650–6.

81. Iversen K, Ihlemann N, Gill SU, et al. Partial Oral versus Intravenous Antibiotic Treatment of Endocarditis. N Engl J Med 2019;380(5):415–24.

82. Wang A. Statement from the International Collaboration on Endocarditis on the current status of surgical outcome in infective endocarditis. Ann Cardiothorac Surg 2019;8(6):678–80.

83. Rodger L, Glockler-Lauf SD, Shojaei E, et al. Clinical Characteristics and Factors Associated With Mortality in First-Episode Infective Endocarditis Among Persons Who Inject Drugs. JAMA Netw Open 2018;1(7):e185220.
84. Kimmel SD, Walley AY, Linas BP, et al. Effect of Publicly Reported Aortic Valve Surgery Outcomes on Valve Surgery in Injection Drug- and Non-Injection Drug-Associated Endocarditis. Clin Infect Dis 2020;71(3):480–7.
85. Leahey PA, LaSalvia MT, Rosenthal ES, et al. High Morbidity and Mortality Among Patients With Sentinel Admission for Injection Drug Use-Related Infective Endocarditis. Open Forum Infect Dis 2019;6(4):ofz089.
86. Baddour LM, Wilson WR, Bayer AS, et al. Infective Endocarditis in Adults: Diagnosis, Antimicrobial Therapy, and Management of Complications: A Scientific Statement for Healthcare Professionals From the American Heart Association. Circulation 2015;132(15):1435–86 [published correction appears in Circulation. 2015 Oct 27;132(17):e215] [published correction appears in Circulation. 2016 Aug 23;134(8):e113] [published correction appears in Circulation. 2018 Jul 31;138(5):e78-e79].
87. Wilson JD, Altieri Dunn SC, Roy P, et al. Inpatient Addiction Medicine Consultation Service Impact on Post-discharge Patient Mortality: a Propensity-Matched Analysis. J Gen Intern Med 2022;37(10):2521–5.
88. Barocas JA, Savinkina A, Adams J, et al. Clinical impact, costs, and cost-effectiveness of hospital-based strategies for addressing the US opioid epidemic: a modelling study. Lancet Public Health 2022;7(1):e56–64.
89. Pollard MS, Tucker JS, Green HD Jr. Changes in adult alcohol use and consequences during the COVID-19 pandemic in the US. JAMA Netw Open 2020; 3:e2022942.
90. Kranzler HR, Soyka M. Diagnosis and pharmacotherapy of alcohol use disorder: a review. JAMA 2018;320:815–24.
91. White AM, Slater ME, Ng G, et al. Trends in alcohol-related emergency department visits in the United States: results from the Nationwide Emergency Department Sample, 2006 to 2014. Alcohol Clin Exp Res 2018;42:352–9.
92. Goldman-Mellor S, Olfson M, Schoenbaum M. Acute injury mortality and all-cause mortality following emergency department presentation for alcohol use disorder. Drug Alcohol Depend 2022;236:109472.
93. Mintz CM, Hartz SM, Fisher SL, et al. A cascade of care for alcohol use disorder: Using 2015-2019 National Survey on Drug Use and Health data to identify gaps in past 12-month care. Alcohol Clin Exp Res 2021;45(6):1276–86.
94. Mason BJ, Quello S, Goodell V, et al. Gabapentin treatment for alcohol dependence: a randomized clinical trial. JAMA Intern Med 2014;174(1):70–7.
95. Samokhvalov AV, Irving HM, Rehm J. Alcohol consumption as a risk factor for pneumonia: a systematic review and meta-analysis. Epidemiol Infect 2010; 138(12):1789–95.
96. Gupta NM, Lindenauer PK, Yu PC, et al. Association Between Alcohol Use Disorders and Outcomes of Patients Hospitalized With Community-Acquired Pneumonia. JAMA Netw Open 2019;2(6):e195172.
97. Gili-Miner M, López-Méndez J, Béjar-Prado L, et al. Alcohol Use Disorders and Community-Acquired Pneumococcal Pneumonia: Associated Mortality, Prolonged Hospital Stay and Increased Hospital Spending. Arch Bronconeumol 2015;51(11):564–70.
98. Morojele NK, Shenoi SV, Shuper PA, et al. Alcohol Use and the Risk of Communicable Diseases. Nutrients 2021;13(10):3317.

99. Rehm J, Samokhvalov AV, Neuman MG, et al. The association between alcohol use, alcohol use disorders and tuberculosis (TB). A systematic review. BMC Publ Health 2009;9:450.

100. Wigger GW, Bouton TC, Jacobson KR, et al. The Impact of Alcohol Use Disorder on Tuberculosis: A Review of the Epidemiology and Potential Immunologic Mechanisms. Front Immunol 2022;13:864817.

101. Mekonen T, Chan GCK, Connor J, et al. Treatment rates for alcohol use disorders: a systematic review and meta-analysis. Addiction 2021;116(10):2617–34.

102. Mintz CM, Hartz SM, Fisher SL, et al. A cascade of care for alcohol use disorder: Using 2015-2019 National Survey on Drug Use and Health data to identify gaps in past 12-month care. Alcohol Clin Exp Res 2021;45(6):1276–86.

103. Maldonado JR, Sher Y, Das S, et al. Prospective Validation Study of the Prediction of Alcohol Withdrawal Severity Scale (PAWSS) in Medically Ill Inpatients: A New Scale for the Prediction of Complicated Alcohol Withdrawal Syndrome. Alcohol Alcohol 2015;50(5):509–18.

104. Wei J, Defries T, Lozada M, et al. An inpatient treatment and discharge planning protocol for alcohol dependence: efficacy in reducing 30-day readmissions and emergency department visits. J Gen Intern Med 2015;30(3):365–70.

105. Singh-Tan S, Torres-Lockhart K, Jakubowski A, et al. Addiction Consult Service and Inpatient Outcomes Among Patients with Alcohol Use Disorder. J Gen Intern Med 2023;38(14):3216–23.

106. Sherbuk JE, McManus KA, McQuade R, et al. Hepatitis C Within a Single Health System: Progression Along the Cascade to Cure Is Higher for Those With Substance Misuse When Linked to a Clinic With Embedded Support Services. Open Forum Infect Dis 2018;5(9):ofy202.

107. Rosecrans A, Harris R, Saxton RE, et al. Mobile low-threshold buprenorphine integrated with infectious disease services. J Subst Abuse Treat 2022;133:108553.

108. CA Bridge. Available at: https://bridgetotreatment.org/tools/resources/. [Accessed 23 January 2024].

109. Taylor JL, Wakeman SE, Walley AY, et al. Substance use disorder bridge clinics: models, evidence, and future directions. Addict Sci Clin Pract 2023;18(1):23.

110. Substance Abuse and Mental Health Services Administration. Available at: https://www.samhsa.gov/find-help/harm-reduction. [Accessed 23 August 2023].

111. Lambdin BH, Davidson PJ, Browne EN, et al. Reduced Emergency Department Visits and Hospitalisation with Use of an Unsanctioned Safe Consumption Site for Injection Drug Use in the United States. J Gen Intern Med 2022;37(15):3853–60.

112. Harris M, Brathwaite R, McGowan CR, et al. 'Care and Prevent': rationale for investigating skin and soft tissue infections and AA amyloidosis among people who inject drugs in London. Harm Reduct J 2018;15(1):23.

113. Aspinall EJ, Nambiar D, Goldberg DJ, et al. Are needle and syringe programmes associated with a reduction in HIV transmission among people who inject drugs: a systematic review and meta-analysis. Int J Epidemiol 2014;43(1):235–48.

114. Bernard CL, Owens DK, Goldhaber-Fiebert JD, et al. Estimation of the cost-effectiveness of HIV prevention portfolios for people who inject drugs in the United States: A model-based analysis. PLoS Med 2017;14(5):e1002312.

115. Hagan H, McGough JP, Thiede H, et al. Reduced injection frequency and increased entry and retention in drug treatment associated with needle-

exchange participation in Seattle drug injectors. J Subst Abuse Treat 2000;19:
247–52.
116. Mostofi N, Collins SE. Impact of Harm Reduction Treatment with or without Pharmacotherapy on Polysubstance Use among People Experiencing Homelessness and Alcohol Use Disorder [published online ahead of print, 2023 May
30]. J Addict Med 2023. https://doi.org/10.1097/ADM.0000000000001182.
117. Marshall BD, Milloy MJ, Wood E, et al. Reduction in overdose mortality after the
opening of North America's first medically supervised safer injecting facility: a
retrospective population-based study. Lancet 2011;377(9775):1429–37.
118. Pinkerton SD. How many HIV infections are prevented by Vancouver Canada's
supervised injection facility? Int J Drug Policy 2011;22(3):179–83.
119. Andresen MA, Boyd N. A cost-benefit and cost-effectiveness analysis of Vancouver's supervised injection facility. Int J Drug Policy 2010;21(1):70–6.
120. Salmon AM, van Beek I, Amin J, et al. The impact of a supervised injecting facility on ambulance call-outs in Sydney, Australia. Addiction 2010;105(4):
676–83.
121. Platt L, Minozzi S, Reed J, et al. Needle syringe programmes and opioid substi-
tution therapy for preventing hepatitis C transmission in people who inject
drugs. Cochrane Database Syst Rev 2017;9(9):CD012021.
122. Fernandes RM, Cary M, Duarte G, et al. Effectiveness of needle and syringe
Programmes in people who inject drugs - An overview of systematic reviews.
BMC Publ Health 2017;17(1):309.
123. Collins SE, Duncan MH, Saxon AJ, et al. Combining behavioral harm-reduction
treatment and extended-release naltrexone for people experiencing homelessness and alcohol use disorder in the USA: a randomised clinical trial. Lancet
Psychiatr 2021;8(4):287–300.
124. Javed Z, Burk K, Facente S, et al. Syringe services programs: a technical package of effective strategies and approaches for Planning, Design, and implementation. Atlanta, GA: US Department of Health and Human Services, National
Center for HIV/AIDS, Viral Hepatitis, STD and TB Prevention, Centers for Disease, Control and Prevention; 2020. p. 2020.
125. HIV Education and Prevention Project of Alameda County. Available at: https://
heppac.org/. [Accessed 23 January 2024].
126. Orenstein, Natalie. 11/2023. Highland Hospital's new vending machine offers
free socks, tampons, and drug test kits. The Oaklandside. Available at:
https://oaklandside.org/2023/11/27/highland-hospital-harm-reduction-vending-
machine-oakland/. [Accessed 23 January 2024].

Coronavirus Disease 2019

Past, Present, and Future

Charlotte Page Wills, MD*, Berenice Perez, MD, Justin Moore, MD

KEYWORDS

- SARS CoV-2 • COVID-19 • COVID variants • Features of COVID-19
- Treatment of COVID-19 • Vulnerable populations • MIS-C • Long COVID

KEY POINTS

- COVID-19 continues to evolve causing significant morbidity and mortality, evaluation involves evaluating for respiratory distress, risk of decompensation, identifying non-respiratory complications and screening for high risk features and comorbidities; antiviral pharmacotherapies may mitigate disease but require careful evaluation for drug-drug interaction prior to adminstration.
- MIS-C is later presenting syndrome in children causing significant illness similar to Kawasaki disease; vulnerable populations at risk for higher rates of severe disease and death include members of minority communities, pregnant patients and patients with mental health disease, substance use disorder, and housing and food insecurity.

INTRODUCTION, PATHOPHYSIOLOGY, AND EPIDEMIOLOGY

Introduction

Coronavirus disease 2019 (COVID-19), caused by severe acute respiratory syndrome coronavirus 2 (SARS-CoV-2), is undoubtedly one of the most impactful diseases experienced in the past century. It has been over four years since the first cluster of cases, millions of people around the world have died from COVID-19 or its complications. Millions more continue to experience the effects of post-acute sequelae of SARS-CoV-2 infection (PASC) or "long COVID." The impact and response to COVID-19 continues to be felt locally and globally and it continues to affect how we deliver care in the Emergency Department (ED). As of August 30, 2023, 770,085,713 documented cases had been reported, with 6,956,173 deaths.[1] While the official US health emergency concluded in May of 2023, as of the summer of 2023, countries across the globe were experiencing a new surge of cases from the newest dominant variant, EG.5 Omicron[2] and a new genetically distinct Omicron descendant BA2.86 had been detected in multiple countries. In all likelihood, more variants will follow and the care of patients

Department of Emergency Medicine, Alameda Health System, Wilma Chan Highland Hospital, Oakland, California, 1411 East 31st Street, Oakland, CA 94602, USA
* Corresponding author.
E-mail address: cwills@alamedahealthsystem.org

Emerg Med Clin N Am 42 (2024) 415–442
https://doi.org/10.1016/j.emc.2024.02.002   **emed.theclinics.com**

with COVID-19 in the ED will continue to evolve along with the virus.[3] This article seeks to offer lessons learned from the pandemic, and to summarize best evidence for current ED management of patients with COVID-19.

Onset and Origins of the Coronavirus Disease 2019 Pandemic

The first cluster of severe pneumonia cases were reported to the World Health Organization (WHO) from the Hubei Province of China on December 31, 2019. Spread from the city of Wuhan to the entire country of China occurred in just 1 month.[4] On January 20, 2020, the Centers for Disease Control and Prevention (CDC) reported the first laboratory confirmed case of SARS-CoV-2 in the United States from a patient in Washington State. By the end of January 2020, SARS-CoV-2 infections had been reported in at least 18 countries. By mid-February 2020, COVID-19 had caused over 1000 deaths, surpassing the number of fatalities from severe acute respiratory syndrome (SARS) caused by SARS-CoV-1. In mid-March 2020, the WHO declared COVID-19 a pandemic. Widespread lockdowns were implemented to slow the spread of disease, straining supply chains for goods including medical supplies and personal protective equipment.

The origin of SARS-CoV-2 remains highly contested and unclear, despite extensive investigation. Zoonotic spread from bats or pangolins is one theory, placing a wet market in Wuhan as the possible point of original contact. Accidental breach from a viral research facility in the same region has also been suggested, as have more nefarious theories like SARS-CoV-2 being a deliberately engineered pathogen (**Box 1**).

Box 1
Terminology pertaining to spread and evolution of severe acute respiratory syndrome coronavirus 2[5–7]

Mutation: a Change in Gene Structure by Alterations, Deletions, or Rearrangements of Bases.

Variant: Virus with altered genetic structure. The WHO characterizes the significance of new variants with both names (Alpha, Beta) and designations (Variant of interest, Variant of Concern) based on transmissibility and virulence factors.

Epistasis: A process where expression of 1 gene influences or modifies the expression of 1 or more other genes. Epistasis is an important driver in the evolution of RNA viruses and in COVID-19.[8]

Antigenic drift: The evolutionary accumulation of mutations in viral proteins selected by host adaptive immune response, which limits the duration of immunity from prior infection and vaccination.[9]

Innate immunity: The first-line immune response against infection, present at birth. Innate immunity prevents viral entry, limits viral propagation, eliminates infected cells, and triggers the adaptive immune response.[6]

Adaptive immunity: The immune response that is triggered by the innate immune response or by vaccination, leading to propagation of select native B and T cells that target specific viral components.[7]

Immune evasion: A strategy to evade a host's immune response, enhancing the chance of transmission to a new host.[10]

Herd immunity: Indirect protection from infection in an individual resulting from a large portion of the surrounding population being immune.[11]

Virulence: Measure of the ability of a pathogen to cause damage in a host.

Serial interval: Time from illness onset in the primary case to illness onset in the secondary case.[12]

Incubation period: Time from transmission to the onset of symptoms.[12]

Pathophysiology of Severe Acute Respiratory Syndrome Coronavirus 2

SARS-CoV-2 is an enveloped double-stranded RNA virus in the Coronaviridae family. Coronaviruses consist of 4 major structural proteins including the membrane protein (M), envelope protein (E), nucleocapsid (N), and spike protein (S). The S protein confers the unique and recognizable structure of the coronavirus. The S protein mediates attachment to angiotensin-converting enzyme to receptors on respiratory epithelium cells and viral entry.[13] The immune response to SARS CoV-2 infection causes a systemic illness with highly variable symptoms and severity. Studies have shown that SARS-CoV-2 can both evade and subvert the innate immune response, allowing initially unabated viral replication, while in some cases triggering a cytokine storm syndrome.[7] Dysregulated interferon and cytokine responses, and a hypercoagulable state can lead to tissue and endothelial damage.[14] This inflammatory state and microvascular damage can manifest as severe pneumonia, cardiac dysrhythmias, thrombosis, gastrointestinal (GI) symptoms, neurologic sequelae, and dermatologic manifestations.

Emergence of the Omicron Variant

Critical SARS-CoV-2 mutations tend to occur on the S protein. RNA viruses in general are more prone to mutation due to the lack of proofreading function.[15] As of September 1, 2023, the CDC lists more than 20 major SARS-CoV-2 variants being monitored (VBM), variants of interest (VOI), and variants of concern (VOC).[16] Continued circulation of disease offers more opportunity for the virus to interact with the host immune system, exerting selective pressure to further mutate.

In November of 2021, the first report appeared of a new variant designated "Omicron" by newly implemented WHO nomenclature. This new variant, while not more virulent, was observed to be much more transmissible than prior VOC. The rapid antigenic drift that gave rise to Omicron was attributed to the large number of mutations in the spike protein, which in turn conferred its enhanced immune evasion. Monoclonal antibody therapies developed for prior variants have proved ineffective to treat acute infections from Omicron and its descendants. However, host T-cell response and adaptive immunity from exposure to prior variants appear to be intact against Omicron. Multiple reports observed lower virulence of Omicron.[17,18] The Omicron BA2 subvariant was found to replicate more efficiently in the nasal turbinates but less efficiently in the lungs, likely contributing to less severe disease and enhanced transmissibility.[19] Overall, with the higher numbers of cases, risk of death from infection with the Omicron variant was found to be 4 times higher than for influenza in the 2022 to 2023 winter respiratory illness season.[20]

Risk for Severe Disease

Despite less severe disease from Omicron in the general population, certain individuals are at higher risk for severe outcomes and require special attention when they present to the ED with acute COVID-19. Severe outcomes are those that require hospitalization, intensive care unit (ICU) admission, intubation, mechanical ventilation, or result in death.[21] Determinants of risk include age, medical comorbidities, vaccination status, and socioeconomic status (**Table 1**). ED providers must consider this list of risk factors in determining which patients are candidates for outpatient antiviral therapy (discussed below). Age remains the most important risk factor for severe disease. When compared with patients aged 18 to 29 years old, the risk of death from COVID is 25 times greater for patients older than 50 years and substantially increases even further after age 65.[21] The medical comorbidities with the strongest association with severe disease are cardiovascular disease, cerebrovascular disease, and pregnancy. Risk of severe disease increases with multiple comorbidities. Individuals who are unvaccinated or not current

Table 1
Risk factors for severe disease[14,21–30]

Risk Factor	Relative Risk
Age 50–64	4.3
Age 65–74	6.7
Age 75–84	8.5
Age 85+	10.6
Unvaccinated status	14.1
Cerebrovascular disease	3.3
Anxiety and fear-related disorders	1.3
Mental health conditions	1.3
Neurocognitive disorders (dementia, Alzheimer's disease)	1.2
Diabetes	2.3
Obesity (BMI $\geq$30 kg/m^2)	1.3
Cardiovascular disease	5.0
Chronic obstructive pulmonary disease (COPD) and bronchiectasis	1.3
Chronic kidney disease	2.6
Chronic liver diseases	2.4
Disabilities	1.6
Human immunodeficiency virus (HIV)	1.8
Pregnancy	3.6
Smoking history	1.5
Cancer	1.5
Solid organ or stem cell transplant	1.5
Systemic glucocorticoid exposure	1.7

with COVID vaccination are also at significantly higher risk of severe disease. Additionally, both adult and pediatric members of minority groups and communities have higher rates of severe disease due to a combination of higher comorbidity burden, lower rates of home testing, and limited access to health care resources.[21]

DIAGNOSIS
Clinical Presentation

In contrast to the severe respiratory distress and hypoxia seen with earlier COVID variants and before vaccines were available, otherwise healthy patients infected with Omicron tend to present with non-severe disease.[31] In such patients, particularly if vaccinated, COVID-19 has become clinically indistinguishable from infection with influenza, respiratory syncytial virus (RSV), and other common respiratory viruses. However, while both hospitalizations and deaths have dropped precipitously worldwide, certain populations, particularly the elderly and unvaccinated, remain at risk for serious disease and death from Omicron infection.

COVID-19 is remarkable in the breadth of symptoms and number of organ systems involved (**Table 2**). However, some symptoms, such as anosmia and dysgeusia, once considered classic and diagnostic for infection with COVID-19 have become less common with the Omicron subvariants. The Omicron sub variants appear to affect the olfactory nerve less frequently.[32] Similarly, there is less involvement of the lower respiratory tract. GI symptoms are still prevalent, as are headache, myalgias, fatigue,

Table 2
Presenting symptoms and complications of coronavirus disease 2019

Organ System	Signs/Symptoms	Disease
Pulmonary	Cough, shortness of breath, hypoxia	Pneumonia, respiratory failure, pulmonary embolism
Cardiac	Palpitations, chest pain, dysrhythmias	Acute coronary syndrome, myocarditis
Gastrointestinal	Abdominal pain, nausea, vomiting, diarrhea	Gastroenteritis, pancreatitis
Neurologic	Headache, confusion, brain fog, weakness, numbness	Long COVID, ischemic stroke
Dermatologic	Rash, itching, urticaria	Vasculitis, "COVID toes"
Genitourinary	Microscopic hematuria and pyuria	Epididymitis, orchitis
Ophthalmologic	Eye redness, discharge	Conjunctivitis
Hematologic	Lymphocytopenia, thrombocytopenia, elevated d-dimer, elevated inflammatory markers	Hypercoagulability, venous thromboembolism, Disseminated intravascular coagulation (DIC)
Vascular	Hypercoagulability	Deep venous thrombosis, pulmonary embolism, ischemic stroke, aortic occlusion

and fever. COVID-19 should still be suspected in patients with fever and respiratory and GI symptoms.[33]

Many patients will present with exacerbations of chronic disease in addition to symptoms from acute COVID-19. Additionally, patients hospitalized for a reason other than COVID-19 infection may incidentally test positive for COVID-19 at the time of admission. It is critical to address and treat conditions which may not be related specifically to infection with COVID-19. Those with exacerbations of pulmonary and cardiovascular disease should generally also receive antiviral therapy for COVID, such as remdesivir.[34] (See below).

Diagnostic Testing

The overall diagnostic approach to suspected COVID-19 has matured with time and with the advent of rapid tests for detection of SARS-CoV-2. Prior to widely available rapid testing, the ED diagnosis of COVID-19 was made on clinical grounds. Clues to acute infection with early SARS-CoV-2 strains included lymphopenia, thrombocytopenia, and elevated C-reactive protein (CRP) in the setting of a normal procalcitonin. Classic chest X-ray findings include a ground glass appearance, small patchy, often bilateral, sometimes nodular consolidations.[35] Lung ultrasound has proven useful in identifying COVID-19 pneumonia, where it typically reveals multifocal B lines and small subpleural consolidations.[35] On chest computed tomography (CT), COVID-19 tends to produce a mix of ground-glass opacities and consolidation, often located peripherally. Pleural effusions are very uncommon in COVID-19.

Diagnostic tests for detection of SARS-CoV-2 are now widely available (**Table 3**). Although the SARS-CoV-2 variants circulating in the fall of 2023 have accumulated numerous S protein mutations not present in the ancestral strain, currently approved diagnostic assays continue to perform well. Rapid nucleic acid amplification panels that simultaneously test for multiple respiratory viruses (most commonly SARS-

Table 3
Diagnostic tests for coronavirus disease 2019

Method	Examples	Specimen Type	Turnaround Time	Comments
Laboratory NAAT (also called molecular tests)	RT-PCR CRISPR Only performed in clinical, research, or public health laboratories.	Nasopharyngeal, mid-turbinate, nasal, or oropharyngeal swab, nasopharyngeal wash; usually collected by health care professional	Generally batched, thus >24 h	Most accurate test type. Sensitivity peaks at day 1–3 of symptomatic illness. Specimen collection/quality affects accuracy. May remain positive for weeks, well beyond symptomatic infection and infectivity (cannot diagnose new infection for 90 d after positive). Sensitivity maintained for new Omicron variants.
Rapid NAAT	Rapid RT-PCR. Now widely used for screening in health care settings. Can be deployed at point of care. Some approved for at-home use.	Same as laboratory NAAT; some commercial systems allow nasal swab self-collection	As short as 15 min	May be less accurate than laboratory NAAT.
Respiratory virus panels	Multiplex PCR for COVID-19, influenza A/B, respiratory syncytial virus	Nasopharyngeal or nasal swab; some commercial systems allow self-collection	Generally available as rapid tests, with turnaround < 1 h	Rapidly evolving technology that will likely become standard of care for diagnosis of acute respiratory virus infection.

Test	Specimen	Time	Comments
Antigen tests	Commercial at-home rapid antigen tests	Nasopharyngeal, nasal swabs only; can be self-collected by patient	Several minutes	Less sensitive than NAAT, but similarly high specificity; most accurate during symptomatic period. Serial testing or follow-up NAAT recommended if negative. Specimen collection/quality affects accuracy. Concern, but limited data, regarding decreased sensitivity for new Omicron variants.
Antibody tests	Immunolobulin (Ig)M and IgG antibodies to S and N proteins	Blood	> 24 h	Test for prior infection or vaccination. Not used to diagnose acute infection (turn positive about 3 wk after illness); Results used to diagnose MISC-C/A, or to monitor population immunity by public health authorities

Abbreviations: CRISPR, clustered regularly interspaced short palindromic repeats; MISC-C/A, multisystem inflammatory syndrome in children/adults; NAAT, nucleic acid amplification test; RT-PCR, reverse transcriptase polymerase chain reaction.

CoV-2, influenza A/B, and RSV) are increasingly available and affordable and may soon become the standard approach to diagnosis in the ED.[38]

Much of the diagnostic workup in COVID-19 is done for severity assessment, risk stratification (see **Tables 1** and **3**), and to evaluate for complications and comorbid disease. Most patients testing positive who are at low risk, minimally symptomatic, and without evidence of respiratory compromise require no additional laboratory testing or diagnostic imaging. Patients who fall into the moderate and severe categories will require additional testing, beginning with chest X-ray. Recommended laboratories include a complete blood count and comprehensive metabolic panel that includes renal and hepatic function. Inflammatory markers such as CRP, d-dimer, and IL-6 may be sent, but are generally used for longer term prognostication in hospitalized patients, rather than immediate ED management. Serum procalcitonin may have a role in risk stratifying for superimposed bacterial infection and the decision to initiate antibacterial treatment, though its utility remains controversial.[36,37]

Advanced imaging should be pursued if more serious complications (pulmonary embolism, stroke, etc) are suspected. Point of care ultrasound can be used not only to detect B lines consistent with COVID pneumonia, but also right heart strain that may indicate pulmonary embolism, cardiac contractility for evidence of cardiac involvement, and intravascular fluid status for the purposes of fluid management and resuscitation.

TREATMENT AND PREVENTION
Management of Coronavirus Disease 2019 in the Emergency Department

Initial ED management of COVID-19 has evolved over the past three years along with the COVID-19 virus itself. While still capable of causing severe disease and death, COVID is now more often managed in a routine fashion, within the wide landscape of diseases and illnesses seen in the ED. Additionally, the many manifestations and complications of COVID-19 are better understood and recognized, and management is increasingly evidence-based. The general approach to managing COVID-19 begins with recognizing the infection, categorizing severity, and assessing patient risk as determined by age, underlying conditions or immunocompromised state, and vaccination status. Severity classification is described in **Table 4** and risk factors for severe disease are listed in **Table 1**.

Admission Versus Outpatient Treatment

The decision to admit versus discharge a patient with COVID-19 is based on multiple factors. Patients with severe COVID as determined by their oxygen requirement, work of breathing, hemodynamics, and potential for decompensation clearly meet criteria for inpatient management. Patients who are managing their symptoms well, have near-normal oxygen saturations, and can quickly seek care if they worsen can be safely discharged from the ED. These patients should be prescribed antiviral therapy if they have a high-risk condition or belong to a vulnerable population. They should be able to isolate as well as understand when to return. If possible, provide the patient with a portable pulse oximetry device with the caution that these may be less accurate with darker skin tone. Follow-up care should be encouraged and this is an ideal use of telehealth from the ED.

The more challenging population includes patients whose oxygen saturations hover around the cutoff of 94% on room air, who have abnormal X-rays but do not meet the 50% involvement required to be considered severe (see **Table 4**), who are relatively stable but have multiple comorbidities, or lack resources to care for themselves at

Table 4
Centers for Disease Control and Prevention classifications of severity of coronavirus disease 2019 infection

Asymptomatic/ Presymptomatic	Mild Illness	Moderate Illness	Severe Illness	Critical Illness
No symptoms, but positive test	Symptoms including fever, cough, sore throat, malaise, headache, muscle pain, nausea, vomiting, diarrhea, disturbance of taste/smell but NO shortness of breath of findings on chest X ray	Evidence of lower respiratory disease with either abnormal imaging or an O_2 sat >94%.[a]	O_2 sat <94%, Pao_2/Fio_2 ratio <300 mm Hg, or lung infiltrates >50%.	Multi-system organ failure, respiratory failure, septic shock.

[a] Occult hypoxemia may easily be missed on pulse oximetry in patients with darker skin tones.
Adapted from Clinical Spectrum of SARS-CoV-2 Infection. https://www.covid19treatmentguidelines.nih.gov/overview/clinical-spectrum/

home or easily return to the ED. These patients can be challenging to craft a safe disposition for and require more consideration.

Multiple clinical calculators have been developed to forecast a patient's trajectory. Although most are designed for use in the inpatient setting, tools such as the Quick COVID Severity Indicator can be used to predict an increased oxygen requirement with information readily available in the ED.[38] The 4 C Mortality Score for COVID-19 predicts in-hospital mortality by incorporating known risk factors including age, number of comorbidities, oxygen saturation, mental status, and laboratory data.[39] This tool is intended for inpatient use, but can be used in the ED to assist with difficult admission decisions. In a recent head-to-head comparison of 6 scoring tools, the 4 C Mortality Calculator performed best in predicting both clinical deterioration and mortality.[40]

At this time, there are no clearly delineated criteria defining which COVID patients should be admitted or discharged. It is ultimately the role of the emergency provider to weigh the patient's clinical condition, potential for progression to severe COVID, available patient resources for supportive care, and local institutional resources.

Pharmacotherapies

There are three antiviral therapies currently approved to treat outpatients with COVID-19: nirmatrelvir/ritonavir (Paxlovid), remdesivir (Veklury), and molnupiravir (Lagevrio) (**Table 5**). Effectiveness of high-titer convalescent plasma is controversial, but can be considered for outpatients not eligible for nirmatrelvir/ritonavir or remdesivir. Targeted monoclonal antibody therapies are no longer recommended as they are largely ineffective against current variants. A large number of medications, proposed to treat the ancestral strain of COVID and early variants, have since been proven ineffective, including ivermectin and hydroxychloroquine (**Box 2**).

The decision to prescribe pharmacotherapy for patients being discharged from the ED begins with identifying those at high risk of progressing to more severe disease (see **Table 1**). Nirmatrelvir/ritonavir is the current first-line treatment for eligible outpatients.[54] Among unvaccinated high-risk outpatients, nirmatrelvir/ritonavir reduced hospitalizations and death by 88% when given within 3 days of symptom onset.[41] Among the alternative therapies, a 3-day course of intravenous remdesivir has a very similar absolute benefit, though it is hampered by the logistics of infusion.[44] Molnupiravir reduces risk of death or hospitalization in high-risk unvaccinated individuals by 30%, at most, and is only approved for non-pregnant patients over age 18.

Caution must be exercised when prescribing nirmatrelvir/ritonavir due to its extensive drug-drug interactions involving the Cytochrome P4503A (CYP3A) pathway. Medications that represent contraindications to nirmatrelvir/ritonavir, or that should be held during therapy, include statins, calcium channel blockers, oral anticoagulants and various over-the-counter medications, and herbal and alternative therapies. Unfortunately, patients who are at high risk for COVID-19 complications and candidates for nirmatrelvir/ritonavir often are taking these medications. Emergency providers should consult a clinical pharmacist, high-quality drug interaction software, or the CDC Current Treatment Guidelines prior to prescribing nirmatrelvir/ritonavir. If an interaction is identified, the emergency providers will need to assess the risks and benefits of holding the patient's medications. For example, simply holding statins during the course of treatment is well-accepted.

At present, there is no role for systemic steroids in the outpatient treatment of mild to moderate COVID-19 infections.[48] Additionally, inhaled steroids are not recommended unless treating underlying conditions or as a usual therapy.[55]

Choice of therapy for patients requiring admission for COVID-19 infection (vs admitted for another process and incidentally COVID-19-positive) depends on the

Table 5
Medications used in the treatment of coronavirus disease 2019 patients

Antivirals	Nirmatrelvir/ritonavir (Paxlovid)[41–43]	300 mg nirmatrelvir/100 mg ritonavir twice Daily for 5 d Moderate renal impairment (eGFR 30–60 mL/min): 150 mg nirmatrelvir/100 mg ritonavir twice daily for 5 d Contraindicated with severe renal impairment (estimated glomerular filtration rate <30 mL/min), end stage renal disease receiving dialysis, severe hepatic impairment (Child-Pugh Class C) Note:Ritonavir is a strong CYP3A inhibitor with potentially severe drug-drug interactions. Prescribers must review medications to check for drug interactions.	Outpatients ≥ 12 y/o and ≥40 kg with mild to moderate COVID-19 at high risk of progression to severe COVID-19 within 72 h of symptom onset.
	Remdesivir (Veklury)[44–46]	Adult dosing: Loading dose 200 mg IV Followed by 100 mg IV daily for 3 d (outpatient) or 5–10 d (inpatient) Pediatric (≥28 d old and ≥3 kg) dosing: Loading dose 5 mg/kg IV Followed by 2.5 mg/kg IV daily for 3 d (outpatient) or 5 d (inpatient) *Check baseline transaminase and prothrombin time prior to initiating. Monitoring should	Outpatients and inpatients ≥28d old and ≥3 kg Outpatients ≥28d old and ≥3 kg with mild to moderate COVID-19 at high risk of progression to severe COVID-19 within 7 d of symptom onset

(continued on next page)

Table 5
(continued)

Molnupiravir (Lagevrio)[47]	continue through the duration of treatment. 800 mg molnupiravir PO twice daily for 5 d	Outpatients ≥18 y/o with mild to moderate COVID-19 at high risk of progression to severe COVID-19 within 5 d of symptom onset *Only recommended in patients when nirmatrelvir/ritonavir and remdesivir are not available or feasible.
Steroids Dexamethasone	6 mg daily up to 10 d *If dexamethasone (preferred) is unavailable these alternatives can be used: • Prednisone 40 mg daily • Methylprednisolone 32 mg daily • Hydrocortisone 160 mg total daily in 2–4 divided doses	All Inpatients requiring supplemental oxygen *Corticosteroids for underlying medical conditions should be continued in patients with COVID-19.[48]
Antithrombotics Unfractionated heparin or low molecular weight heparin	Prophylactic heparin dosing recommended for all nonpregnant adult inpatients with COVID-19 unless contraindications exist Therapeutic heparin dosing recommended in the following: • Evidence of venous thromboembolism • Without evidence of venous thromboembolism, but D-dimer levels above upper limit of normal with low-flow O_2 requirement, non-ICU setting and without increased bleeding risk	Inpatient only

Interleukin-6 Inhibitors	Tocilizumab (Actemra)[34,49]	Preferred immunomodulator: 8 mg/kg IV (max 800 mg per dose)	Inpatients requiring more than nasal cannula oxygen or rapidly increasing oxygen needs or signs of hyperinflammatory response
	Sarilumab (Kevzara)[34]	Third line if preferred or alternative immunomodulator unavailable: 400 mg IV once daily *Only commercially available in subcutaneous (SubQ) formulation	*Only add 1 immunomodulator in addition to dexamethasone.
Janus kinase inhibitors	Baricitinib (Olumiant)[50]	Preferred immunomodulator: 4 mg PO daily. Requires dose adjustment for eGFR<60.	**Remdesivir may be added in addition in patients who are immunocompromised, ongoing viral replication or ≤10 d from symptom onset
	Tofacitinib (Xeljanz)[51]	Third line if preferred or alternative immunomodulator unavailable: 10 mg PO twice daily. Requires dose adjustment for eGFR < 60	Inpatient only
T-cell costimulationsu modulator	Abatacept (Orencia)[52]	Alternative to first-line immunomodulator in patients not on mechanical ventilation or extracorporeal membrane oxygenation (ECMO): 10 mg/kg/dose IV ×1 (max 1000 mg per dose)	
Tumor necrosis factor (TNF) inhibitor	Infliximab (Remicade)[53]	Alternative to first-line immunomodulator in patients not on mechanical ventilation or ECMO: 5 mg/kg/IV x1 dose	

Box 2
Medications not recommended for treatment of coronavirus disease 2019

- Ivermectin
- Hydroxychloroquine
- Chloroquine
- Metformin
- Fluvoxamine
- Colchicine
- Azithromycin
- Nitazoxanide
- Lopinavir/ritonavir

---

severity of disease as indicated by degree of hypoxemia, increasing oxygen requirement, or involvement of multiple organ systems (see **Table 4**). Hypoxemia (pulse oximetry <94% requiring supplemental oxygen) is the indication for treatment with systemic glucocorticoids, most commonly dexamethasone (see **Table 5**). [56]

Patients admitted with COVID-19 are typically also treated with antithrombotic therapy. COVID-19 infection induces a prothrombotic state, with complications from this seen in the acute setting and for weeks beyond. Depending on severity of illness and level of care required, inpatients may receive either prophylactic or therapeutic doses of antithrombotics such as low-molecular weight heparin or unfractionated heparin. The use of anticoagulants or antiplatelets is not recommended for preventative measures in COVID-19, unless within the standard of care treatment of another specific condition.[57] Also, there is no evidence to support outpatient anticoagulation including patients discharged from the ED with COVID-19, unless another specific condition is being treated.[58,59]

Lastly, severe cases with evidence of rapidly progressive oxygen requirements and/or hyperinflammatory response may qualify for treatment with one of many immuno-modulating agents such as interleukin-6 (IL-6) antagonists, including tocilizumab (preferred) and sarilumab, a Janus kinase inhibitor, baricitinib (preferred) or tofacitinib, a T-cell costimulation modulator, abatacept, or a tumor necrosis factor (TNF) inhibitor, infliximab.[34] These therapies may all be given in conjunction with steroid therapy. These therapies are reserved for severe COVID-19 cases being managed in the ICU and generally are not initiated in the ED.

Non-pharmacologic Therapies

It is crucial that emergency providers be able to manage hypoxemia and hemodynamic instability in acutely ill COVID patients. Non-pharmacologic treatment strategies are described in **Table 6**.

Supplemental oxygen in non-intubated patients with COVID-19 should be initiated when the SpO_2 falls below 92%, with a target of 92% to 96%. In critically ill patients, an SpO_2 goal of less than 92% and greater than 96% is not beneficial and may cause harm.[60,61] It is important to recognize that in patients with darkly pigmented skin, SpO_2 may overestimate actual arterial oxygen saturation.[71] Black patients who may be hypoxemic should have at least one arterial blood gas measurement to determine whether SpO_2 is correlating with arterial oxygen saturation. Escalating oxygen therapy begins

Table 6
Non-pharmacologic emergency department management of severe coronavirus disease 2019 infection

Oxygenation strategies in non-intubated patients	Start supplemental oxygen if SpO_2 is < 92% to maintain SpO_2 between 92% and 96%. Escalating oxygen therapy: • Low-flow oxygen Delivery (nasal Cannula, simple face mask non-rebreather mask) • High-Flow Nasal Cannula (HFNC) • Non-invasive Ventilation (NIV) • Supplemental oxygen typically begins with low-flow delivery, but should be escalated to HFNC or NIV if needed to maintain target SpO_2. Awake Prone Positioning • Use in patients with persistent hypoxemia receiving supplemental oxygen via HFNC or NIV who can independently adjust to a prone position without the need for sedation. • Should not be used in patients meeting criteria for mechanical ventilation. • Encourage prone positioning for at least 6–8 h per day.	SpO_2 < 92% may be harmful, and SpO_2 > 96% has not been shown to be beneficial.[60,61] Most of the evidence suggests that prone positioning reduces intubation rates, with no effect on mortality.[64] The benefit appears to be greater in patients receiving HFNC or NIV than those on low-flow oxygen.[65] A longer duration of prone positioning is associated with lower intubation rates in patients on HFNC.[66,67]
Mechanical ventilation Strategies	Initial Ventilator Management • Assist Control/Volume Control • Low tidal volume (4–8 mL/kg predicted body weight. • Set respiratory rate to match baseline minute ventilation. • Target plateau pressure of <30 cm H_2O. • Initial positive end expiratory pressure (PEEP) 5 cm H_2O with Fio_2 of 1.0, then titrate PEEP and Fio_2 using the acute respiratory distress syndrome (ARDS) Net protocol to achieve SpO_2 goal[68] • Goal SpO_2 88%–96%	In patients with ARDS, low tidal volume ventilation has been shown to improve mortality and the number of ventilator-free days.[69]

(continued on next page)

Table 6
(continued)

Hemodynamic strategies	Fluid Management • A conservative fluid strategy is preferred to a liberal strategy • Buffered balanced crystalloids are preferred over colloids • 0.9% saline is a reasonable alternative Vasopressors • Titrate to meet a target mean arterial pressure (MAP) of 60–65 mm Hg • The first-line agent is norepinephrine • Second-line agents are vasopressin and epinephrine • In patients with cardiac dysfunction, dobutamine can be added to norepinephrine • Dopamine is not recommended	Direct evidence is lacking on optimal fluid management in patients with COVID-19. Recommendations are based on evidence in patients with ARDS. In a study of 1000 patients randomized to a conservative vs liberal fluid strategy, the conservative strategy improved oxygen index, lung injury score, number of ventilator-free days, and number of intensive care unit (ICU) days.[70] Direct evidence is lacking on the use of vasopressors in patients with COVID-19 and shock. Recommendations reflect general recommendations for septic shock.

with low-flow delivery systems, which can achieve an FiO_2 of up to 70%. Oxygen by nasal cannula at a rate of 6 L per minute (LPM) can deliver an FiO_2 of about 40%; a simple face mask at 10 LPM delivers an FiO_2 of about 55%; and a non-rebreather mask at 15 LPM can achieve an FiO_2 of about 70%.

However, in patients with lung injury from severe COVID pneumonia and acute respiratory distress syndrome (ARDS), because of alveolar fluid and collapse, delivery of an Fio_2 above 50% alone may not improve oxygenation, and the addition of positive end expiratory pressure (PEEP) is generally required. PEEP allows atelectatic alveoli to open and participate in oxygenation, reducing V/Q mismatch. PEEP can be provided by switching the patient from a low-flow oxygen delivery system to a high-flow nasal cannula or non-invasive ventilation (NIV), including continuous positive airway pressure and bilevel positive airway pressure (BiPAP). High-flow nasal cannula (HFNC) at an oxygen flow rate of 40 to 60 LPM can deliver an Fio_2 of approximately 100%.[62] HFNC is best tolerated when the air delivered is warmed and humidified. HFNC will provide 1 cm H_2O of PEEP for every 10 LPM increment. Non-invasive ventilation (NIV) can provide higher levels of PEEP than HFNC.[63]

Awake prone positioning is another strategy to address hypoxemia in patients with COVID-19. It improves ventilation and decreases atelectasis of dependent portions of the lungs and facilitates drainage of secretions. Most of the evidence suggests that prone positioning in COVID patients on HFNC or NIV reduces intubation rates with no effect on mortality.[64,65] Patients should be able to independently adjust to and tolerate the prone position without the need for sedation. Evidence suggests that the prone position should be maintained for at least 6 to 8 hours per day.[66,67]

In patients with persistent hypoxemia due to COVID pneumonia, immediate escalation to mechanical ventilation is no longer recommended. Rather, it is advised to escalate first to HFNC and then to NIV if the patient requires additional support.[59] Such an approach has been shown to reduce the need for mechanical ventilation. The decision whether and when to intubate for respiratory failure depends on the patient's work of breathing and mental status and the judgment that decompensated respiratory failure is ensuing. Once the patient is intubated, ventilator management should follow the low tidal volume ventilation (LTVV) strategy, recommended for patients with ARDS, which is associated with lower mortality and fewer days on the ventilator.[59,69] The ARDSNet protocol can be used to determine initial ventilator settings and to make adjustments to meet pH, plateau pressure, and oxygenation goals (see **Table 5**).

While there is no direct evidence on optimal fluid management in the setting of severe COVID-19, it seems reasonable to apply what is known from prior studies of ARDS patients. Since increased capillary permeability contributes to ARDS, a conservative fluid management approach has been proposed. This approach targets a central venous pressure (CVP) of 4 to 8 mm Hg, provided mean arterial pressure is >60 mm Hg and urine output is adequate, generally favoring pressors over fluid boluses to maintain blood pressure. In a large trial, ARDS patients randomized to such a conservative fluid strategy, versus usual care, had lower lung injury scores and fewer days on the ventilator and in the ICU.[72] Thus, for emergency providers involved in the initial care of severe COVID pneumonia, the imperative is to avoid unnecessary IV fluid administration and a positive fluid balance, and to begin vasopressors for shock once the CVP is >4 to 8.

The choice of vasopressor for shock in patients with COVID-19 does not differ substantially from other causes of septic shock; when required, norepinephrine is the vasopressor of choice.[73]

Coronavirus Disease in Pregnancy

Similar to infection with other viral pneumonias, pregnant patients with COVID-19 are at increased risk for severe disease and prenatal complications. These include pre-eclampsia, eclampsia, and infections requiring antibiotics.[74] This risk has persisted with Omicron and is most pronounced in patients who are symptomatic and unvaccinated and those who are obese. Further, rates of pregnancy loss and COVID-19 in the neonate were higher in lower income patients.[75]

Pregnant patients with moderate and severe COVID-19 infection should be admitted for inpatient therapy. The pulse oximetry threshold for hypoxia is 95% rather than 94% to account for additional oxygen demands from the fetus and higher risk of respiratory compromise.[76] Admitted pregnant patients are treated for COVID-19 with remdesivir and steroids. The Society for Maternal-Fetal Medicine currently recommends outpatient treatment with nirmatrelvir/ritonavir or remdesivir for 3 days in asymptomatic and mildly symptomatic pregnant patients. Molnupiravir is not recommended in pregnancy.[77]

Vaccination is strongly recommended in pregnancy as it significantly protects against severe disease. To date, there are no documented cases of vaccine-associated pregnancy complications, congenital anomalies, or other sequelae.[78–80]

Coronavirus Disease in Children

Children have accounted for approximately 20% of COVID-19 cases in the United States to date, but rates of severe disease have been low. Most children will do well with supportive care only, and nonhospitalized children do not need any specific therapy. However, severe disease is possible, especially in those with risk factors. Risk factors for progression to acute severe COVID-19 disease are included in **Tables 7**. It is the responsibility of emergency providers to identify any high-risk conditions when evaluating even well-appearing children with acute COVID-19.

Studies of children requiring admission with the Omicron variant found they tended to be younger and have more underlying health conditions. Fever, sore throat, vomiting, and seizures were the most common symptoms.[82,83] Children who were obese and unvaccinated were at particular risk of adverse outcomes.

Antiviral medications are not recommended for asymptomatic, mild, or moderate disease.[84] For children ≥12 years of age with mild to moderate COVID-19 and at risk for

Table 7
Risk factors in children for progression to severe disease

High Risk	Moderate Risk	Unknown Risk
BMI>95%	Sickle Cell Disease	Mild asthma
Immunosuppressive disorder	Poorly controlled diabetes	Overweight
Neurodevelopmental disorder	Chronic kidney disease	Well-controlled diabetes
Medical complexity (eg, tracheostomy)	Chronic liver disease	
Severe congenital or acquired heart disease	Nonsevere cardiac, neurologic, or metabolic disease	
Multiple moderate or severe chronic diseases	Age <1 y	
Pregnancy		

progression to severe disease (see **Table 7**), the American Academy of Pediatrics recommends a 5-day course of nirmatrelvir/ritonavir (Paxlovid) if they are within 5 days of symptom onset.[85] For children $\geq$28 days old (and $\geq$3 kg in weight) with severe COVID-19, a 5 to 10-day remdesivir infusion is recommended.[84] Molnupiravir is not approved in children.[85] Vaccination is recommended in all children. Myocarditis is a recognized rare complication of COVID-19 mRNA vaccinations, predominantly affecting young adults and adolescent males with an estimated rate of 12.6 cases per one million doses. Most patients had a mild course with complete resolution of symptoms.[86]

Multisystem Inflammatory Syndrome in Children

Multisystem inflammatory syndrome in children (MIS-C) is a severe hyperinflammatory response typically seen 2 to 6 weeks after infection with COVID-19 (see **Table 8**). It occurs in less than 1% of infected children. MIS-C is a separate entity from severe COVID and can be distinguished by the presence of cardiac dysfunction. MIS-C exhibits significant similarities to Kawasaki disease (KD), as both conditions can present with conjunctivitis, mucocutaneous rash, lymphadenopathy, and cardiac involvement.[87] In the ED, it can be difficult to differentiate between MIS-C and KD. MIS-C typically affects older children (age 5–13) than KD (age <5), and has more prominent GI and cardiac symptoms. Although KD and MIS-C can both lead to coronary artery aneurysms, MIS-C is more prone to manifest with reduced left ventricular function. Children at increased risk for MIS-C included males, those of Hispanic/Latino or Non-Hispanic Black race/

Table 8
Signs and symptoms of multisystem inflammatory syndrome in children[81]

Organ System	Signs/Symptoms	Disease
Pulmonary	Hypoxia, respiratory distress, cough	Pulmonary edema, pulmonary infiltrates
Cardiac	Hypotension or shock, tachycardia, elevated troponin/N-terminal pro b-type natriuretic peptide	Coronary artery aneurysms, cardiac dysfunction, pericardial effusion, myocarditis, atrioventricular block
Gastrointestinal	Vomiting, abdominal pain, diarrhea	
Renal	Dehydration	Acute kidney injury
Dermatologic	Rash, mucocutaneous involvement, swollen hands or feet	
Hematologic	Bleeding or coagulopathy (elevated prothrombin time, partial thromboplastin time, D-dimer, or abnormal fibrinogen), thrombocytopenia, lymphopenia, lymphadenopathy	
Ophthalmologic	Conjunctival hyperemia	
Neurologic	Confusion, headache, seizures	
Inflammatory	Elevated erythrocyte sedimentation rate, C-reactive protein, procalcitonin, ferritin, lactic acid dehydrogenase , IL-6, or neutrophils. Decreased lymphocytes	

ethnicity, younger than 13 years, and with obesity.[2,88] Unlike severe acute COVID-19, MIS-C more often affects children without comorbidities. Approximately 80% of children with MIS-C will require ICU care and the mortality is 1%.[59]

Post Acute Sequelae of Coronavirus Disease 2019 Infection

Since early in the pandemic, COVID-19 has been notorious for its clinical tenacity and lingering symptoms. One of the earliest reports of post-acute sequelae of COVID-19 infections (PASC), more commonly known as "long COVID," was from Italy in the spring of 2020. Authors reported that weeks after hospital discharge, 87.4% of patients still complained of at least one symptom, most commonly fatigue or dyspnea.[89] At this juncture in the pandemic 3 years later, PASC remains incompletely defined and poorly understood. The WHO is in the process of generating a global consensus formal definition. Over 4% of patients previously infected with Omicron met proposed criteria for the syndrome.[90]

The National Institute of Health's RECOVER Initiative published data from over 9700 participants to characterize features of the syndrome. Fatigue was the most commonly reported symptom, with an additional 200 symptoms reported, that were felt to be debilitating and life-altering by the participants, spanning all organ systems. These include headache, fever/sweats/chills, post exertional malaise, palpitations, GI disturbances, dizziness, and persistent alterations in taste and smell.[91] New onset illnesses included type 2 diabetes, thrombotic and cardiovascular disease, and postural orthostatic tachycardia syndrome.[92] Risk factors include experiencing a severe case of COVID-19 infection, female sex, older age, and multiple comorbidities.[93] Vaccination does appear to be protective against PASC.[94]

PASC is a diagnosis to be considered in ED for patients presenting with persistent and debilitating symptoms without clear cause following COVID-19 infection. While treatment remains largely supportive based on individual symptoms, these patients should be counseled and referred for further evaluation, if possible to a center with expertise in PASC.

CONSIDERATIONS FOR FUTURE SURGES
Non-pharmacologic Preventative Measures

COVID-19 represents the widest global transmission of a disease in human history. Adding further insult, the WHO estimates between 80,000 and 160,000 health care workers died from COVID-19 as of September 2021.[95] Meanwhile, new variants of COVID-19 have improved transmissibility and shorter incubation periods and serial intervals compared to the ancestral strain. As a result, individuals now frequently transmit disease before they are symptomatic and up to 4 days after.[96] Optimizing nonpharmacologic measures that limit spread of the virus would appear to be a key to protecting patients and maintaining the integrity of the health care workforce. Nowhere are these measures more important than in the ED.

Factors to consider include mobility, masking, ventilation, testing, vaccination, and exposure of vulnerable populations. The interplay of these clearly moderate the spread of the disease. Nonpharmacologic interventions in aggregate and across populations have been demonstrated to decrease the incidence and mortality of COVID-19.[97] However, their comparative impact at both population and individual levels remains uncertain, and evidence is often conflicting and a source of controversy.

Numerous studies have established that transmission of COVID-19 can occur both via droplets and aerosols (airborne transmission). Airborne transmission can also be "long distance" in indoor settings when air replacement cycles are inadequate.[98]

This ability of the virus has led to so-called "superspreader events." Unventilated enclosed spaces likely do increase transmission of COVID-19. In health care settings, devices to manage airborne dispersal such as enclosed boxes for intubation and barriers to separate patients have met with mixed results.[99,100] However, portable high-efficiency particulate air filters, recommended by the CDC and now widely deployed in US EDs during surge conditions, have been shown to reduce COVID-19 transmission by up to 65% in an experimental model.[101]

Masking in health care settings can be viewed as a strategy to both protect health care workers from becoming infected and to protect patients from one another and from potentially infected health care workers. With the realization that COVID-19 can be transmitted via aerosols, N-95 and comparable respirators have become standard in many health care systems when caring for patients with active disease and for aerosol-generating procedures. CDC recommendations last updated in May 2023 continue to call for masking of patients with COVID-19 for source control, as well use of masks, respirators, and barrier face coverings and/or eye protection for the health care providers. In fact, the efficacy of masks is surprisingly difficult to prove. Meta-analyses of generally low-quality studies of both COVID-19 and other respiratory viruses have found only weak evidence of a small benefit from masking overall, with a possible small benefit conferred by N-95 type masks over surgical masks.[102,103] However, studies have noted greater compliance with surgical masks than N-95 type respirators.[104]

Hand hygiene remains a cornerstone of infection prevention of all infectious diseases including COVID-19, and reduction in transmission of respiratory viruses like COVID-19 through hand hygiene is well supported.[102] Results of laboratory studies have been mixed as to whether SARS CoV-2 remains viable and transmissible for a significant period on inanimate surfaces.[105] Thus, extensive environmental cleaning has been deemphasized as an important non-pharmacologic preventive measure. The CDC and WHO do continue to recommend that COVID-19 patients be placed in individual rooms and that health care workers use gowns, as well as gloves and masks, during close contact with these patients.[21] Finally, an important concept for ED infection control policies, that the CDC now stresses, is that nonpharmacologic measures should be deployed flexibly, based on rapidly changing local conditions, as opposed to the use of broad mandates.

Caring for Vulnerable Populations

The COVID-19 pandemic has both exposed and amplified myriad disparities existing within health care. Adult and pediatric patients and health care workers identifying as

---

Box 3
Vulnerable populations

- Minority groups
  - Indigenous
  - Hispanic/Latino
  - Pacific Islander
  - Non-Hispanic/Black

- Homelessness

- Unemployment

- Incarceration

- Substance use disorder

- Poverty

members of minority groups have died in disproportionate numbers. Other vulnerable populations at risk include people with mental health disease, substance use disorders, and housing and food insecurity (**Box 3**). Identifying a patient as a member of a vulnerable population is a crucial step in implementing care. It can influence pharmacotherapy, the decision to admit for inpatient treatment, follow-up care, counseling, and mobilization of additional resources like housing and social work. Patients who belong to vulnerable populations should all be advised to get vaccinated if not already vaccinated.

CLINICS CARE POINTS

- COVID-19 continues to mutate; new variants show increased transmissibility and enhanced immune evasion.
- Vaccination and prior infection are protective against serious infection.
- Patients at high risk for severe disease include those who are unvaccinated, elderly, pregnant, immunocompromised, have medical comorbidities, and members of minority and vulnerable groups.
- Antiviral therapies should be initiated promptly in those with risk factors.
- Steroid therapy for COVID-19 is reserved for hospitalized patients.
- MIS-C should be suspected in children presenting with Kawasaki disease-like symptoms in the setting of recent infection with COVID-19.
- Nonpharmacologic measures can be employed to mitigate transmission of disease.

DISCLOSURE

Drs C.P. Wills, B. Perez and J. Moore have no relevant commercial or financial conflict of interest or funding sources.

REFERENCES

1. WHO Coronavirus (COVID-19) Dashboard. Available at: https://covid19.who.int. [Accessed 4 November 2023].
2. CDC. COVID Data Tracker. Centers for Disease Control and Prevention. 2020. Available at: https://covid.cdc.gov/covid-data-tracker. [Accessed 4 November 2023].
3. Risk Assessment Summary for SARS CoV-2 Sublineage BA.2.86 | CDC. 2023. Available at: https://www.cdc.gov/respiratory-viruses/whats-new/covid-19-variant.html. [Accessed 4 November 2023].
4. Wu Z, McGoogan JM. Characteristics of and Important Lessons From the Coronavirus Disease 2019 (COVID-19) Outbreak in China: Summary of a Report of 72 314 Cases From the Chinese Center for Disease Control and Prevention. JAMA 2020;323(13):1239–42.
5. Eldred S. Coronavirus FAQ: Help me with omicron vocab. What's immune evasion? Epistasis?. Available at: NPR 2021; https://www.npr.org/sections/goatsandsoda/2021/12/03/1061219646/coronavirus-faq-help-me-with-omicron-vocab-whats-immune-evasion-epistasis. [Accessed 4 November 2023].
6. Diamond MS, Kanneganti TD. Innate immunity: the first line of defense against SARS-CoV-2. Nat Immunol 2022;23(2):165–76.
7. Sette A, Crotty S. Adaptive immunity to SARS-CoV-2 and COVID-19. Cell 2021; 184(4):861–80.

8. Alemrajabi M, Macias Calix K, Assis R. Epistasis-Driven Evolution of the SARS-CoV-2 Secondary Structure. J Mol Evol 2022;90(6):429–37.

9. Yewdell JW. Antigenic drift: Understanding COVID-19. Immunity 2021;54(12): 2681–7.

10. Immune evasion - Latest research and news | Nature. Available at: https://www.nature.com/subjects/immune-evasion. [Accessed 4 November 2023].

11. Coronavirus disease (COVID-19): Herd immunity, lockdowns and COVID-19. Available at: https://www.who.int/emergencies/diseases/novel-coronavirus-2019/question-and-answers-hub/q-a-detail/herd-immunity-lockdowns-and-covid-19?gclid=Cj0KCQjwgNanBhDUARIsAAeIcAtHmaadPCFc_tP_KSU8VDzTXb2yekIDs ZK6hhqc5eCiQjiGEVPl4BUaAukrEALw_wcB. [Accessed 4 November 2023].

12. Alene M, Yismaw L, Assemie MA, et al. Serial interval and incubation period of COVID-19: a systematic review and meta-analysis. BMC Infect Dis 2021; 21(1):257.

13. Boopathi S, Poma AB, Kolandaivel P. Novel 2019 coronavirus structure, mechanism of action, antiviral drug promises and rule out against its treatment. J Biomol Struct Dyn 2020;1–10. https://doi.org/10.1080/07391102.2020. 1758788.

14. Starkey T, Ionescu MC, Tilby M, et al. A population-scale temporal case–control evaluation of COVID-19 disease phenotype and related outcome rates in patients with cancer in England (UKCCP). Sci Rep 2023;13(1):11327.

15. On the Evolutionary Trajectory of SARS-CoV-2: Host Immunity as a Driver of Adaptation in RNA Viruses - PMC. Available at: https://www.ncbi.nlm.nih.gov/pmc/articles/PMC9866609/. [Accessed 4 November 2023].

16. CDC. Coronavirus Disease 2019 (COVID-19). Centers for Disease Control and Prevention. 2020. Available at: https://www.cdc.gov/coronavirus/2019-ncov/variants/variant-classifications.html. [Accessed 4 November 2023].

17. Tabatabai M, Juarez PD, Matthews-Juarez P, et al. An Analysis of COVID-19 Mortality During the Dominancy of Alpha, Delta, and Omicron in the USA. J Prim Care Community Health 2023;14. https://doi.org/10.1177/21501319231170164. 21501319231170164.

18. Shuai H, Chan JFW, Hu B, et al. Attenuated replication and pathogenicity of SARS-CoV-2 B.1.1.529 Omicron. Nature 2022;603(7902):693–9.

19. Chan JFW, Hu B, Chai Y, et al. Virological features and pathogenicity of SARS-CoV-2 Omicron BA.2. Cell Rep Med 2022;3(9):100743.

20. Goldstein E. Mortality associated with Omicron and influenza infections in France before and during the COVID-19 pandemic. Epidemiology and Infection. 2023. Available at: https://www.google.com/search?client=safari&rls=en&q=Goldstein+E.+Mortality+associated+with+Omicron+and+influenza+infections+in+France+before+and+during+the+COVID-19+pandemic.+Epidemiology+and+Infection.+Published+online+2023%3A1-22.+doi%3A10.1017%2Fs095026882 3001358&ie=UTF-8&oe=UTF-8. [Accessed 4 November 2023].

21. CDC. Healthcare Workers. Centers for Disease Control and Prevention. 2020. Available at: https://www.cdc.gov/coronavirus/2019-ncov/hcp/clinical-care/underlyingconditions.html. [Accessed 4 November 2023].

22. Dzinamarira T, Murewanhema G, Chitungo I, et al. Risk of mortality in HIV-infected COVID-19 patients: A systematic review and meta-analysis. J Infect Public Health 2022;15(6):654–61.

23. Oakes MC, Kernberg AS, Carter EB, et al. Pregnancy as a risk factor for severe coronavirus disease 2019 using standardized clinical criteria. Am J Obstet Gynecol Mfm 2021;3(3):100319.

24. Chattopadhyay S, Malayil L, Kaukab S, et al. The predisposition of smokers to COVID-19 infection: A mini-review of global perspectives. Heliyon 2023;9(7): e17783.

25. Jdiaa SS, Mansour R, El Alayli A, et al. COVID–19 and chronic kidney disease: an updated overview of reviews. J Nephrol 2022;35(1):69–85.

26. Matsushita K, Ding N, Kou M, et al. The Relationship of COVID-19 Severity with Cardiovascular Disease and Its Traditional Risk Factors: A Systematic Review and Meta-Analysis. Glob Heart 2020;15(1):64. https://doi.org/10.5334/gh.814.

27. de Almeida-Pititto B, Dualib PM, Zajdenverg L, et al. Severity and mortality of COVID 19 in patients with diabetes, hypertension and cardiovascular disease: a meta-analysis. Diabetol Metab Syndr 2020;12(1):75.

28. Kolla E, Weill A, Zaidan M, et al. COVID-19 Hospitalization in Solid Organ Transplant Recipients on Immunosuppressive Therapy. JAMA Netw Open 2023;6(11): e2342006.

29. Ward D, Gørtz S, Ernst MT, et al. The effect of immunosuppressants on the prognosis of SARS-CoV-2 infection. Eur Respir J 2022;59(4). https://doi.org/10.1183/13993003.00769-2021.

30. Johnson AG, Linde L, Ali AR, et al. COVID-19 Incidence and Mortality Among Unvaccinated and Vaccinated Persons Aged ≥12 Years by Receipt of Bivalent Booster Doses and Time Since Vaccination — 24 U.S. Jurisdictions, October 3, 2021–December 24, 2022. MMWR Morb Mortal Wkly Rep 2023;72. https://doi.org/10.15585/mmwr.mm7206a3.

31. The effect of SARS-CoV-2 variant on respiratory features and mortality | Scientific Reports. Available at: https://www.nature.com/articles/s41598-023-31761-y. [Accessed 4 November 2023].

32. von Bartheld CS, Wang L. Prevalence of Olfactory Dysfunction with the Omicron Variant of SARS-CoV-2: A Systematic Review and Meta-analysis. medRxiv 2023. https://doi.org/10.1101/2022.12.16.22283582.

33. Menni C, Valdes AM, Polidori L, et al. Symptom prevalence, duration, and risk of hospital admission in individuals infected with SARS-CoV-2 during periods of omicron and delta variant dominance: a prospective observational study from the ZOE COVID Study. Lancet Lond Engl 2022;399(10335):1618–24.

34. Hospitalized Adults: Therapeutic Management. COVID-19 Treatment Guidelines. Available at: https://www.covid19treatmentguidelines.nih.gov/management/clinical-management-of-adults/hospitalized-adults–therapeutic-management/. [Accessed 4 November 2023].

35. Caroselli C, Blaivas M, Marcosignori M, et al. Early Lung Ultrasound Findings in Patients With COVID-19 Pneumonia: A Retrospective Multicenter Study of 479 Patients. J Ultrasound Med 2022;41(10):2547–56.

36. Kaal A, Snel L, Dane M, et al. Diagnostic yield of bacteriological tests and predictors of severe outcome in adult patients with COVID-19 presenting to the emergency department. Emerg Med J EMJ 2021;38(9):685–91.

37. Dolci A, Robbiano C, Aloisio E, et al. Searching for a role of procalcitonin determination in COVID-19: a study on a selected cohort of hospitalized patients. Clin Chem Lab Med 2020;59(2):433–40.

38. Haimovich AD, Ravindra NG, Stoytchev S, et al. Development and Validation of the Quick COVID-19 Severity Index: A Prognostic Tool for Early Clinical Decompensation. Ann Emerg Med 2020;76(4):442–53.

39. Knight SR, Ho A, Pius R, et al. Risk stratification of patients admitted to hospital with covid-19 using the ISARIC WHO Clinical Characterisation Protocol: development and validation of the 4C Mortality Score. BMJ 2020;370:m3339.

40. de Santos Castro PÁ, Martín-Rodríguez F, Arribas LTP, et al. Head-to-head comparison of six warning scores to predict mortality and clinical impairment in COVID-19 patients in emergency department. Intern Emerg Med 2023. https://doi.org/10.1007/s11739-023-03381-x.

41. Hammond J, Leister-Tebbe H, Gardner A, et al. Oral Nirmatrelvir for High-Risk, Nonhospitalized Adults with Covid-19. N Engl J Med 2022;386(15):1397–408.

42. Dosing Information | PAXLOVID™ (nirmatrelvir tablets; ritonavir tablets). Available at: https://www.paxlovidhcp.com/dosing. [Accessed 16 January 2024].

43. Ritonavir-Boosted Nirmatrelvir (Paxlovid). COVID-19 Treatment Guidelines. Available at: https://www.covid19treatmentguidelines.nih.gov/therapies/antivirals-including-antibody-products/ritonavir-boosted-nirmatrelvir–paxlovid-/. [Accessed 16 January 2024].

44. Table: Remdesivir Clinical Data. COVID-19 Treatment Guidelines. Available at: https://www.covid19treatmentguidelines.nih.gov/tables/remdesivir-data/. [Accessed 16 January 2024].

45. VEKLURY® (remdesivir) Dosing and Administration | HCP. Available at: https://www.vekluryhcp.com/dosing-and-admin/. [Accessed 16 January 2024].

46. Remdesivir. COVID-19 Treatment. Guidelines. Available at: https://www.covid19treatmentguidelines.nih.gov/therapies/antivirals-including-antibody-products/remdesivir/. [Accessed 16 January 2024].

47. Molnupiravir. COVID-19 Treatment Guidelines. Available at: https://www.covid19treatmentguidelines.nih.gov/therapies/antivirals-including-antibody-products/molnupiravir/. [Accessed 16 January 2024].

48. Systemic Corticosteroids. COVID-19 Treatment Guidelines. Available at: https://www.covid19treatmentguidelines.nih.gov/therapies/immunomodulators/systemic-corticosteroids/. [Accessed 16 January 2024].

49. Dosing for COVID-19 Treatment | ACTEMRA® (tocilizumab). actemra. Available at: https://www.actemrahcp.com/coronavirus/dosing-and-monitoring/dosing-schedule.html. [Accessed 16 January 2024].

50. Epocrates Web Results. Available at: https://www.epocrates.com/online/results?query=baricitinib%20adult%20dosing. [Accessed 16 January 2024].

51. Xeljanz: Dosing, contraindications, side effects, and pill pictures - epocrates online. Available at: https://www.epocrates.com/online/drugs/6514/xeljanz#adult-dosing. [Accessed 16 January 2024].

52. Orencia: Dosing, contraindications, side effects, and pill pictures - epocrates online. Available at: https://www.epocrates.com/online/drugs/4307/orencia#adult-dosing. [Accessed 16 January 2024].

53. Remicade: Dosing, contraindications, side effects, and pill pictures - epocrates online. Available at: https://www.epocrates.com/online/drugs/2173/remicade#adult-dosing. [Accessed 16 January 2024].

54. Reis S, Metzendorf MI, Kuehn R, et al. Nirmatrelvir combined with ritonavir for preventing and treating COVID-19. Cochrane Database Syst Rev 2022;9(9):CD015395.

55. Ramakrishnan S, Nicolau DV, Langford B, et al. Inhaled budesonide in the treatment of early COVID-19 (STOIC): a phase 2, open-label, randomised controlled trial. Lancet Respir Med 2021;9(7):763–72.

56. IDSA Guidelines on the Treatment and Management of Patients with COVID-19. Available at: https://www.idsociety.org/practice-guideline/covid-19-guideline-treatment-and-management/. [Accessed 4 November 2023].

57. Antithrombotic Therapy. COVID-19 Treatment Guidelines. Available at: https://www.covid19treatmentguidelines.nih.gov/therapies/antithrombotic-therapy/. [Accessed 16 January 2024].

58. Ramacciotti E, Barile Agati L, Calderaro D, et al. Rivaroxaban versus no anticoagulation for post-discharge thromboprophylaxis after hospitalisation for COVID-19 (MICHELLE): an open-label, multicentre, randomised, controlled trial. Lancet Lond Engl 2022;399(10319):50–9.

59. Coronavirus Disease 2019 (COVID-19) Treatment Guidelines. Available at: https://www.covid19treatmentguidelines.nih.gov/.

60. Chu DK, Kim LHY, Young PJ, et al. Mortality and morbidity in acutely ill adults treated with liberal versus conservative oxygen therapy (IOTA): a systematic review and meta-analysis. Lancet Lond Engl 2018;391(10131):1693–705.

61. Barrot L, Asfar P, Mauny F, et al. Liberal or Conservative Oxygen Therapy for Acute Respiratory Distress Syndrome. N Engl J Med 2020;382(11):999–1008.

62. Walls RM, Murphy MF, Barker TD, et al. The Walls Manual of Emergency Airway Management, 5th ed, 2022, Lippincott Williams & Wilkins.

63. Frat JP, Coudroy R, Marjanovic N, et al. High-flow nasal oxygen therapy and noninvasive ventilation in the management of acute hypoxemic respiratory failure. Ann Transl Med 2017;5(14):297. https://doi.org/10.21037/atm.2017.06.52.

64. Weatherald J, Parhar KKS, Duhailib ZA, et al. Efficacy of awake prone positioning in patients with covid-19 related hypoxemic respiratory failure: systematic review and meta-analysis of randomized trials. BMJ 2022;379:e071966.

65. Li J, Luo J, Pavlov I, et al. Awake prone positioning for non-intubated patients with COVID-19-related acute hypoxaemic respiratory failure: a systematic review and meta-analysis. Lancet Respir Med 2022;10(6):573–83.

66. Ehrmann S, Li J, Ibarra-Estrada M, et al. Awake prone positioning for COVID-19 acute hypoxaemic respiratory failure: a randomised, controlled, multinational, open-label meta-trial. Lancet Respir Med 2021;9(12):1387–95.

67. Ibarra-Estrada M, Li J, Pavlov I, et al. Factors for success of awake prone positioning in patients with COVID-19-induced acute hypoxemic respiratory failure: analysis of a randomized controlled trial. Crit Care 2022;26(1):84.

68. NHLBI ARDS Network | Tools. Available at: http://www.ardsnet.org/tools.shtml. [Accessed 16 January 2024].

69. Acute Respiratory Distress Syndrome Network, Brower RG, Matthay MA, et al. Ventilation with lower tidal volumes as compared with traditional tidal volumes for acute lung injury and the acute respiratory distress syndrome. N Engl J Med 2000;342(18):1301–8.

70. ARDS Clinical Network. Prospective, Randomized, Multi-Center Trial of Higher End-expiratory Lung Volume/Lower FiO2 versus Lower End-expiratory Lung Volume/Higher FiO2 Ventilation in Acute Lung Injury and Acute Respiratory Distress Syndrome. Available at: http://www.ardsnet.org/files/alveoliV1_1999-07-20.pdf. [Accessed 16 January 2024].

71. Fawzy A, Wu TD, Wang K, et al. Clinical Outcomes Associated With Overestimation of Oxygen Saturation by Pulse Oximetry in Patients Hospitalized With COVID-19. JAMA Netw Open 2023;6(8):e2330856.

72. Comparison of Two Fluid-Management Strategies in Acute Lung Injury | NEJM. Available at: https://www.nejm.org/doi/full/10.1056/nejmoa062200. [Accessed 16 January 2024].

73. Alhazzani W, Møller MH, Arabi YM, et al. Surviving Sepsis Campaign: guidelines on the management of critically ill adults with Coronavirus Disease 2019 (COVID-19). Intensive Care Med 2020;46(5):854–87.

74. Pregnancy outcomes and vaccine effectiveness during the period of omicron as the variant of concern, INTERCOVID-2022: a multinational, observational study - PubMed. Available at: https://pubmed.ncbi.nlm.nih.gov/36669520/. [Accessed 4 November 2023].

75. Simbar M, Nazarpour S, Sheidaei A. Evaluation of pregnancy outcomes in mothers with COVID-19 infection: a systematic review and meta-analysis. J Obstet Gynaecol J Inst Obstet Gynaecol 2023;43(1):2162867.

76. Eid J, Stahl D, Costantine MM, et al. Oxygen saturation in pregnant individuals with COVID-19: time for re-appraisal? Am J Obstet Gynecol 2022;226(6):813–6.

77. COVID_treatment_table_6-21-22_(final).pdf. Available at: https://s3.amazonaws.com/cdn.smfm.org/media/3526/COVID_treatment_table_6-21-22_%28final%29.pdf. [Accessed 4 November 2023].

78. Effectiveness and safety of COVID-19 vaccine in pregnant women: A systematic review with meta-analysis - PubMed. Available at: https://pubmed.ncbi.nlm.nih.gov/36444098/. [Accessed 4 November 2023].

79. Grünebaum A, Dudenhausen J, Chervenak FA. Covid and pregnancy in the United States - an update as of August 2022. J Perinat Med 2023;51(1):34–8.

80. Prabhu M, Riley LE. Coronavirus Disease 2019 (COVID-19) Vaccination in Pregnancy. Obstet Gynecol 2023;141(3):473–82.

81. Molloy EJ, Nakra N, Gale C, et al. Multisystem inflammatory syndrome in children (MIS-C) and neonates (MIS-N) associated with COVID-19: optimizing definition and management. Pediatr Res 2023;93(6):1499–508.

82. Differences in SARS-CoV-2 Clinical Manifestations and Disease Severity in Children and Adolescents by Infecting Variant - PMC. Available at: https://www.ncbi.nlm.nih.gov/pmc/articles/PMC9622241/. [Accessed 4 November 2023].

83. Shoji K, Akiyama T, Tsuzuki S, et al. Clinical characteristics of COVID-19 in hospitalized children during the Omicron variant predominant period. J Infect Chemother 2022;28(11):1531–5.

84. Chiotos K, Hayes M, Kimberlin DW, et al. Multicenter interim guidance on use of antivirals for children with COVID-19/SARS-CoV-2. J Pediatr Infect Dis Soc 2020;piaa115. https://doi.org/10.1093/jpids/piaa115.

85. Management Strategies in Children and Adolescents with Mild to Moderate COVID-19. Available at: https://www.aap.org/en/pages/2019-novel-coronavirus-covid-19-infections/clinical-guidance/outpatient-covid-19-management-strategies-in-children-and-adolescents/. [Accessed 4 September 2023].

86. Myocarditis With COVID-19 mRNA Vaccines | Circulation. Available at: https://www.ahajournals.org/doi/10.1161/CIRCULATIONAHA.121.056135. [Accessed 4 November 2023].

87. Characterizing the differences between multisystem inflammatory syndrome in children and Kawasaki disease - PubMed. Available at: https://pubmed.ncbi.nlm.nih.gov/34226639/. [Accessed 4 November 2023].

88. Characteristics, Outcomes, and Severity Risk Factors Associated With SARS-CoV-2 Infection Among Children in the US National COVID Cohort Collaborative | Pediatrics | JAMA Network Open | JAMA Network. Available at: https://jamanetwork.com/journals/jamanetworkopen/fullarticle/2788844. [Accessed 4 November 2023].

89. Persistent Symptoms in Patients After Acute COVID-19 | Critical Care Medicine | JAMA | JAMA Network. Available at: https://jamanetwork.com/journals/jama/fullarticle/2768351. [Accessed 4 November 2023].

90. Antonelli M, Pujol JC, Spector TD, et al. Risk of long COVID associated with delta versus omicron variants of SARS-CoV-2. Lancet Lond Engl 2022; 399(10343):2263–4.

91. Thaweethai T, Jolley SE, Karlson EW, et al. Development of a Definition of Post-acute Sequelae of SARS-CoV-2 Infection. JAMA 2023;329(22):1934–46.

92. Davis HE, McCorkell L, Vogel JM, et al. Long COVID: major findings, mechanisms and recommendations. Nat Rev Microbiol 2023;21(3):133–46.

93. Age, sex and previous comorbidities as risk factors not associated with SARS-CoV-2 infection for long COVID-19: a systematic review and meta-analysis - PubMed. Available at: https://pubmed.ncbi.nlm.nih.gov/36555931/. [Accessed 4 November 2023].

94. Watanabe A, Iwagami M, Yasuhara J, et al. Protective effect of COVID-19 vaccination against long COVID syndrome: A systematic review and meta-analysis. Vaccine 2023;41(11):1783–90.

95. The impact of COVID-19 on health and care workers: a closer look at deaths. Available at: https://www.who.int/publications/i/item/WHO-HWF-WorkingPaper-2021.1. [Accessed 2 December 2023].

96. Transmission of SARS-CoV-2: Implications for infection prevention precautions. 2020. Available at: https://www.who.int/news-room/commentaries/transmission-of-sars-cov-2-implications-for-infection-prevention-precautions. [Accessed 4 September 2023].

97. Delaugerre C, Foissac F, Abdoul H, et al. Prevention of SARS-CoV-2 transmission during a large, live, indoor gathering (SPRING): a non-inferiority, randomised, controlled trial. Lancet Infect Dis 2022;22(3):341–8.

98. Duval D, Palmer JC, Tudge I, et al. Long distance airborne transmission of SARS-CoV-2: rapid systematic review. BMJ 2022;377:e068743.

99. Sorbello M, Rosenblatt W, Hofmeyr R, et al. Aerosol boxes and barrier enclosures for airway management in COVID-19 patients: a scoping review and narrative synthesis. Br J Anaesth 2020;125(6):880–94.

100. Cheng A, Pirie J, Lin Y, et al. Aerosol Box Use in Reducing Health Care Worker Contamination During Airway Procedures (AIRWAY Study): A Simulation-Based Randomized Clinical Trial. JAMA Netw Open 2023;6(4):e237894.

101. Lindsley WG, Derk RC, Coyle JP, et al. Efficacy of Portable Air Cleaners and Masking for Reducing Indoor Exposure to Simulated Exhaled SARS-CoV-2 Aerosols — United States, 2021. MMWR Morb Mortal Wkly Rep 2021;70. https://doi.org/10.15585/mmwr.mm7027e1.

102. Jefferson T, Dooley L, Ferroni E, et al. Physical interventions to interrupt or reduce the spread of respiratory viruses. Cochrane Database Syst Rev 2023; 1(1):CD006207.

103. Chou R, Dana T. Major Update: Masks for Prevention of SARS-CoV-2 in Health Care and Community Settings-Final Update of a Living, Rapid Review. Ann Intern Med 2023;176(6):827–35.

104. Medical Masks Versus N95 Respirators for Preventing COVID-19 Among Health Care Workers : A Randomized Trial - PubMed. Available at: https://pubmed.ncbi.nlm.nih.gov/36442064/. [Accessed 4 November 2023].

105. Sammartino JC, Colaneri M, Bassoli C, et al. Real-life lack of evidence of viable SARS-CoV-2 transmission via inanimate surfaces: The SURFACE study. J Infect Public Health 2023;16(5):736–40.

Optimizing Antimicrobial Stewardship in the Emergency Department

Julia Sapozhnikov, PharmD[a], Fritzie S. Albarillo, MD, BSN[b],
Michael S. Pulia, MD, PhD[c],*

KEYWORDS

- Antimicrobial stewardship • Clinical decision support
- Pharmacists Emergency medicine • Diagnostic stewardship

KEY POINTS

- The emergency department is a unique and essential setting for antimicrobial stewardship initiatives.
- Antimicrobial stewardship is a patient safety (eg, adverse drug reactions) and public health imperative because of rising rates of bacterial resistance.
- Emergency department antibiotic stewardship interventions should take into consideration the work system and target infection-specific factors that drive inappropriate prescribing.
- Education-based stewardship interventions alone rarely result in sustainable behavior change and are not recommended.
- Clinical decision support tools embedded in the electronic health record (eg, antibiotic order sets) and pharmacist-led interventions (eg, culture follow-up and prospective antibiotic review) are the most effective ways to improve antibiotic prescribing in the emergency department.
- Innovative rapid pathogen detection assays and host response biomarkers hold promise for identifying bacterial infection, but there is insufficient evidence currently to designate any of these tests as standard of care.

INTRODUCTION TO ANTIMICROBIAL STEWARDSHIP

Antimicrobial stewardship (AMS), within a health care context, refers to efforts aimed at optimizing antimicrobial utilization. The primary focus of AMS is on antibacterial agents given the well-established causal link between utilization and bacteria

[a] Medical Science Liaison, Karius Inc, 975 Island Drive, Redwood City, CA 94065, USA;
[b] Department of Medicine, Infectious Diseases Division, Loyola University Medical Center, Loyola University Medical Center is 2160 South First Avenue, Maywood, IL 60153, USA;
[c] BerbeeWalsh Department of Emergency Medicine, University of Wisconsin School of Medicine and Public Health, 800 University Bay Drive, Suite 300, Madison, WI 53705, USA
* Corresponding author.
E-mail address: mspulia@medicine.wisc.edu
Twitter: @DrMichaelPulia (M.S.P.)

Emerg Med Clin N Am 42 (2024) 443–459
https://doi.org/10.1016/j.emc.2024.02.003
0733-8627/24/© 2024 Elsevier Inc. All rights reserved.

resistance; however, antiviral and antifungal agents are also within the scope of antimicrobial stewardship programs (ASPs). Antimicrobial resistance (AMR) is now a worldwide phenomenon accelerated by the overuse of antibiotics, and is considered a public health threat by the Centers for Disease Control and Prevention (CDC) and the World Health Organization.[1,2] In 2019, resistant bacterial infections were associated with nearly 5 million deaths worldwide, and in the United States, more than 2.8 million AMR-related infections occur annually leading to 35,000 deaths.[3] There is mounting evidence to support that AMS can lead to reduction in antimicrobial use and AMR.[4,5] Highlighting the critical need for AMS, approximately 50% of hospitalized patients receive at least one antibiotic during their hospital stay, and up to 50% of these antibiotics are deemed unnecessary.[6–8]

At a more granular level, the goal of AMS is to identify patients who have bacterial infections requiring treatment, while avoiding treatment in those who do not, to optimize selection of antimicrobials, their dosing and route, and duration of therapy, so as to optimize clinical outcomes while curtailing adverse consequences of antimicrobial exposure.[6] AMS programs have been shown to improve patient safety outcomes including proper evaluation of antibiotic allergies, prevention of kidney injury, and adequate treatment of infections to improve clinical outcomes. Reduction in *Clostridioides difficile* infection (CDI) is another major benefit of effective AMS.[9] Antibiotic use can lead to alteration of the intestinal microbiota leading to disruption of the gut microbiome and overgrowth of pathogenic organisms, such as *C difficile*. CDI is considered a major health threat by the CDC. In 2017, there were 223,900 hospitalized patients secondary to CDI leading to 12,900 deaths, primarily among older adults.[3]

KEY ROLE OF THE EMERGENCY DEPARTMENT IN ANTIMICROBIAL STEWARDSHIP

As recognized by a 2020 policy statement from the American College of Emergency Physicians, AMS is an important quality-of-care imperative in which all emergency providers and emergency departments (ED) should engage.[10] The ED plays a central role in the health care system by serving as a bridge between the ambulatory care, long-term care, and inpatient care settings. In addition to steadily increasing patient volumes, the ED often functions as the de facto setting where acute, undifferentiated patients undergo rapid diagnostic evaluation. A significant portion of acute ambulatory conditions are diagnosed and treated in the ED, patients in long-term care setting are often evaluated in the ED for potential infections, and most unscheduled admissions originate from the ED. As such, the ED is responsible for assigning an initial diagnosis for patients transitioning across health care settings. Correct diagnosis of a bacterial infection is the component of AMS that is furthest upstream, because efforts to optimize antibiotic selection, dose, and duration presume a correct diagnosis was made to justify antibiotic initiation. Failure to properly diagnosis and initiate antibiotic therapy in patients with bacterial infections can result in infection progression and adverse outcomes. Conversely, overuse of antibiotics in patients without true infections can also result in patient harm and worsening AMR at the hospital and community level. Additionally, decisions to initiate antibiotic therapy in the ED result in diagnostic and therapeutic inertia that can result in continuation of unnecessary antibiotics in downstream care settings.[11–13] This highlights the importance of the ED as a key setting for AMS, where diagnostic and management decisions directly impact antibiotic use across the entire health care continuum.

BARRIERS TO ANTIMICROBIAL STEWARDSHIP IN THE EMERGENCY DEPARTMENT

As a work system, the ED presents unique challenges to implementation of quality improvement initiatives and AMS is no exception. ED providers treat patients in a crowded, noisy environment, under incredible time pressure while simultaneously engaging in high-risk and high-density decision making with incomplete information. This often necessitates the use of cognitive heuristics that can increase the risk of diagnostic and therapeutic errors. Examples that pertain to ED AMS include attributing vague weakness to a urinary tract infection (UTI) in older adults, failing to recognize an important antibiotic dose adjustment for patients with renal impairment, or initiating antibiotic therapy without recognizing a history of AMR and broadening coverage. It is incumbent on those seeking to implement stewardship in the ED to consider the unique work system elements and ensure that interventions address actual drivers of suboptimal prescribing as characterized in the qualitative and mixed-methods literature. Specific guidance on successful implementation is available from research that characterizes barriers and how to overcome them, using a frontline provider perspective. Common drivers of antibiotic overuse and misuse include diagnostic uncertainty, perceived patient preferences for antibiotics, concern about adverse outcomes, and medicolegal liability.[14–19] Although patient preference is often offered up as a driver by providers, the available literature does not indicate this is a widespread phenomenon nor that overprescribing of antibiotics improves satisfaction.[20,21] Interventions should also be infection specific and thoughtfully integrated into existing ED workflows/care pathways. Lack of knowledge about when to withhold antibiotics and correct antibiotic selection does not seem to be a primary driver, and as such educational interventions alone are unlikely to succeed as an ED-focused intervention.

ROLE OF EMERGENCY PROVIDERS IN ANTIMICROBIAL STEWARDSHIP

Emergency providers make multiple diagnostic and management decisions that impact AMS. In addition to making an initial diagnosis and empiric antibiotic selection, emergency providers are tasked with collecting appropriate microbiologic specimens that allow downstream providers to confirm the presence of a bacterial infection and tailor or de-escalate antibiotic therapy according to isolate susceptibility. Specific recommendations for obtaining infection-specific (eg, urinary, sputum) cultures are covered elsewhere in this issue. Blood cultures should generally be obtained whenever there is a suspicion of bacteremia, a working diagnosis of sepsis, critical illness related to suspected infection, and immunocompromised status. Blood cultures should also be strongly considered when initiating broad-spectrum antibiotic therapy, to promote and facilitate downstream antibiotic de-escalation.

Beyond ED patient care, emergency providers should participate in AMS intervention design and implementation, at the ED and institutional level. For example, this includes representation on the hospital AMS and sepsis committees. An ED AMS champion would ideally have protected nonclinical time to participate in quality improvement initiatives, committee work, and the design and implementation ED-specific AMS interventions. Informatics support for this role is also critical because it generally involves generating metrics from electronic health record data and benchmarking prescribing patterns to enable audit and feedback activities aimed at improving antibiotic prescribing by outlier providers.

ROLE OF INFECTIOUS DISEASE PHYSICIANS IN EMERGENCY DEPARTMENT ANTIBIOTIC STEWARDSHIP

In conjunction with an ED AMS champion, infectious diseases (ID) physicians can help guide ED AMS activities and improve success. The literature highlights the following potential roles for the ID specialist: timely ID consultation in the ED, development of guidelines and treatment algorithms, evaluating antimicrobial prescriptions to assess for compliance with local guidelines, providing audit and feedback intervention, and education. Dinh and colleagues performed a quasiexperimental study following implementation of a dedicated ID physician (0.2 full-time equivalent) in the ED of a tertiary university hospital in France.[8,22–25] The ID physician reviewed and provided feedback on antimicrobial prescriptions, developed treatment guidelines, provided educational courses, and reviewed microbiology data. The study showed significant decreases in overall and guideline-discordant antimicrobial prescribing.[24]

EMERGENCY DEPARTMENT PHARMACISTS AND BEDSIDE ANTIBIOTIC STEWARDSHIP

The role of a pharmacist within the ED has expanded over time to include the provision of comprehensive clinical services.[26] The presence of an ED clinical pharmacists is increasing and is often considered an integral component of multidisciplinary ED practice.[27] ED pharmacists are uniquely positioned to be able to impact antimicrobial prescribing from various angles. Evidence-based AMS interventions include spectrum assessment, optimizing time to antibiotic administration, allergy assessment, and dose optimization.

ED clinical pharmacists can assist providers in antibiotic selection based on a variety of factors. They have knowledge of the spectrum of activity of antimicrobials, drug formulations, dosing, and drug-interactions, allowing them to ensure that the right antibiotics are ordered on the right patient. ED pharmacists can perform activities that busy ED providers may not, such as reviewing a patient's electronic health record for previous microbiologic results or antimicrobial history to evaluate risk factors for resistance organisms. Clinical pharmacists are able to serve as a physician extender by reviewing microbiologic culture data in real time and proactively communicating with providers to assist with decision making regarding the spectrum of antibiotic regimens.[28–30] ED pharmacist may also take into consideration clinical acuity, source of infection, renal function, and local susceptibilities patterns.[31] Studies have demonstrated the impact that pharmacists have had on improving initial antimicrobial selection, streamlining, and resolving bug-drug mismatches in the ED.[32–34] Improved outcomes have been shown across various indications and infectious syndromes including sepsis, pneumonia, intra-abdominal infections (IAIs), UTIs, and trauma/fracture prophylaxis.[28,33,35–39] A recent study of ED patients with community-acquired pneumonia (CAP) and IAI found that just the presence of a pharmacist significantly increased guideline-concordant antibiotic prescribing in ED and subsequent inpatient orders.[35] Similarly, a systematic review and meta-analysis of 24 studies demonstrated that appropriate prescribing of antibiotics was more likely with pharmacist intervention, particularly in patients with pneumonia and UTI (odds ratio, 3.47; 95% confidence interval, 2.39–5.03).[40]

Early and appropriate antimicrobial administration is associated with improved clinical outcomes in patients with sepsis and is a recommended practice by the Surviving Sepsis Campaign.[41] The involvement of an ED pharmacist has been shown to reduce time to antimicrobial administration in patients presenting with sepsis.,[33,42] with one study showing a median 16-minute reduction in time to antibiotic administration.[33] Prospective verification of intravenous antibiotics by an ED pharmacist can also reduce time to appropriate antibiotic therapy in noncritically ill patients, including pneumonia, UTI, skin and soft tissue infections, and IAI.[43] In addition, ED pharmacists may impact time to administration by admixing antibiotics, priming lines, programming medication pumps, and facilitating rapid delivery of medications not stocked in the ED, as needed.[42] ED pharmacists are also available for bedside questions, such as compatibility with lines or other medications.

The ED pharmacists' role can also include conducting allergy assessments, a critical AMS activity. Patients labeled with β-lactam allergy receive more costly, toxic, broad-spectrum, and, at times, less effective antibiotics.[44] The ED is an ideal place to assess allergies because it is often the first point of contact for hospitalized patients. Pharmacists have the knowledge, skills, and time to be able to perform an allergy assessment. A retrospective, quasiexperimental study of 380 patients showed that a pharmacist-led penicillin allergy assessment and interview increased the use of guideline-concordant antibiotics and decreased the use of fluoroquinolones in the ED setting.[44] Further studies should investigate novel strategies involving ED pharmacists to improve allergy assessment, such as participation in allergy delabeling.[45]

One of the most common activities that ED pharmacists participate in is providing dosing recommendations for empiric antibiotics.[36] Dose optimization in the ED is challenging, because host factors impacting pharmacokinetic and pharmacodynamic properties are not known. When selecting an antimicrobial and dosing regimen, in addition to age and weight, pharmacists evaluate renal and hepatic clearance, site of infection, other concomitant medications, and properties of the antimicrobial.[46] Furthermore, patients with sepsis may have various pharmacokinetic derangements that impact dosing including altered protein binding, volume of distribution, renal clearance, and oral absorption. Clinical pharmacists are best equipped to consider all these factors. DeWitt and coworkers[47] demonstrated that antibiotic orders were more likely to have appropriate doses when the ED pharmacist was present (95% vs 74%; odds ratio, 6.9; 95% confidence interval, 2.5–18.8), and this impact was even more profound in patients with renal impairment. Many ED order sets have the option to place an antibiotic order as "pharmacist to dose," allowing pharmacists to make dosing decisions independently.[28]

Lastly, ED pharmacists can conduct patient and health care provider education.[48] ED pharmacists can counsel patients on new medications, including antimicrobials.[49] Information might include the purpose of the medication and expected benefits, proper administration, common side effects, monitoring parameters, potential drug-drug interactions, and warnings or precautions to be aware of. ED pharmacists routinely provide antimicrobial-related education to nursing staff, including sequence of infusions and commonly encountered side effects.[36]

INFECTIOUS DISEASE PHARMACISTS AND EMERGENCY DEPARTMENT ANTIBIOTIC STEWARDSHIP PROGRAMS

High ED staff turnover rates, rotating schedules, and crowding are just some of the barriers to sustained system-based AMS in the ED.[30] Although ID clinical pharmacists traditionally spend their time on inpatient interventions, there is a growing focus on AMS efforts that occur in the ED and outpatient setting and during transitions of care. In their call to action, May and colleagues[46] outline several strategies that can be implemented in the ED. Examples of resources that can help ED providers in making antimicrobial-related decisions include clinical guidelines/pathways, order sets[50,51] and other clinical decision support systems (CDSS), formulary restrictions, education, and ED-specific antibiograms. CDSS are discussed further later. ID pharmacists can play an integral part in the development and implementation of these types of AMS activities in the ED.

ID pharmacists collaborate with microbiology departments to create antibiograms for the inpatient and outpatient settings. Because the ED lies at the intersection between the two, institutions may create ED-specific antibiograms to more accurately reflect the susceptibility patterns in this heterogeneous population.[52,53] Resistance patterns in isolates from ED patients may vary significantly from that of hospitalized patients, particularly for UTIs, and this information has been used to improve ED antimicrobial utilization.[52–58] ED-specific antibiograms should be incorporated into CDSS platforms to assist providers at the point of clinical decision-making.[46]

ID pharmacists are usually involved in developing empiric therapy guidelines or clinical pathway and can tailor guidelines and pathways to specific units, such as the ED, by considering ED-specific susceptibility data and patient populations. Incorporating guideline-concordant recommendations into the electronic health record can aid ED providers in ordering first-line antimicrobials more readily.[8] Order sets and clinical pathways can be integrated in CDSS platforms to aid providers during decision-making. For example, best practice alerts may appear when restricted antimicrobials are ordered or when new microbiologic results are available.[30] These types of interventions have been studied for multiple infection types. A multicenter prospective preintervention/postintervention study of UTIs in the ED found that incorporating recommendations in CDSS platforms improved antibiotic selection.[59] CDSS strategies have been shown to reduce antimicrobial prescriptions for acute bronchitis by 14%.[60] A study of ED patients with CAP demonstrated feasibility and potential benefit of real-time CDSS in aiding physicians' antimicrobial prescribing in this population.[61] ID pharmacists may be involved in sepsis committees, contributing to the standardization of order sets to increase appropriateness and decrease time to antibiotics related to sepsis care. To sustain success, they should seek to avoid alert fatigue and information overload. Ultimately, guideline creation and CDSS implementation should be multidisciplinary, involving ID pharmacists and ED stakeholders.[30]

ID pharmacists are well positioned to lead AMS education efforts, although these are not recommended as a stand-alone intervention, and are best combined with other AMS interventions.[62] Common education strategies include prospective audit and feedback, seminars, grand rounds, academic detailing, peer comparison, and learning modules.[27,62] ID pharmacists can collaborate with an ED champion to facilitate education for new-hires and staff annually on various AMS updates including local resistance patterns, new clinical guidelines, or quality improvement initiatives. Continued education of staff promotes dialogue and increases visibility of AMS efforts in the ED setting.[30] Multifaceted approaches in the ED (ie, clinical guidelines in combination with behavioral interventions) have been effective for a variety of infection types, including pharyngitis, asymptomatic bacteriuria, and UTIs.[8,63–65] One study showed guideline-adherent treatment of CAP, skin and soft tissue infections, and UTIs was increased with pharmacist-driven implementation of integrated clinical algorithms.[66] To improve successful uptake of any ED-focused AMS initiatives, ID pharmacists should include ED stakeholders at all stages of implementation.

CLINICAL DECISION SUPPORT SYSTEMS TO IMPROVE EMERGENCY DEPARTMENT STEWARDSHIP

CDSS are electronic tools that receive data, such as medication orders and administration, and microbiology results from the electronic health record. CDSS provide opportunities for clinicians to streamline AMS interventions. They are recommended by the 2016 Infectious Disease Society of America and Society for Healthcare Epidemiology of America as a tool in improving antimicrobial prescribing.[67,68] Several studies have shown that use of CDSS in the ED has led to decrease in antimicrobial use, improving empiric antibiotic selection,[69] and compliance to guidelines.[59] Using a CDSS, real-time alerts can be customized to aid clinicians in streamlining antimicrobial therapy, such as drug-bug mismatch, double anaerobic coverage, and identification of multidrug-resistant organisms.[68] Monitoring and tracking antimicrobial usage, and susceptibility patterns of organisms via antibiograms can also be developed through CDSS.[68] Hajesmaeel-Gohari and colleagues[70] reviewed 11 publications evaluating the utility of Computerized Physician Order Entry and CDSS in decreasing adverse drug events in the ED. The authors found that with the use of these tools, there is significant reduction in the rates of erroneous prescriptions/doses, excessive doses, adverse drug events, and inappropriate prescription.[70]

DIAGNOSTIC STEWARDSHIP THROUGH ADVANCES IN INFECTIOUS DISEASE DIAGNOSTICS

Diagnostic stewardship (DS), as applied to ID, is considered a synergistic adjunct to AMS.[71,72] The triple aim of DS has been described as "ordering the right test, for the right patient, at the right time."[73] This is achieved by improving the ordering, performing, and reporting of diagnostic tests to increase the likelihood that the provider will reach the correct diagnosis.[71,74] As previously discussed, accurate identification of bacterial infection is the first step of AMS, one that often occurs in the ED. Rapid expansion of the ID diagnostic options available to emergency providers highlights how critical DS is to overall AMS efforts. This must include balancing considerations, such as sample collection feasibility, turnaround times, diagnostic performance, clinical impact, and cost/benefit ratios. Here we discuss some of the recent advances in ID diagnostics from an AMS/DS lens.

Rapid Pathogen Detection

Because of the fast-paced nature of the ED, rapid diagnostic tools are essential to provide prompt and appropriate interventions for patients. Numerous rapid diagnostic tools have been developed and implemented mostly for inpatient use, but their utility in the ED is promising because of their rapid turnaround time for detection of pathogens, which can improve prompt initiation of therapy and de-escalation of unnecessary broad-spectrum therapy, or discontinuation of antibiotics altogether.

Upper respiratory tract infections are one of the leading causes of ED visits. Although almost entirely caused by viruses, up to 52% of these patients receive antibiotics. In pharyngitis, group A streptococcus, which accounts for only 5% to 15% of cases, is the only indication for antibiotics.[75,76] There are several studies demonstrating improved diagnostic accuracy for group A streptococcus using rapid antigen detection test or polymerase chain reaction (PCR).[77-79]

Lower respiratory tract infections (LTRIs), including acute bronchitis and CAP, are among the most common ED diagnoses. Bronchitis is generally considered to be viral by definition and even CAP is more commonly caused by viruses than bacteria.[80,81] The overuse of antibiotics in LTRI is typically caused by the challenges distinguishing between bacterial and viral causes. Rapid urine antigen testing for detection of *Streptococcus pneumoniae* and *Legionella pneumophila* have specificity rates of 98% and 97.1%, respectively, and stand to improve antibiotic prescribing.[82] However, a recent systematic review reported the portion of bacterial CAP cases caused by *S pneumoniae* as between 33% and 50%, whereas *Legionella* was much less common at 3% to 8%.[83] Real-time PCR-based assays for detection of influenza A/B and respiratory syncytial virus from nasopharyngeal swabs also have high specificity rates of 97.9% and 97%,[82] respectively, which improve antibiotic prescribing.[84,85]

Multiplex PCR assays can detect multiple respiratory pathogens from a single specimen, with rapid turnaround times. An example is the original BioFire FilmArray respiratory panel, Food and Drug Administration (FDA)-approved in May 2011, which can detect 15 respiratory viruses within approximately 1 hour. Rappo and colleagues[86] evaluated the use of this assay in the ED of a tertiary care center. Compared with usual care with standard microbiologic process, respiratory panel lead to decreased time to diagnosis of viral causes including influenza, and was associated with significantly lower odds ratios for hospitalization, length of stay, duration of antimicrobial utilization, and number chest radiographs.[86] In 2017, the panel was expanded to detect a total of 21 pathogens (17 viruses and 4 bacteria) with shorter turnaround time of 45 minutes. In October 2020, the FDA issued an Emergency Use Authorization for BioFire RP2.1-EZ Panel that included detection of SARS-CoV-2.

The FilmArray Pneumonia panel (PNA panel) is a multiplex PCR test that detects 18 bacterial targets, 8 viral targets, and 7 AMR genes. It requires a high-quality sputum sample or lower respiratory tract specimen (from bronchoscopy) and has a turnaround time of about 1 hour. For 15 of the bacterial targets, the test provides a semiquantitative result that may distinguish colonization versus true infection. Buchan and colleagues[87] evaluated the use of the PNA panel in 259 adult patients admitted with LTRIs, for its diagnostic test characteristics and potential impact on AMS. The panel showed positive percent agreement and negative percent agreement values of 96.2% and 98.1%, respectively, when compared with routine bacterial sputum cultures.[87] Furthermore, the authors concluded that with the use of this panel, there is potential for antibiotic streamlining in 70.7% of cases, with de-escalation or discontinuation of antibiotics in 48.2% of cases.[87]

Rapid PCR-based tests capable of detecting multiple pathogens have also been developed to facilitate diagnosis of infectious diarrhea, abscess pathogen (ie, methicillin-resistant *Staphylococcus aureus*),[88] and central nervous system infections. Examples include gastrointestinal panel and meningitis/encephalitis panel. Beal and colleagues[89] compared the utility of gastrointestinal panel with conventional stool culture. The gastrointestinal panel detected a broader range of pathogens than conventional stool culture, decreased need for imaging studies, reduced need for antibiotics, and resulted in a shorter length of stay.[89] The use of the meningitis/encephalitis panel in 79 ED patients with suspected central nervous system infection was evaluated by Ena and colleagues.[90] Although 58% of patients had clinical and cerebrospinal fluid findings concerning for central nervous system infection, only 30% had an infection confirmed by cerebrospinal fluid culture. The time difference between meningitis/encephalitis panel and cerebrospinal fluid culture results was 3.2 days and meningitis/encephalitis panel results led to antimicrobial adjustments in 59% of patients.[90]

Host Response Biomarkers

The ability to rapidly identify which patients have bacterial infections as opposed to viral or infectious mimics, remains a significant diagnostic challenge for emergency providers. Signs and symptoms of infectious and noninfectious substantially overlap, which can lead to inappropriate antibiotic use. Traditional host response biomarkers, such as leukocyte count and C-reactive protein, in isolation, lack sufficient discriminatory performance for viral versus bacterial infection to definitively guide antibiotic prescribing. Procalcitonin is FDA approved to help providers differentiate viral from bacterial LRTI; however, the most recent American Thoracic Society/Infectious Diseases Society of America CAP guideline does not recommend use of procalcitonin plus clinical judgment to guide initiation of antibiotics for CAP. This recommendation was driven by one large study demonstrating negative initial procalcitonin values in inpatients with subsequently confirmed bacterial CAP.[91,92] However, a recently published Infectious Diseases Society of America CAP clinical pathway recommends the use of procalcitonin in the context of hospital AMS guidelines.[93] Although procalcitonin should not be used for all patients with CAP, whether or not it can be successfully used to guide antibiotic initiation in specific clinical scenarios, such as healthy, low-acuity patients with a questionable pulmonary infiltrate on chest radiograph or those with confirmed viral CAP, is a matter of ongoing debate and inquiry.[94,95] A variety of next-generation host response biomarkers are being developed with the goal of improving rapid identification of true bacterial infections, including in the setting of sepsis.[96–99] Although data on the diagnostic performance and potential management impact are promising, there is not yet clinical effectiveness data to support their adoption. We anticipate this will change in the coming years and that one or more of these assays will be incorporated into best practice guidelines for ID diagnosis in the ED.

Diagnostic Stewardship for Urine Testing

Appropriate urine testing is a core AMS focus of DS because accurate UTI diagnosis involves several significant challenges. It is particularly challenging to assess patients with impaired ability to provide a history (eg, cognitive impairment, delirium) and there tends to be an overreliance on urinalysis (UA), a test that has a high false-positive rate.[100] DS around UA and urine culture test ordering and results interpretation thus stands to reduce overdiagnosis and subsequent overtreatment of UTI.[74] Most urine cultures should be ordered for patients with symptoms. Symptomatic UTI must first be distinguished from sexually transmitted infections, overactive bladder, and other conditions, which can mimic certain symptoms.[71] Provider education has been reported to reduce the number of urine cultures, although education alone may not change prescribing behavior.[101] Other so-called preanalytic strategies to reduce culture ordering, and thus overdiagnosis, include requiring an indication to place a urine culture order or holding cultures for processing until requested.[74,102] Another successful preanalytic strategy that has been described is to remove prechecked UA and urine culture orders from order sets, particularly for abdominal pain and psychiatric conditions.[103,104] DS analytical strategies take place at the point of test performance, typically in the laboratory. For UTI diagnosis, an analytical strategy is limiting "reflex" urine cultures to those meeting criteria for pyuria.[105] Postanalytic strategies for UTI DS include suppression or modification of culture results reporting, inclusion of help text to facilitate interpretation of contaminated cultures/skin flora, or incorporating evidence-based guideline recommendations in CDSS triggered at the time of UA and/or urine culture order placement.[59,106,107] These strategies should be considered, piloted, and refined by ED pharmacists to reduce overdiagnosis of UTIs or other infections and ultimately improve antimicrobial use.

Culture Follow-Up Optimization

About a one-third of all antimicrobials prescribed in the outpatient or ED setting are considered inappropriate, according to an estimation by the CDC.[108] Part of antibiotic stewardship in the ED should include appropriate follow-up once cultures and other diagnostic test results have returned. Failure to follow up on culture results can result in delays in appropriate treatment, antibiotic overuse, and poor clinical outcomes.[109] Yet successful culture follow-up (CFU) is challenging in the ED given the intermittent nature of providers' shifts and is often fraught with inconsistent management and documentation.[109] Formal CFU programs have been described, and represent yet another way to successfully expand AMS efforts into the ED settings and bridge transitions of care.[110] CFU programs most commonly focus on urine cultures, but also are used for follow-up on testing involving sexually transmitted infections, skin and soft tissue infections, bloodstream infections, and respiratory tract infections.[31,111] Physicians, ED pharmacists, and advanced practice providers all have the skills and knowledge required to perform CFU duties.[110,112] ED pharmacist-led CFU programs have been shown to decrease ED visits and admissions, treatment failure rates, and time to patient contact, and increase appropriateness of antimicrobial regimens in various studies.[48,110,113–115] For example, in one study of 180 ED urine cultures an ED pharmacist doing CFU identified inappropriate treatment in 23% of cases, with successful intervention in 83% of these.[38] A large health system of 13 EDs published their experience with a pharmacist-driven CFU program where approximately 40% of patients discharged with cultures pending required intervention (most often initiation of antibiotic therapy).[109] There is also published data on the positive impact of adding a clinical ED pharmacist to advanced practice providers- and physician-led CFU programs, particularly in terms of improving antibiotic selection, dose, and duration.[110,114,116,117] These innovative partnerships improve antimicrobial prescribing in patients discharged from the ED, especially when resources are limited.

SUMMARY

Antibiotic stewardship is a core component of ED practice and impacts patient safety, clinical outcomes, and public health. The unique characteristics of ED practice, including crowding, time pressure, and diagnostic uncertainty, need to be considered when implementing antibiotic stewardship interventions in this setting. Rapid advances in pathogen detection and host response biomarkers promise to revolutionize the diagnosis of ID in the ED, but such tests are not yet considered standard of care. At present, clinical decision support embedded in the electronic health record and pharmacist-led interventions are the two most effective ways to improve antibiotic prescribing in the ED.

DISCLOSURE

Dr J. Sapozhnikov is an employee of Karius, Inc. Drs F.S. Albarillo and M.S. Pulia have no relevant commercial or financial conflict of interest or funding sources related to this work.

REFERENCES

1. Centers for Disease Control and Prevention. About antibiotic resistance. Available at: 2022 https://www.cdc.gov/drugresistance/about.html. [Accessed 30 June 2023].
2. World Health Organization. Antimicrobial resistance. Available at: https://www.who.int/news-room/fact-sheets/detail/antimicrobial-resistance. [Accessed 30 June 2023].
3. Centers for Disease Control and Prevention, Antibiotic Resistance Threats in the United States 2019, Available at: https://www.cdc.gov/drugresistance/pdf/threats-report/2019-ar-threats-report-508.pdf. (Accessed 1 March 2024).
4. Morris AM, Bai A, Burry L, et al. Long-term effects of phased implementation of antimicrobial stewardship in academic ICUs: 2007-2015. Crit Care Med 2019; 47(2):159–66.
5. Yong MK, Buising KL, Cheng AC, et al. Improved susceptibility of gram-negative bacteria in an intensive care unit following implementation of a

computerized antibiotic decision support system. J Antimicrob Chemother 2010;65(5):1062–9.

6. Dellit TH, Owens RC, McGowan JE Jr, et al. Infectious Diseases Society of America and the Society for Healthcare Epidemiology of America guidelines for developing an institutional program to enhance antimicrobial stewardship. Clin Infect Dis 2007;44(2):159–77.

7. Magill SS, Edwards JR, Beldavs ZG, et al. Prevalence of antimicrobial use in US acute care hospitals, May-September 2011. JAMA 2014;312(14):1438–46.

8. Hecker MT, Fox CJ, Son AH, et al. Effect of a stewardship intervention on adherence to uncomplicated cystitis and pyelonephritis guidelines in an emergency department setting. PLoS One 2014;9(2). https://doi.org/10.1371/journal.pone.0087899.

9. Valiquette L, Cossette B, Garant MP, et al. Impact of a reduction in the use of high-risk antibiotics on the course of an epidemic of Clostridium difficile-associated disease caused by the hypervirulent NAP1/027 strain. Clin Infect Dis 2007;45(Suppl 2):S112–21.

10. ACEP Antimicrobial Stewardship Policy Statement. Available at: https://www.acep.org/patient-care/policy-statements/antimicrobial-stewardship/. [Accessed 3 August 2020].

11. Gupta A, Petty L, Gandhi T, et al. Overdiagnosis of urinary tract infection linked to overdiagnosis of pneumonia: a multihospital cohort study. BMJ Qual Saf 2022;31(5):383–6.

12. Kooda K, Bellolio F, Dierkhising R, et al. Defining antibiotic inertia: application of a focused clinical scenario survey to illuminate a new target for antimicrobial stewardship during transitions of care. Clin Infect Dis 2022;74(11):2050–2.

13. Kiyatkin D, Bessman E, McKenzie R. Impact of antibiotic choices made in the emergency department on appropriateness of antibiotic treatment of urinary tract infections in hospitalized patients. J Hosp Med 2016;11(3):181–4.

14. May L, Gudger G, Armstrong P, et al. Multisite exploration of clinical decision making for antibiotic use by emergency medicine providers using quantitative and qualitative methods. Infect Control Hosp Epidemiol 2014;35(9):1114–25.

15. Pulia MS, Schwei RJ, Hesse SP, et al. Characterizing barriers to antibiotic stewardship for skin and soft-tissue infections in the emergency department using a systems engineering framework. Antimicrob Steward Healthc Epidemiol ASHE 2022;2(1):e180.

16. Valmadrid LC, Schwei RJ, Maginot E, et al. The impact of health care provider relationships and communication dynamics on urinary tract infection management and antibiotic utilization for long-term care facility residents treated in the emergency department: a qualitative study. Am J Infect Control 2021;49(2):198–205.

17. Chan YY, Bin Ibrahim MA, Wong CM, et al. Determinants of antibiotic prescribing for upper respiratory tract infections in an emergency department with good primary care access: a qualitative analysis. Epidemiol Infect 2019;147. https://doi.org/10.1017/S095026881800331X.

18. Goulopoulos A, Rofe O, Kong D, et al. Attitudes and beliefs of Australian emergency department clinicians on antimicrobial stewardship in the emergency department: a qualitative study. Emerg Med Australas EMA 2019;31(5):787–96.

19. Stefan MS, Spitzer KA, Zulfiqar S, et al. Uncertainty as a critical determinant of antibiotic prescribing in patients with an asthma exacerbation: a qualitative study. J Asthma 2022;59(2):352–61.

20. Pulia MS, Hesse S, Schwei RJ, et al. Inappropriate antibiotic prescribing for respiratory conditions does not improve Press Ganey patient satisfaction scores in the emergency department. Open Forum Infect Dis 2020;7(6):ofaa214.
21. Ong S, Nakase J, Moran GJ, et al. Antibiotic use for emergency department patients with upper respiratory infections: prescribing practices, patient expectations, and patient satisfaction. Ann Emerg Med 2007;50(3):213–20.
22. Borde JP, Kern WV, Hug M, et al. Implementation of an intensified antibiotic stewardship programme targeting third-generation cephalosporin and fluoroquinolone use in an emergency medicine department. Emerg Med J 2015; 32(7):509–15.
23. Ostrowsky B, Sharma S, DeFino M, et al. Antimicrobial stewardship and automated pharmacy technology improve antibiotic appropriateness for community-acquired pneumonia. Infect Control Hosp Epidemiol 2013;34(6): 566–72.
24. Dinh A, Duran C, Davido B, et al. Impact of an antimicrobial stewardship programme to optimize antimicrobial use for outpatients at an emergency department. J Hosp Infect 2017;97(3):288–93.
25. Jorgensen SCJ, Yeung SL, Zurayk M, et al. Leveraging antimicrobial stewardship in the emergency department to improve the quality of urinary tract infection management and outcomes. Open Forum Infect Dis 2018;5(6). https://doi.org/10.1093/ofid/ofy101.
26. Randolph TC. Expansion of pharmacists' responsibilities in an emergency department. Am J Health Syst Pharm 2009;66(16):1484–7.
27. Pulia M, Redwood R, May L. Antimicrobial stewardship in the emergency department. Emerg Med Clin North Am 2018;36(4):853–72.
28. DeFrates SR, Weant KA, Seamon JP, et al. Emergency pharmacist impact on health care-associated pneumonia empiric therapy. J Pharm Pr 2013;26(2): 125–30.
29. Acquisto NM, Baker SN. Antimicrobial stewardship in the emergency department. J Pharm Pr 2011;24(2):196–202.
30. Trinh TD, Klinker KP. Antimicrobial stewardship in the emergency department. Infect Ther 2015;4(Suppl 1):39–50.
31. Wymore ES, Casanova TJ, Broekemeier RL, et al. Clinical pharmacist's daily role in the emergency department of a community hospital. Am J Health-Syst Pharm AJHP 2008;65(5):395–6, 398-399.
32. Davis LC, Covey RB, Weston JS, et al. Pharmacist-driven antimicrobial optimization in the emergency department. Am J Health Syst Pharm 2016;73(5 Suppl 1):S49–56.
33. Moussavi K, Nikitenko V. Pharmacist impact on time to antibiotic administration in patients with sepsis in an ED. Am J Emerg Med 2016;34(11):2117–21.
34. Rech MA, Adams W, Smetana KS, et al. PHarmacist Avoidance or Reductions in Medical Costs in Patients Presenting the EMergency Department: PHARM-EM Study. Crit Care Explor 2021;3(4):e0406.
35. Kulwicki BD, Brandt KL, Wolf LM, et al. Impact of an emergency medicine pharmacist on empiric antibiotic prescribing for pneumonia and intra-abdominal infections. Am J Emerg Med 2019;37(5):839–44.
36. Weant KA, Baker SN. Emergency medicine pharmacists and sepsis management. J Pharm Pr 2013;26(4):401–5.
37. Faine BA, Mohr N, Dietrich J, et al. Antimicrobial therapy for pneumonia in the emergency department: the impact of clinical pharmacists on appropriateness. West J Emerg Med 2017;18(5):856–63.

38. Lingenfelter E, Drapkin Z, Fritz K, et al. ED pharmacist monitoring of provider antibiotic selection aids appropriate treatment for outpatient UTI. Am J Emerg Med 2016;34(8):1600–3.

39. Harvey S, Brad Hall A, Wilson K. Impact of an emergency medicine pharmacist on initial antibiotic prophylaxis for open fractures in trauma patients. Am J Emerg Med 2018;36(2):290–3.

40. Kooda K, Canterbury E, Bellolio F. Impact of pharmacist-led antimicrobial stewardship on appropriate antibiotic prescribing in the emergency department: a systematic review and meta-analysis. Ann Emerg Med 2022;79(4):374–87.

41. Evans L, Rhodes A, Alhazzani W, et al. Surviving Sepsis Campaign: international guidelines for management of sepsis and septic shock 2021. Crit Care Med 2021;49(11):e1063–143.

42. Flynn JD, McConeghy KW, Flannery AH, et al. Utilization of pharmacist responders as a component of a multidisciplinary sepsis bundle. Ann Pharmacother 2014;48(9):1145–51.

43. Hunt A, Nakajima S, Hall Zimmerman L, et al. Impact of prospective verification of intravenous antibiotics in an ED. Am J Emerg Med 2016. https://doi.org/10.1016/j.ajem.2016.09.004.

44. Campbell S, Hauler G, Immler EL, et al. Pharmacist-led penicillin allergy assessment in the emergency department reduced empiric fluoroquinolone use. Clin Infect Dis 2020;71(9):e506–8.

45. Alqurashi W, Saux NL, Vyles D, et al. De-labelling penicillin allergy in the emergency department. J Allergy Clin Immunol 2023;151(2):AB66.

46. May L, Cosgrove S, L'Archeveque M, et al. A call to action for antimicrobial stewardship in the emergency department: approaches and strategies. Ann Emerg Med 2013;62(1):69–77.e2.

47. DeWitt KM, Weiss SJ, Rankin S, et al. Impact of an emergency medicine pharmacist on antibiotic dosing adjustment. Am J Emerg Med 2016;34(6):980–4.

48. Baker SN, Acquisto NM, Ashley ED, et al. Pharmacist-managed antimicrobial stewardship program for patients discharged from the emergency department. J Pharm Pr 2012;25(2):190–4.

49. Cohen V, Jellinek SP, Hatch A, et al. Effect of clinical pharmacists on care in the emergency department: a systematic review. Am J Health-Syst Pharm AJHP 2009;66(15):1353–61.

50. Seitz RM, Wiley Z, Francois CF, et al. Improved empiric antibiotic prescribing for common infectious disease diagnoses using order sets with built-in clinical decision support in the emergency department. Infect Control Hosp Epidemiol 2021;1–2. https://doi.org/10.1017/ice.2021.73.

51. Vuong L, Kenney RM, Thomson JM, et al. Implementation of indication-based antibiotic order sentences improves antibiotic use in emergency departments. Am J Emerg Med 2023. https://doi.org/10.1016/j.ajem.2023.03.048.

52. Peyko V, Daves A, Eggleston M. Comparing an emergency department–specific antibiogram versus hospital-wide antibiogram and therapeutic dilemmas for uncomplicated cystitis. Infect Dis Clin Pract 2019;27(3):155–9.

53. Zatorski C, Jordan JA, Cosgrove SE, et al. Comparison of antibiotic susceptibility of Escherichia coli in urinary isolates from an emergency department with other institutional susceptibility data. Am J Health-Syst Pharm AJHP 2015;72(24):2176–80.

54. Hudepohl NJ, Cunha CB, Mermel LA. Antibiotic prescribing for urinary tract infections in the emergency department based on local antibiotic resistance

patterns: implications for antimicrobial stewardship. Infect Control Hosp Epidemiol 2016;37(3):359–60.

55. Smith SC, Bazzoli C, Chung I, et al. Antimicrobial susceptibility of *Escherichia coli* in uncomplicated cystitis in the emergency department: is the hospital antibiogram an effective treatment guide? Acad Emerg Med 2015;22(8):998–1000.
56. Jorgensen S, Zurayk M, Yeung S, et al. Emergency department urinary antibiograms differ by specific patient group. J Clin Microbiol 2017;55(9):2629–36.
57. Rosa R, Abbo LM, Raney K, et al. Antimicrobial resistance in urinary tract infections at a large urban ED: factors contributing to empiric treatment failure. Am J Emerg Med 2017;35(3):397–401.
58. Fleming VH, White BP, Southwood R. Resistance of *Escherichia coli* urinary isolates in ED-treated patients from a community hospital. Am J Emerg Med 2014; 32(8):864–70.
59. Demonchy E, Dufour JC, Gaudart J, et al. Impact of a computerized decision support system on compliance with guidelines on antibiotics prescribed for urinary tract infections in emergency departments: a multicentre prospective before-and-after controlled interventional study. J Antimicrob Chemother 2014; 69(10):2857–63.
60. Gonzales R, Anderer T, McCulloch CE, et al. A cluster randomized trial of decision support strategies for reducing antibiotic use in acute bronchitis. JAMA Intern Med 2013;173(4):267–73.
61. Dean NC, Jones BE, Jones JP, et al. Impact of an electronic clinical decision support tool for emergency department patients with pneumonia. Ann Emerg Med 2015;66(5):511–20.
62. Satterfield J, Miesner AR, Percival KM. The role of education in antimicrobial stewardship. J Hosp Infect 2020;105(2):130–41.
63. Percival KM, Valenti KM, Schmittling SE, et al. Impact of an antimicrobial stewardship intervention on urinary tract infection treatment in the ED. Am J Emerg Med 2015;33(9):1129–33.
64. Flottorp S, Oxman AD, Håvelsrud K, et al. Cluster randomised controlled trial of tailored interventions to improve the management of urinary tract infections in women and sore throat. BMJ 2002;325(7360):367.
65. Hecker MT, Son AH, Murphy NN, et al. Impact of syndrome-specific antimicrobial stewardship interventions on use of and resistance to fluoroquinolones: an interrupted time series analysis. Am J Infect Control 2019;47(8):869–75.
66. Stoll K, Feltz E, Ebert S. Pharmacist-driven implementation of outpatient antibiotic prescribing algorithms improves guideline adherence in the emergency department. J Pharm Pract 2021;34(6):875–81.
67. Barlam TF, Cosgrove SE, Abbo LM, et al. Implementing an antibiotic stewardship program: guidelines by the Infectious Diseases Society of America and the Society for Healthcare Epidemiology of America. Clin Infect Dis 2016; 62(10):e51–77.
68. Albarillo FS, Labuszewski L, Lopez J, et al. Use of a clinical decision support system (CDSS) to improve antimicrobial stewardship efforts at a single academic medical center. Germs 2019;9(2):106–9.
69. Harrington N, Sierzenski P, Taylor K, et al. Enhancing antimicrobial stewardship for pneumonia in the emergency department utilizing a clinical decision support tool. Open Forum Infect Dis 2015;2(suppl_1):1431.
70. Hajesmaeel-Gohari S, Bahaadinbeigy K, Tajoddini S, et al. Effect of computerized physician order entry and clinical decision support system on adverse

drug events prevention in the emergency department: a systematic review. J Pharm Technol JPT 2021;37(1):53–61.

71. Morgan DJ, Malani P, Diekema DJ. Diagnostic stewardship—leveraging the laboratory to improve antimicrobial use. JAMA 2017;318(7):607.

72. Claeys KC, Johnson MD. Leveraging diagnostic stewardship within antimicrobial stewardship programmes. Drugs Context 2023;12. 2022-2029-5.

73. Zakhour J, Haddad SF, Kerbage A, et al. Diagnostic stewardship in infectious diseases: a continuum of antimicrobial stewardship in the fight against antimicrobial resistance. Int J Antimicrob Agents 2023;62(1):106816.

74. Goebel MC, Trautner BW, Grigoryan L. The five Ds of outpatient antibiotic stewardship for urinary tract infections. Clin Microbiol Rev 2021;34(4):e0000320.

75. Cooper RJ, Hoffman JR, Bartlett JG, et al. Principles of appropriate antibiotic use for acute pharyngitis in adults: background. Ann Intern Med 2001;134(6):509–17.

76. Stone S, Gonzales R, Maselli J, et al. Antibiotic prescribing for patients with colds, upper respiratory tract infections, and bronchitis: a national study of hospital-based emergency departments. Ann Emerg Med 2000;36(4):320–7.

77. Rao A, Berg B, Quezada T, et al. Diagnosis and antibiotic treatment of group a streptococcal pharyngitis in children in a primary care setting: impact of point-of-care polymerase chain reaction. BMC Pediatr 2019;19(1):24.

78. Orda U, Mitra B, Orda S, et al. Point of care testing for group A streptococci in patients presenting with pharyngitis will improve appropriate antibiotic prescription. Emerg Med Australas 2016;28(2):199–204.

79. Cardoso DM, Gilio AE, Hsin SH, et al. Impact of the rapid antigen detection test in diagnosis and treatment of acute pharyngotonsillitis in a pediatric emergency room. Rev Paul Pediatr 2013;31(1):4–9.

80. Clark TW, jo Medina M, Batham S, et al. Adults hospitalised with acute respiratory illness rarely have detectable bacteria in the absence of COPD or pneumonia; viral infection predominates in a large prospective UK sample. J Infect 2014;69(5):507–15.

81. Papi A, Bellettato CM, Braccioni F, et al. Infections and airway inflammation in chronic obstructive pulmonary disease severe exacerbations. Am J Respir Crit Care Med 2006;173(10):1114–21.

82. Bouzid D, Zanella MC, Kerneis S, et al. Rapid diagnostic tests for infectious diseases in the emergency department. Clin Microbiol Infect 2021;27(2):182–91.

83. Shoar S, Musher DM. Etiology of community-acquired pneumonia in adults: a systematic review. Pneumonia 2020;12(1):11.

84. Lee JJ, Verbakel JY, Goyder CR, et al. The clinical utility of point-of-care tests for influenza in ambulatory care: a systematic review and meta-analysis. Clin Infect Dis 2019;69(1):24–33.

85. Stamm BD, Tamerius J, Reddy S, et al. The influence of rapid influenza diagnostic testing on clinician decision-making for patients with acute respiratory infection in urgent care. Clin Infect Dis 2023;76(11):1942–8.

86. Rappo U, Schuetz AN, Jenkins SG, et al. Impact of early detection of respiratory viruses by multiplex PCR assay on clinical outcomes in adult patients. J Clin Microbiol 2016;54(8):2096–103.

87. Buchan BW, Windham S, Balada-Llasat JM, et al. Practical comparison of the BioFire FilmArray pneumonia panel to routine diagnostic methods and potential impact on antimicrobial stewardship in adult hospitalized patients with lower respiratory tract infections. J Clin Microbiol 2020;58(7). e00135-20.

88. May L, Dissen E, Smith M, et al. Clinical decisionmaking and antibiotic use in patients with abscesses after rapid point-of-care MRSA/MSSA testing in the emergency department. Ann Emerg Med 2011;58(4):S292–3.

89. Beal SG, Tremblay EE, Toffel S, et al. A gastrointestinal PCR panel improves clinical management and lowers health care costs. J Clin Microbiol 2018;56(1). 014577-17.

90. Ena J, Afonso-Carrillo RG, Bou-Collado M, et al. Evaluation of FilmArray ME panel for the rapid diagnosis of meningitis-encephalitis in emergency departments. Intern Emerg Med 2021;16(5):1289–95.

91. Metlay JP, Waterer GW, Long AC, et al. Diagnosis and treatment of adults with community-acquired pneumonia. An official clinical practice guideline of the American Thoracic Society and Infectious Diseases Society of America. Am J Respir Crit Care Med 2019;200(7):e45–67.

92. Self WH, Balk RA, Grijalva CG, et al. Procalcitonin as a marker of etiology in adults hospitalized with community-acquired pneumonia. Clin Infect Dis 2017; 65(2):183–90.

93. IDSA Community-Acquired Pneumonia (CAP) Clinical Pathway Algorithm. Available at: https://www.idsociety.org/globalassets/idsa/practice-guidelines/community-acquired-pneumonia-in-adults/cap-clinical-pathway-overview.pdf. [Accessed 1 February 2024].

94. Pulia MS, Lindenauer PK. Annals for hospitalists inpatient notes: a critical look at procalcitonin testing in pneumonia. Ann Intern Med 2021;174(6). HO2-HO3.

95. Tsalik EL, Rouphael NG, Sadikot RT, et al. Efficacy and safety of azithromycin versus placebo to treat lower respiratory tract infections associated with low procalcitonin: a randomised, placebo-controlled, double-blind, non-inferiority trial. Lancet Infect Dis 2023;23(4):484–95.

96. Atallah J, Mansour MK. Implications of using host response-based molecular diagnostics on the management of bacterial and viral infections: a review. Front Med 2022;9:805107.

97. Klein A, Shapira M, Lipman-Arens S, et al. Diagnostic accuracy of a real-time host-protein test for infection. Pediatrics 2023;e2022060441. https://doi.org/10.1542/peds.2022-060441.

98. Shapiro NI, Filbin MR, Hou PC, et al. Diagnostic accuracy of a bacterial and viral biomarker point-of-care test in the outpatient setting. JAMA Netw Open 2022; 5(10):e2234588.

99. O'Neal HRJ, Sheybani R, Caffery TS, et al. Assessment of a cellular host response test as a sepsis diagnostic for those with suspected infection in the emergency department. Crit Care Explor 2021;3(6):e0460.

100. Claeys KC, Blanco N, Morgan DJ, et al. Advances and challenges in the diagnosis and treatment of urinary tract infections: the need for diagnostic stewardship. Curr Infect Dis Rep 2019;21(4):11.

101. Chironda B, Clancy S, Powis JE. Optimizing urine culture collection in the emergency department using frontline ownership interventions. Clin Infect Dis 2014; 59(7):1038–9.

102. Stagg A, Lutz H, Kirpalaney S, et al. Impact of two-step urine culture ordering in the emergency department: a time series analysis. BMJ Qual Saf 2018;27(2): 140–7.

103. Dietz J, Lo TS, Hammer K, et al. Impact of eliminating reflex urine cultures on performed urine cultures and antibiotic use. Am J Infect Control 2016;44(12): 1750–1.

104. Jaeger C, Waymack J, Sullivan P, et al. Refining reflex urine culture testing in the ED. Am J Emerg Med 2019;37(7):1380–2.
105. Coughlin RF, Peaper D, Rothenberg C, et al. Electronic health record-assisted reflex urine culture testing improves emergency department diagnostic efficiency. Am J Med Qual 2020;35(3):252–7.
106. Cunney R, Aziz HA, Schubert D, et al. Interpretative reporting and selective antimicrobial susceptibility release in non-critical microbiology results. J Antimicrob Chemother 2000;45(5):705–8.
107. Daley P, Garcia D, Inayatullah R, et al. Modified reporting of positive urine cultures to reduce inappropriate treatment of asymptomatic bacteriuria among nonpregnant, noncatheterized inpatients: a randomized controlled trial. Infect Control Hosp Epidemiol 2018;39(7):814–9.
108. Fleming-Dutra KE, Hersh AL, Shapiro DJ, et al. Prevalence of inappropriate antibiotic prescriptions among US ambulatory care visits, 2010-2011. JAMA 2016; 315(17):1864–73.
109. Wu JY, Balmat R, Kahle ML, et al. Evaluation of a health system-wide pharmacist-driven emergency department laboratory follow-up and antimicrobial management program. Am J Emerg Med 2020;38(12):2591–5.
110. Dumkow LE, Kenney RM, MacDonald NC, et al. Impact of a multidisciplinary culture follow-up program of antimicrobial therapy in the emergency department. Infect Ther 2014;3(1):45–53.
111. Shealy SC, Alexander C, Hardison TG, et al. Pharmacist-driven culture and sexually transmitted infection testing follow-up program in the emergency department. Pharm Basel Switz 2020;8(2):72.
112. Almulhim AS, Aldayyen A, Yenina K, et al. Optimization of antibiotic selection in the emergency department for urine culture follow ups, a retrospective pre-post intervention study: clinical pharmacist efforts. J Pharm Policy Pract 2019;12:8.
113. Miller K, McGraw MA, Tomsey A, et al. Pharmacist addition to the post-ED visit review of discharge antimicrobial regimens. Am J Emerg Med 2014;32(10): 1270–4.
114. Randolph TC, Parker A, Meyer L, et al. Effect of a pharmacist-managed culture review process on antimicrobial therapy in an emergency department. Am J Health Syst Pharm 2011;68(10):916–9.
115. Olson A, Feih J, Feldman R, et al. Involvement of pharmacist-reviewed urine cultures and sexually transmitted infections in the emergency department reduces time to antimicrobial optimization. Am J Health-Syst Pharm AJHP 2020; 77(Supplement_2):S54–8.
116. Rainess RA, Patel VV, Cavanaugh JB, et al. Evaluating the addition of a clinical pharmacist service to a midlevel provider-driven culture follow-up program in a community emergency department. J Pharm Technol JPT 2021;37(3):140–6.
117. Bao H, Dubrovskaya Y, Jen SP, et al. Novel multidisciplinary approach for outpatient antimicrobial stewardship using an emergency department follow-up program. J Pharm Pract 2023;36(2):329–35.

Managing Antimicrobial Resistance in the Emergency Department

Julianne Yeary, PharmD, BCCCP, BCEMP[a],*,
Larissa Hacker, PharmD, BCIDP[b], Stephen Y. Liang, MD, MPHS[c]

KEYWORDS

- Infectious diseases • Emergency department • Multi-drug resistant organisms
- Antimicrobial resistance • Antibiotics

KEY POINTS

- A basic awareness and understanding of antimicrobial resistance and prevailing mechanisms can aid emergency physicians in providing appropriate care to patients with infection due to a multidrug-resistant organism (MDRO).
- Empiric antibiotic coverage of MDROs should be considered for patients recently treated for MDRO infection in the past 3 to 6 months and presenting with similar or recurrent infectious symptoms.
- Newer broad-spectrum antibiotics should be reserved for critically ill patients whereby there is a high likelihood of infection with an MDRO.

INTRODUCTION TO ANTIMICROBIAL RESISTANCE

Antimicrobial resistance remains an ongoing global crisis, contributing more than 2.8 million infections and more than 35,000 deaths annually in the U.S.[1] As frontline health care settings, emergency departments (ED) play an important role in recognizing and managing patients at high risk for infection due to multi-drug resistant organisms (MDRO). Timely and appropriate antimicrobial therapy can impact morbidity and mortality associated with these infections. Conversely, inappropriate selection and administration of antibiotics can lead to adverse events, patient harm, and greater antimicrobial resistance.[2]

In addition to broadening the spectrum of empirical coverage for individuals at high risk of MDROs, emergency clinicians are often responsible for the initial

---

[a] Department of Pharmacy, Barnes Jewish Hospital, 1 Barnes Jewish Place, St Louis, MO 63110, USA; [b] Department of Pharmacy, UW Health, 600 Highland Avenue, Madison, WI 53792, USA; [c] Department of Emergency Medicine and Division of Infectious Diseases, John T. Milliken Department of Medicine, Washington University School of Medicine, St. Louis, MO 63110, USA
* Corresponding author.
E-mail address: julianne.yeary@bjc.org

Emerg Med Clin N Am 42 (2024) 461–483
https://doi.org/10.1016/j.emc.2024.02.005
0733-8627/24/© 2024 Elsevier Inc. All rights reserved.

emed.theclinics.com

management of patients who present to the ED due to positive cultures. The most challenging among these cases are those whose culture and susceptibility results indicate a resistant organism. As such, it is critical for emergency clinicians to understand the current landscape of bacterial resistance and appropriate treatment options. Toward that aim, this article presents a deep dive review on the epidemiology of MDRO infections, describes current mechanisms of antimicrobial resistance in gram-negative and gram-positive bacteria, outlines optimal antibiotic therapy covering MDROs in emergency care, and provides an overview of several newer antibiotics now available in the U.S.

THE SCOPE OF THE PROBLEM

Infections due to MDROs have steadily increased in the U.S. over the last 3 decades. Consequently, emergency clinicians are likely to encounter and provide care to patients with MDRO infection in practice (**Table 1**).[3] Given the uncommon nature of these infections, empirical treatment using newer antibiotics should ideally be reserved for patients recently (within 3–6 months) treated for MDRO infection and presenting with similar or recurrent infectious symptoms. As the rise in MDRO infections is entwined with inappropriate antimicrobial prescribing, it is imperative to reserve the use of newer antibiotics to treat confirmed culture-positive MDRO infections wherever possible.

Table 1
Incidence of MDROs in the United States reported from 2017[4]

| MDRO | Incidence Rates per 10,000 Hospitalizations | | |
	Overall	Community Acquired	Hospital Acquired
ESBL	57.12	49.66	7.46
CRE	3.79	2.78	1.01
CRAB	2.47	1.67	0.80
DTR Pseudomonas	9.43	6.66	2.76
VRE	15.76	10.47	5.29
MRSA	93.68	80.25	13.44

ANTIMICROBIAL RESISTANCE MECHANISMS AND ANTIBIOTIC SELECTION
Beta-lactamases

Beta-lactamases are enzymes that inactivate beta-lactam antibiotics by opening the beta-lactam ring. They are commonly classified by their amino acid structure (Ambler system).[4–8] **Table 2** describes the types and features of several beta-lactamases commonly encountered in clinical practice.

Extended-spectrum beta-lactamase enterobacterales
Extended-spectrum beta-lactamase (ESBL) includes all enzymes that hydrolyze oxyimino-cephalosporins (cefotaxime and ceftazidime). All ESBL are plasmid-mediated, meaning these enzymes are encoded by plasmids and are not inducible in the presence of antimicrobials.[25] Acquisition of these plasmids by gram-negative organisms, most commonly Enterobacterales (eg, *Escherichia coli, Klebsiella pneumoniae, Klebsiella oxytoxa*), confers resistance against penicillins, most cephalosporins, and aztreonam. Although routine ESBL testing is not performed widely, non-susceptibility to ceftriaxone is often used as a proxy for ESBL production (**Table 3**).[26]

Table 2
Beta-lactamase classification and features

Ambler Class	Enzyme Type	Examples	Possible Substrates	Host Organisms	Beta-Lactamase Inhibitors
A	Extended-spectrum beta-lactamase (ESBL)	TEM SHV CTX-M	Penicillin, amoxicillin, piperacillin, narrow-spectrum cephalosporins (cefazolin, cefuroxime), ceftriaxone, aztreonam	Enterobacteriaceae and nonfermenting gram-negative bacilli	Avibactam, vaborbactam, relebactam, tazobactam, durlobactam, clavulanic acid, sulbactam
	Carbapenemase	KPC	Same as ESBL plus carbapenems		Avibactam, vaborbactam, relebactam, durlobactam
B	Metallo-beta-lactamase	NDM VIM IMP	All beta-lactams except for aztreonam		EDTA, divalent cation chelators
C	Cephalosporinase	AmpC	Same as ESBL plus cephamycins	*Hafnia alvei, Enterobacter cloacae, Citrobacter freundii, Klebsiella aerogenes, Yersinia enterocolitica* and *Pseudomonas aeruginosa*	Avibactam vaborbactam, relebactam, durlobactam
D	Carbapenemase	OXA-48	Same as ESBL plus carbapenems	Enterobacteriaceae and nonfermenting gram-negative bacilli	Avibactam, relebactam, durlobactam, clavulanic acid, sulbactam

Table 3
Example of an ESBL-producing organism phenotype[9]

	Ampicillin	Amp-Sulbactam	Ceftriaxone	Meropenem	Aztreonam	Ciprofloxacin	Nitrofurantoin
E. Coli	R	S	R	S	R	S	S

This is an example phenotype of an organism that harbors ESBL. Please refer to local antibiogram or susceptibility testing to determine appropriate empiric treatment.

Optimal antibiotic therapy to treat ESBL infections include[11]:

- Uncomplicated cystitis:
  - *(Preferred)* Nitrofurantoin or trimethoprim-sulfamethoxazole (TMP-SMX)
  - *(Alternative)* Single-dose aminoglycosides, oral fosfomycin (*E coli* only), carbapenems, levofloxacin, or ciprofloxacin
  - If cefepime or piperacillin-tazobactam was initiated as empirical therapy and later identified as an ESBL-E and clinical improvement occurs, no change or extension of antibiotic therapy is necessary
- Pyelonephritis and complicated UTI:
  - *(Preferred)* TMP-SMX, ciprofloxacin, or levofloxacin
  - *(Alternative)* Ertapenem, meropenem, imipenem-cilastatin, or aminoglycosides
- Infections outside of the urinary system:
  - *(Preferred)* Carbapenem
    - *(Critically ill and/or experiencing hypoalbuminemia):* meropenem or imipenem-cilastatin
  - Can consider transitioning to oral fluoroquinolone or TMP-SMX
  - Piperacillin-tazobactam and cefepime are not suggested for treatment, even if susceptibility to agent is demonstrated

AmpC beta-lactamase-producing enterobacterales

AmpC beta-lactamases inactivate cephalosporins and are produced by a variety of gram-negative organisms, as production can arise from inducible chromosomal resistance in the presence of certain antibiotics (aminopenicillins, narrow spectrum cephalosporins, and cephamycins).[27] Antibiotic susceptibility testing of AmpC producing organisms may initially demonstrate sensitivity to cephalosporins; however, resistance on repeat testing after exposure to these inducers can occur. Similar to ESBL, AmpC can also be plasma mediated with the tip-off being demonstrated resistance to ceftriaxone on susceptibility testing.

Common inducible AmpC producers, often referred to as the "HECK-Yes" organisms include: *Hafnia alvei, Enterobacter cloacae, Citrobacter freundii, Klebsiella aerogenes,* and *Yersinia enterocolitica.* IDSA guidelines suggest that only *Enterobacter cloacae, K aerogenes* and *Citrobacter freundii* are organisms at moderate to high risk for becoming clinically significant AmpC producers (**Table 4**).[11]

Optimal antibiotic therapy to treat AmpC infections include:[11]

- Uncomplicated cystitis with <u>any</u> AmpC producer:
  - *(Preferred)* Nitrofurantoin OR TMP-SMX
  - Ceftriaxone (if susceptible)
  - *(Alternative)* Single-dose aminoglycoside, ciprofloxacin OR levofloxacin
- Invasive infection
  - Cefepime MIC less than 4 mcg/mL*: cefepime.
  - Cefepime MIC ≥4 mcg/mL*: carbapenem
    - *Refer to local antibiogram if MIC is not available*
  - TMP-SMX or fluoroquinolone after:
    - Susceptibility demonstrated
    - Patient is hemodynamically stable
    - Reasonable source control has occurred
    - Concerns about insufficient intestinal absorption are not present
  - Avoid oral step-down to nitrofurantoin, fosfomycin, doxycycline, or amoxicillin-clavulanate for bloodstream infections

Table 4
Example of an AmpC-producing organism phenotype[10]

	Ampicillin	Amp-Sulbactam	Ceftriaxone	Meropenem	Aztreonam	Ciprofloxacin	Nitrofurantoin
E. Cloacae	R	R	R	S	R	S	S

*This is an example phenotype of an organism that harbors an AmpC beta-lactamase. Please refer to local antibiogram or susceptibility testing to determine appropriate empiric treatment.

Carbapenem-resistant enterobacteriaceae

Any Enterobacteriaceae resistant to at least one carbapenem antibiotic or identified as producing a carbapenemase is termed a carbapenem-resistant Enterobacteriaceae (CRE). The most common carbapenemases in the U.S. are *K. pneumoniae* carbapenemases (KPCs) with *E. coli* also ranked high. Carbapenemase enzymes exhibit different levels of resistance to beta-lactamase inhibitors including KPC can be inhibited by avibactam, relebactam, and vaborbactam, OXA-48 can be inhibited by avibactam, while NDM cannot be inhibited by the newer beta-lactamase inhibitor agents (**Table 5**).[28,29]

Optimal antibiotic therapy targeting infection with a CRE include:[11]

- If susceptibility to meropenem and imipenem (MIC ≤ 1 μg/mL): the use of extended infusion meropenem is suggested (unless carbapenemases identified)
- Uncomplicated cystitis
    - *(Preferred)* Nitrofurantoin, TMP-SMX, ciprofloxacin, or levofloxacin
    - *(Alternative)* single dose aminoglycoside, fosfomycin (*E. Coli* only), colistin, ceftazidime-avibactam, meropenem-vaborbactam, imipenem-cilastatin-relebactam, or cefiderocol
- Complicated UTI and pyelonephritis
    - *(Preferred if susceptibility demonstrated)* TMP-SMX, ciprofloxacin, or levofloxacin
    - *(Preferred)* Ceftazidime-avibactam, meropenem-vaborbactam, imipenem-cilastatin-relebactam, and cefiderocol
    - *(Alternative)* aminoglycoside
- Infections outside of the urinary tract
    - Carbapenemase testing results are not available or negative
        - *(Preferred)* Ceftazidime-avibactam, meropenem-vaborbactam, and imipenem-cilastatin-relebactam
    - Empiric treatment
        - For patients with CRE infections with recent (previous 12 months) medical care received in countries with a relatively high prevalence of metallo-β-lactamase-producing organisms or who have previously had a clinical or surveillance culture whereby a metallo-β-lactamase-producing isolate was identified, preferred treatment options include:
            - Ceftazidime-avibactam plus aztreonam, or cefiderocol as monotherapy while awaiting susceptibility
    - Confirmed KPC
        - *(Preferred)* Ceftazidime-avibactam, meropenem-vaborbactam, OR imipenem-cilastatin-relebactam
        - *(Alternative)* cefiderocol
    - Confirmed NDM
        - *(Preferred)* Cefiderocol or Ceftazidime/avibactam plus azetronam
        - *(Alternative)* tigecycline or eravacycline
            Not recommended as monotherapy for the treatment of UTIs or blood stream infections
    - OXA-48 like carbapenemase identified
        - *(Preferred)* Ceftazidime-avibactam
        - *(Alternative)* Cefiderocol

Difficult-To-Treat Resistant Pseudomonas aeruginosa

P aeruginosa with difficult to treat resistance is defined as exhibiting nonsusceptibility to all of the following antibiotics: piperacillin-tazobactam, ceftazidime, cefepime,

Table 5
Example of a CRE phenotype

	Piperacillin-Tazobactam	Cefepime	Meropenem	Meropenem-Vaborbactam	Ceftazidime-Avibactam	Ciprofloxacin	Nitrofurantoin
K. Pneumoniae	R	R	R	S	S	S	S

*This is an example phenotype of an organism that harbors a carbapenemase. Please refer to local antibiogram or susceptibility testing to determine appropriate empiric treatment.

aztreonam, meropenem, imipenem-cilastatin, ciprofloxacin, and levofloxacin.[26] The main 3 mechanisms of resistance in *Pseudomonas* include AmpC beta lactamase production, loss of porins, and induction of efflux pumps (**Tables 6 and 7**).[7,30]

Carbapenem-resistant Acinetobacter baumannii

Carbapenem-resistant *A baumannii* (CRAB) is most commonly isolated from the respiratory tract or wounds, and can be challenging to differentiate as a true pathogen or colonizer. *A baumannii* exhibits resistance to most antibiotics through mechanisms including metallo- and serine beta lactamases the modification of 16S rRNA methyltransferases or upregulation of efflux pumps.[31] Sulbactam has proven success in overcoming resistance in *A baumannii*, however it remains unclear the full extent of the mechanisms of resistance in this species (**Table 8**).[32]

Optimal antibiotic therapy to treat CRAB infection include:[11]

- Combination with high-dose ampicillin-sulbactam (9gm IV q8h more than 4 hours OR 27 g IV q24 h continuous infusion) plus at least one other agent
  - High dose ampicillin-sulbactam (even if CRAB isolate is not susceptible to ampicillin-sulbactam, it is still reasonable to consider in combination therapy)
  - Minocycline
  - Tigecycline
  - Polymyxin B
  - Cefiderocol should be limited to CRAB infections refractory to other antibiotics or intolerance to other agents precludes their use and be used in combination
  - *Sulbactam-durlobactam* (newer agent, see later in discussion regarding the additional details)

Stenotrophomonas maltophilia

Stenotrophomonas maltphilia is a gram-negative bacillus that is ubiquitous in water environments. It is generally less pathogenic than other nosocomial organism, however it has virulence factors leading to difficulty to treat in certain hosts when it is a true pathogen.[33] *S. maltophilia* can harbor resistance genes such as metallo- and serine beta lactamases, intrinsic resistance to aminoglycosides, and efflux pumps that reduce the activity of tetracyclines and fluoroquinolones.[34] Similar to CRAB, combination therapy is recommended with limited options for treatment (**Table 9**).[31]

Treatment of choice:[11]

- Combination therapy with at least 2 active agents until clinical improvement: TMP-SMX, minocycline, tigecycline, cefiderocol, or levofloxacin

Table 6
New beta lactam-beta-lactamase inhibitor activity against MDR *Pseudomonas* resistance mechanisms

Agents	Stable Against AmpC Overproduction	Stable Against Loss of Porins	Stable Against Efflux Pumps
Ceftolozane-tazobactam	+ (ceftolozane)	+ (ceftolozane)	+ (ceftolozane)
Ceftazidime- avibactam	+ (avibactam)	-	-
Meropenem- vaborbactam	+ (vaborbactam)	- (OprM)[a]	- (MexAB)[a]
Imipenem/cilastatin/relebactam	+ (relebactam)	- (OprD)[a]	+
Cefiderocol	+	+	+

[a] MexAB-OprM is a common efflux pump in *P. aeruginosa* and oprD protein is a common porin channel for imipenem efflux.

Table 7
Example of a DTR *Pseudomonas* phenotype

	Piperacillin-Tazobactam	Cefepime	Ceftazidime	Meropenem	Aztreonam	Ciprofloxacin	Tobramycin
P. aeruginosa	R	R	R	R	R	R	S

Infectious Source	Preferred	Alternative
Uncomplicated Cystitis	Ceftolozane-tazobactam Ceftazidime-avibactam	Cefiderocol Single dose Tobramycin or Amikacin
Pyelonephritis and cUTIs Infectious outside of the urinary tract	Imipenem-cilastatin-relebactam	Cefiderocol

This is an example phenotype of an organism that harbors *P. aeruginosa* resistance mechanisms. Please refer to local antibiogram or susceptibility testing to determine appropriate empiric treatment.
Treatment of choice[11]

Table 8
Example of a CRAB phenotype

	Ampicillin-Sulbactam	Meropenem	Ceftazidime	Levofloxacin	Gentamicin	TMP-SMX	Cefepime
A. Baumanni	R	R	R	R	R	R	R

This is an example phenotype of an organism that harbors CRAB resistance mechanisms. Please refer to local antibiogram or susceptibility testing to determine appropriate empiric treatment.

Table 9
Example of an _S. maltophilia_ phenotype[12]

	Ceftazidime	Levofloxacin	TMP-SMX	Minocycline
S. maltophilia	R	R	S	S

This is an example phenotype of an organism that harbors _S. maltophilia_ resistance mechanisms. Please refer to local antibiogram or susceptibility testing to determine appropriate empiric treatment.

- _(Clinical instability or intolerance or inactivity toward the above agents)_ Ceftazidime-avibactam plus aztreonam

Vancomycin-resistant Enterococcus

Vancomycin-resistant enterococci (VRE) are a leading cause of health care associated infections with limited treatment options. Enterococci are commensal organisms in the gastrointestinal tract; therefore, the risk for VRE colonization commonly arises through exposure to antimicrobials. _Enterococcus faecium_ has the biggest risk of developing resistance, whereas _Enterobacter faecalis_ commonly retains susceptibility to ampicillin. All enterococci have intrinsic resistance to all cephalosporins, anti-staphylococcal penicillins, aminoglycosides, and TMP-SMX, leading to few options for treatment when resistance develops (**Tables 10 and 11**).[35]

Methicillin-resistant Staphylococcus aureus

S aureus is a leading cause of bacteremia, cellulitis, and endocarditis. MRSA spread through health care and community settings is declining overtime but remains very high with more than 300,000 estimated cases in hospitalized patients in 2017.[36] Choice of treatment may depend on infection severity, availability, cost, and patient factors rather than resistance.

Table 10
Antibiotic options for VRE based on site of infection[13–18]

	Cystitis[d]	Pyelonephritis	Blood	Endocarditis[a]	Intraabdominal[c]	CNS
Nitrofurantoin	X					
Amoxicillin[b]	X					
Ampicillin[b]	X	X	X	X	X	X
Fosfomycin	X					
Linezolid	X	X	X	X	X	X
Daptomycin			X[e]	X[e]	X[e]	

Disclaimer: off-label treatment with oritavancin and tigecycline can be used if susceptible but would encourage an infectious disease consult.[17,18].
[a] Please refer to the infective endocarditis guideline for synergy options based on susceptibility and valve type.
[b] Confirm susceptibility before use. Would not recommend empirically.
[c] Not recommended to cover VRE empirically in intraabdominal infections unless the patient is high risk such as a liver transplant recipient with an intra-abdominal infection originating in the hepatobiliary tree or patient known to be colonized with VRE.
[d] Frequent colonizer or cause of asymptomatic bacteriuria. Once GI colonization, eradication is not possible and hence it may frequently appear in the urinary system.
[e] 8 to 12 mg/kg/day if normal renal function dosing recommendation.

Table 11
Example of a VRE phenotype

	Ampicillin	Vancomycin	Levofloxacin	Tetracycline	Linezolid	Daptomycin	Nitrofurantoin
E. Faceium	R	R	R	R	S	S	S

This is an example an organism that harbors *E. faecium* resistance mechanisms. Please refer to local antibiogram or susceptibility testing to determine appropriate empirical treatment.

Table 12
Antibiotic options for MRSA based on site of infection[14,15,19–24]

	SSTI	Bacteremia	Endocarditis[a]	Intraabdominal	Pneumonia	Meningitis
TMP-SMX	X[b]					X
Doxycycline	X[b]					
Clindamycin[c]	X				X	
Linezolid	X	X	X	X	X	X
Vancomycin	X	X	X	X	X	X
Daptomycin	X	X	X	X		
Telavancin	X	X				
Oritavancin	X					
Dalbavancin	X					
Ceftaroline	X[d]					

[a] Please refer to the infective endocarditis guideline for synergy options based on susceptibility and valve type.
[b] For moderate to severe purulent SSTI only.
[c] Can be used empirically if clindamycin resistance is < 10-15% at the institution. Confirm susceptibility before use.
[d] Ceftaroline is only FDA approved for SSTI, but may be used in conjunction with daptomycin or vancomycin as salvage therapy for persistently positive MRSA bacteremia[25].

Beta-lactam resistance in *S aureus* is mediated by penicillin binding protein 2a (PBP2a) production.[37] Vancomycin resistance is rare, and it is generally not recommended to empirically cover for vancomycin-resistant *S aureus* (VISA) **(Tables 12 and 13)**.[19]

Oritavancin

Oritavancin is structurally similar to vancomycin but differs by having properties against vancomycin-resistant strains (hydrophobic tail and inhibition of transpeptidation).[38–40] It has activity against MRSA, Streptococcus species, and vancomycin-susceptible *E.faecalis*. The half-life of oritavancin is long (200–300 hours), which provides a complete course of SSTI with one dose. Oritavancin was found to be noninferior to vancomycin in SSTI for early clinical response (82.3% vs 28.9% SOLO I; 80.1% vs 82.9% SOLO II). Adverse events included nausea and headache, with no difference in serious adverse events reported (4.4%–7.4%). Other infectious sources have been retrospectively reviewed for off-label indications including osteomyelitis, endocarditis, bacteremia, and prosthetic joint infection. Implications of oritavancin include drug-drug interactions (warfarin) and affect coagulation tests including prolonged prothrombin time and activated partial thromboplastin time (aPTT) due to interaction with phospholipid reagent.

Table 13
Example of an MRSA phenotype

	Oxacillin	Vancomycin	Nitrofurantoin	Rifampin	SMP-TMX	Linezolid	Daptomycin
S. Aureus	R	S	S	S	S	S	S

This is an example phenotype of MRSA. Please refer to local antibiogram or susceptibility testing to determine appropriate empiric treatment.

Table 14
A quick guide to newer broad-spectrum antibiotics with activity against MDROs

Drug	Indications	Spectrum	Notes	Trial Data
Ceftolozane/Tazobactam [Zerbaxa][44–49]	1.5 g–3g q8h* • cUTI • cIAI (+Metro) • Pneumonia *requires renal adjustment	Gram [-] ENT PSA (resistance increasing) *Ineffective against ESBL, Enterococcus, & anaerobes* Limited efficacy against Staph or Strep	Increased affinity for PSA PBPs, greater stability vs AmpC hydrolysis Ceftolozane has similar activity to ceftazidime but with heavier side change preventing hydrolysis	*ASPECT-cIAI (n = 993)* + Metro -non-inferior vs mero for clinical cure (83% vs 87.3%)	*ASPECT-cUTI (n = 1083)* • higher micro eradication (80.4%) vs levo (72.1%) *ASPECT-NP (n = 726)* • Noninferior vs mero 28-d mortality (24% vs 25.3%)
Ceftazidime/Avibactam [Avicaz][50–52]	2.5 g q8h * • cUTI • cIAI (+Metro) • HAP *requires renal adjustment	Gram [-] ENT +/– PSA ESBL Steno *No coverage of Staphylococcus, Streptococcus or Enterococcus*	Potent inhibition of ESBL, AmpC beta-lactamase by avibactam *No increased coverage of PSA or Acineto*	*RECLAIM (n = 1066)* + Metro -non-inferior to mero for clinical cure at 28 d in cIAI (81.6% vs 85.1%)	*REPRISE (n = 302)* • Ceftaz-R ENT and PSA cUTIs and cIAIs • cUTI: 79% micro response • similar clinical cure rates vs BAT (91% vs 91%) *REPROVE (n = 726)* • noninferior to mero (68.8% vs 73% for clinical cure) for HAP
Meropenem/ Vaborbactam [Vabomere][53–55]	4gm q8h * -cUTI *requires renal adjustment	KPC-producing CRE PSA (mero susceptible)	Vaborbactam protects from degradation by certain serine beta-lactamases (KPC) If PSA culture resistant to meropenem – Vabomere has limited efficacy	*TANGO-I (n = 545)* • Phase III vs zosyn cUTI • noninferior (overall success) *TANGO-II (n = 77)* • cUTI, HAP, VAP, BSI, cIAI • superior vs BAT in CRE (n = 47) • clinical cure rates (59.4% vs 26.7%) *BAT: carbapenem, aminoglycoside, polymixin B, colistin, tigecycline or ceftazidime-avibactam*	

(continued on next page)

Table 14
(continued)

Drug	Indications	Spectrum	Notes	Trial Data
Imipenem/Cilastatin-Relebactam [Recarbrio][56–58]	1.25 gm q6h* • cUTI • cIAI • HAP/VAP *requires renal adjustment	PSA ESBL	Potent inhibition of AmpC beta-lactamase by relebactam (similar to avibactam) *Limited benefit with CRE unless produce KPC*	*RESTORE-IMI 1* (n = 47) • vs imipenem/colistin combo • HAP, cIAI, or cUTI • 71% vs 70% favorable overall response *RESTORE-IMI 2* (n-537) • HAP & VAP vs zosyn • noninferior 28 all-cause mortality (15.9% vs 21.3%)
Cefepime/Enmetazobactam[59]	0.5-2gm q8h* - cUTI *requires renal adjustment	PSA ESBL *Limited CRE data*	Enmetazobactam restores activity against ESBL producers (more potent than tazobactam)	*ALIUM* (n = 678) • vs Zosyn for cUTI and pyelo; similar clinical cure rates (92.5% vs 88.9%) [met noninferiority] • higher rate of micro eradication (82.9% vs 64.9%) • ESBL: 73.7% vs 51.5% clinical cure and micro eradication
Cefiderocol [Fetroja][60–64]	2gm q8h* -cUTI -HAP/VAP *requires renal adjustment	ENT PSA Acineto *No Gram positive or Anaerobe coverage*	Enhanced penetration by siderophore transport (iron complex), greater stability vs AmpC hydrolysis (KPCs, OXA-48, and metallo-beta lactamases)	*APEKS-cUTI* (n = 448) • Phase II; noninferior to Imi (clin and micro response 73% vs 55%) *CREDIBLE-CR* (n = 152) • vs BAT in CRE (HAP, VAP, HCAP, bacteremia); similar clinical and microbiological efficacy; higher mortality in the Acineto group treated with cefiderocol *Falcone, et al* (n = 124) • vs colistin • Acinetobacter infections • Higher 30-d mortality in the colistin group (55.8% vs 34%, *P* = .018) *APEKS-NP* (n = 300) • vs mero GNB nosocomial PNA (HAP or VAP); found noninferiority of mortality at day 14 (12.4% vs 11.6%)

Drug	Dose/Indications	Coverage	Notes	Trial Data
Plazomicin [Zemdri][65,66] (aminoglycoside)	15 mg/kg once daily* -cUTI *requires renal adjustment	CRE ESBL Gentamicin-resistant E.coli	Blocks interactions and inactivation by most of the AG-modifying enzymes among CREs *More potent than other AGs against KPC-producing ENT *Limited data against PSA and Acineto*	EPIC (n = 600) • superior vs mero in cUTI & acute pyelo • 78.5% (vs 68.9%) composite cure in cUTI and 85.7% (vs 71.8%) in pyelo CARE (n = 39) • invasive CRE (BSI, VAP, HAP, cUTI) vs colistin PLUS mero or tigecycline • mITT pop n = 37 • lower 28-d mortality (11.8% vs 40%)
Eravacycline [Xerava][67–70] ("4th Generation" tetracycline)	1 mg/kg q12 h -cIAI	Acineto ESBL CRE No PSA coverage *In-vitro MRSA and Enterococcus*	10x higher affinity for ribosomal binding	IGNITE 1 (n = 541) • vs erta cIAI • Noninferior in clinical response (86.8% vs 87.6%) • Similar clinical failure rates (19 vs 11) IGNITE 4 (n = 500) • vs Mero cIAI • Noninferior in clinical response (90.8% vs 91.2%) IGNITE 2 & 3 (n = 908) • vs Levo or Erta cUTI • did not meet noninferiority for clinical cure/micro eradication • (60.4% vs 66.9% vs levo & 84.8% vs 94.8% vs erta)
Sulbactam-Durlobactam[71–73]	1gm/1gm q6h* • cUTI • HABP/VAP • BSI *requires renal adjustment	Acineto Limited data against ENT	Double beta-lactamase coverage Durlobactam active against A, C, and D beta-lactamases	Sagan, et al (n = 80) • cUTI • With imipenem vs imipenem alone • similar overall success (76.6% vs 81%) ATTACK (n = 207) • HABP/VAP • +IMI vs colistin • non-inferior to colistin for 28-d all-cause mortality (12% vs 32.3%)

Abbreviations: Acineto, Acinetobacter; AG, aminoglycosides; BAT, best available therapy; cIAI, complicated intra-abdominal infection, CRE, carbapenemase-resistant Enterobacteriaceae; cUTI, complicated Urinary Tract Infection; ENT, enterobacteriaceae, GNB, gram negative bacteria; HAP, hospital-acquired pneumonia; Imi, imipenem; Levo, levofloxacin, Mero, meropenem; Metro, metronidazole; mITT, microbiologic intention to treat group; MDR, multidrug resistant; NP, nosocomial pneumonia; PSA, Pseudomonas; Pyelo, pyelonephritis; Zosyn, piperacillin/tazobactam.

Dalbavancin

Dalbavancin is considered a semisynthetic lipoglycopeptide and has a high potency against MRSA.[41–43] It is susceptible to other gram-positive bacteremia including Streptococcus species and vancomycin-susceptible *E. faecalis*. Important properties include a long duration of action (half life of 346 hours) and no drug-drug interactions. Dalbavancin has been evaluated in two phase 3, noninferiority, randomized controlled trials in SSTI versus vancomycin (DISCOVER-1 and DISCOVER-2). Noninferiority was met in both trials of early clinical response (83.3% vs 81.8%, DISCOVER-1 & 76.8% vs 78.3%, DISCOVER-2). Adverse events included nausea and headache, with minimal serious adverse events observed (2.6% vs 4%). Dalbavancin has also been evaluated in a number of other disease states, including osteomyelitis, endocarditis, bacteremia, and prosthetic join infections with osteomyelitis. Another randomized controlled trial of dalbavancin compared with the standard of care in osteomyelitis found noninferiority of clinical response (97% vs 88%).

Oritavancin and dalbavancin are only FDA approved for SSTI but may be used off-label in special populations in the ED, such as injection drug users or patients that have poor health care access to outpatient parenteral antimicrobial therapy (OPAT) with serious infections (**Table 14**).[74]

SUMMARY

Empiric broad-spectrum antibiotic therapy to treat serious infection is common in emergency medicine as the source of an infection may not be known nor microbiological culture data may be be available. Empiric treatment of MDRO infections should be approached with caution and guided by the most likely pathogens based on the differential diagnosis, severity of the illness, suspected source of infection, patient specific factors, and local antibiotic susceptibility patterns. Newer broad-spectrum antibiotics should be reserved for critically ill patients whereby there is a high likelihood of infection with an MDRO, such as a recent infection with a carbapenem-resistant organism in the last 6 months, antibiotic exposures within the last 30 days, and local susceptibility profiles for the likely pathogen.[61]

CLINICS CARE POINTS

- A basic awareness and understanding of antimicrobial resistance and prevailing mechanisms can aid emergency clinicians in providing appropriate care to patients with infections due to a multidrug-resistant organism (MDRO).
- Empiric antibiotic coverage of MDROs should be considered for patients recently treated for MDRO infection in the past 3 to 6 months and presenting with similar or recurrent infectious symptoms.
- Newer broad-spectrum antibiotics should be reserved for critically ill patients whereby there is a high likelihood of infection with an MDRO.

DISCLOSURE

The authors report no conflicts of interest or funding relevant to the preparation of this article. SYL received support through the Foundation for Barnes-Jewish Hospital, United States and the Washington University Institute of Clinical and Translational Sciences which is, in part, supported by the NIH, United States/National

Center for Advancing Translational Sciences (NCATS), Clinical and Translational Science Award (CTSA) program (UL1TR002345).

REFERENCES

1. CDC. Antibiotic resistance threats in the United States, 2019. Atlanta, GA: U.S. Department of Health and Human Services, CDC; 2019. [Accessed 4 June 2023].
2. Denny KJ, Gartside JG, Alcorn K, et al. Appropriateness of antibiotic prescribing in the Emergency Department. J Antimicrob Chemother 2019;74(2):515–20. https://doi.org/10.1093/JAC/DKY447.
3. Jernigan JA, Hatfield KM, Wolford H, et al. Multidrug-Resistant Bacterial Infections in U.S. Hospitalized Patients, 2012–2017. NEJM 2020;382(14):1309–19.
4. Jacoby GA, Munoz-Price LS. The New β-Lactamases. NEJM 2005;352(4):380–91.
5. Bush K, Jacoby GA. Updated functional classification of beta-lactamases. Antimicrob Agents Chemother 2010;54(3):969–76.
6. Shapiro AB, Moussa SH, McLeod SM, et al. Durlobactam, a New Diazabicyclooctane β-Lactamase Inhibitor for the Treatment of Acinetobacter Infections in Combination With Sulbactam. Front Microbiol 2021;12:1953.
7. Yahav D, Giske CG, Gramatniece A, et al. New β-Lactam-β-Lactamase Inhibitor Combinations. Clin Microbiol Rev 2020;34(1):1–61.
8. Zumla A. Mandell, Douglas, and Bennett's principles and practice of infectious diseases. Lancet Infect Dis 2015;20(8):264–5.
9. Kumar D, Singh Amit K, Mohammad RA, et al. Antimicrobial Susceptibility Profile of Extended Spectrum β-Lactamase (ESBL) Producing Escherichia coli from Various Clinical Samples. Infect Dis Res Treat 2014;7–8.
10. Khari FIM, Karunakaran R, Rosli R, et al. Genotypic and Phenotypic Detection of AmpC β-lactamases in Enterobacter spp. Isolated from a Teaching Hospital in Malaysia. PLoS One 2016;11(3):150643.
11. Tamma PD, Aitken SL, Bonomo RA, et al. Infectious Diseases Society of America 2023 Guidance on the Treatment of Antimicrobial Resistant Gram-Negative Infections. Clin Infect Dis 2023. ciad428. Accessed June 12, 2023.
12. Bostanghadiri N, Ghalavand Z, Fallah F, et al. Characterization of Phenotypic and Genotypic Diversity of Stenotrophomonas maltophilia Strains Isolated From Selected Hospitals in Iran. Front Microbiol 2019;10(MAY).
13. Gupta K, Hooton TM, Naber KG, et al. International Clinical Practice Guidelines for the Treatment of Acute Uncomplicated Cystitis and Pyelonephritis in Women: A 2010 Update by the Infectious Diseases Society of America and the European Society for Microbiology and Infectious Diseases. Clin Infet Dis 2011;52(5):e103–20.
14. Baddour LM, Wilson WR, Bayer AS, et al. Infective Endocarditis in Adults: Diagnosis, Antimicrobial Therapy, and Management of Complications. Circulation 2015;132(15):1435–86.
15. Solomkin JS, Mazuski JE, Bradley JS, et al. Diagnosis and Management of Complicated Intra-abdominal Infection in Adults and Children: Guidelines by the Surgical Infection Society and the Infectious Diseases Society of America. Clinl Infects Dis 2010;50(2):133–64.
16. O'Driscoll T, Crank CW. Vancomycin-resistant enterococcal infections: epidemiology, clinical manifestations, and optimal management. Infect Drug Resist 2015;8:217.

17. DAPTOmycin - Lexicomp. Available at: https://online.lexi.com/lco/action/doc/retrieve/docid/uofwisconsin_f/3680586?cesid=9Ow5mwUfFGI&searchUrl=%2Flco%2Faction%2Fsearch%3Fq%3DDAPTOmycin%26t%3Dname%26acs%3Dtrue%26acq%3Ddapt#. [Accessed 12 June 2023].

18. Johnson JA, Feeney ER, Kubiak DW, et al. Prolonged Use of Oritavancin for Vancomycin-Resistant Enterococcus faecium Prosthetic Valve Endocarditis. Open Forum Infect Dis 2015;2(4):1–5.

19. Liu C, Bayer A, Cosgrove SE, et al. Clinical practice guidelines by the infectious diseases society of america for the treatment of methicillin-resistant Staphylococcus aureus infections in adults and children: executive summary. Clin Infect Dis 2011;52(3):285–92.

20. Stevens DL, Bisno AL, Chambers HF, et al. Practice guidelines for the diagnosis and management of skin and soft tissue infections: 2014 update by the infectious diseases society of America. Clinl Infect Dis 2014;59(2).

21. Kalil AC, Metersky ML, Klompas M, et al. Management of Adults With Hospital-acquired and Ventilator-associated Pneumonia: 2016 Clinical Practice Guidelines by the Infectious Diseases Society of America and the American Thoracic Society. Clin Infect Dis 2016;63(5):e61–111.

22. Metlay JP, Waterer GW, Long AC, et al. Diagnosis and Treatment of Adults with Community-acquired Pneumonia. An Official Clinical Practice Guideline of the American Thoracic Society and Infectious Diseases Society of America. Am J Respir Crit Care Med 2019;200(7):e45–67.

23. Tunkel AR, Hartman BJ, Kaplan SL, et al. Practice Guidelines for Bacterial Meningitis CID. Published online 2004;1267.

24. Burnett YJ, Echevarria K, Traugott KA. Ceftaroline as Salvage Monotherapy for Persistent MRSA Bacteremia. Ann Pharmacother 2016;50(12):1051–9.

25. Livermore DM. Defining an extended-spectrum β-lactamase. Clinical Microbiology and Infection 2008;14(SUPPL. 1):3–10.

26. IDSA Guidance on the Treatment of Antimicrobial-Resistant Gram-Negative Infections: Version 1.0. Accessed June 4, 2023.

27. Jacoby GA. AmpC B-Lactamases. Clin Microbiol Rev 2009;22(1):161–82.

28. Iovleva A, Doi Y. Carbapenem-Resistant Enterobacteriaceae. Clin Lab Med 2017;37(2):303–15.

29. Shields RK, Doi Y. Aztreonam Combination Therapy: An Answer to Metallo-β-Lactamase–Producing Gram-Negative Bacteria? Clin Infect Dis 2020;71(4):1099.

30. Henrichfreise B, Wiegand I, Pfister W, Wiedemann B. Resistance Mechanisms of Multiresistant Pseudomonas aeruginosa Strains from Germany and Correlation with Hypermutation. Antimicrob Agents Chemother 2007;51(11):4062.

31. IDSA Guidance on the Treatment of Antimicrobial-Resistant Gram-Negative Infections: Version 2.0. Accessed June 4, 2023.

32. Levin AS. Multiresistant Acinetobacter infections: a role for sulbactam combinations in overcoming an emerging worldwide problem. Clinical Microbiology and Infection 2002;8(3):144–53.

33. Paez JIG, Costa SF. Risk factors associated with mortality of infections caused by Stenotrophomonas maltophilia: a systematic review. J Hosp Infect 2008;70(2):101–8.

34. Li XZ, Li J, Li XZ, Li J. Antimicrobial Resistance in Stenotrophomonas maltophilia: Mechanisms and Clinical Implications. Antimicrobial Drug Resistance 2017;937–58. Published online.

35. Cairns KA, Udy AA, Peel TN, et al. Therapeutics for Vancomycin-Resistant Enterococcal Bloodstream Infections. Clin Microbiol Rev 2023;36(2):e0005922.

36. Methicillin-resistant staphylococcus aureus. www.cdc.gov/DrugResistance/Biggest-Threats.html. [Accessed 4 June 2023].

37. Peacock SJ, Paterson GK. Mechanisms of Methicillin Resistance in Staphylococcus aureus. Annu Rev Biochem 2015;84:577–601.

38. Ralph Corey G, Good S, Jiang H, et al. Single-Dose Oritavancin Versus 7–10 Days of Vancomycin in the Treatment of Gram-Positive Acute Bacterial Skin and Skin Structure Infections: The SOLO II Noninferiority Study. Clinical Infectious Diseases 2015;60(2):254–62.

39. Corey GR, Kabler H, Mehra P, et al. Single-Dose Oritavancin in the Treatment of Acute Bacterial Skin Infections. NEJM 2014;370(23):2180–90.

40. Bassetti M, Labate L, Vena A, Giacobbe DR. Role or oritavancin and dalbavancin in acute bacterial skin and skin structure infections and other potential indications. Curr Opin Infect Dis 2021;34(2):96–108.

41. Rappo U, Puttagunta S, Shevchenko V, et al. Dalbavancin for the Treatment of Osteomyelitis in Adult Patients: A Randomized Clinical Trial of Efficacy and Safety. Open Forum Infect Dis 2018;6(1).

42. Dunne MW, Puttagunta S, Giordano P, et al. A Randomized Clinical Trial of Single-Dose Versus Weekly Dalbavancin for Treatment of Acute Bacterial Skin and Skin Structure Infection. CID 2016;62(5):545–51.

43. Boucher HW, Wilcox M, Talbot GH, et al. Once-Weekly Dalbavancin versus Daily Conventional Therapy for Skin Infection. NEJM 2014;370(23):2169–79.

44. van Duin D, Bonomo RA. Ceftazidime/Avibactam and Ceftolozane/Tazobactam: Second-generation β-Lactam/β-Lactamase Inhibitor Combinations. CID 2016;63(2):234–41.

45. Sun Y, Fan J, Chen G, et al. A phase III, multicenter, double-blind, randomized clinical trial to evaluate the efficacy and safety of ceftolozane/tazobactam plus metronidazole versus meropenem in Chinese participants with complicated intra-abdominal infections. International Journal of Infectious Diseases 2022;123:157–65.

46. Lucasti C, Hershberger E, Miller B, et al. Multicenter, double-blind, randomized, phase II trial to assess the safety and efficacy of ceftolozane-tazobactam plus metronidazole compared with meropenem in adult patients with complicated intra-abdominal infections. Antimicrob Agents Chemother 2014;58(9):5350–7.

47. Solomkin J, Hershberger E, Miller B, et al. Ceftolozane/Tazobactam Plus Metronidazole for Complicated Intra-abdominal Infections in an Era of Multidrug Resistance: Results From a Randomized, Double-Blind, Phase 3 Trial (ASPECT-cIAI). Clinical Infectious Diseases 2015;60(10):1462–71.

48. Wagenlehner FM, Umeh O, Steenbergen J, et al. Ceftolozane-tazobactam compared with levofloxacin in the treatment of complicated urinary-tract infections, including pyelonephritis: a randomised, double-blind, phase 3 trial (ASPECT-cUTI). The Lancet 2015;385(9981):1949–56.

49. Kollef MH, Nováček M, Kivistik Ü, et al. Ceftolozane–tazobactam versus meropenem for treatment of nosocomial pneumonia (ASPECT-NP): a randomised, controlled, double-blind, phase 3, non-inferiority trial. Lancet Infect Dis 2019;19(12):1299–311.

50. Mazuski JE, Gasink LB, Armstrong J, et al. Efficacy and Safety of Ceftazidime-Avibactam Plus Metronidazole Versus Meropenem in the Treatment of Complicated Intra-abdominal Infection: Results From a Randomized, Controlled, Double-Blind, Phase 3 Program. CID 2016;62(11):1380–9.

51. Carmeli Y, Armstrong J, Laud PJ, et al. Ceftazidime-avibactam or best available therapy in patients with ceftazidime-resistant Enterobacteriaceae and Pseudomonas

aeruginosa complicated urinary tract infections or complicated intra-abdominal infections (REPRISE): a randomised, pathogen-directed, phase 3 study. Lancet Infect Dis 2016;16(6):661–73.

52. Torres A, Zhong N, Pachl J, et al. Ceftazidime-avibactam versus meropenem in nosocomial pneumonia, including ventilator-associated pneumonia (REPROVE): a randomised, double-blind, phase 3 non-inferiority trial. Lancet Infect Dis 2018;18(3):285–95.

53. Petty LA, Henig O, Patel TS, et al. Overview of meropenem-vaborbactam and newer antimicrobial agents for the treatment of carbapenem-resistant Enterobacteriaceae. Infect Drug Resist 2018;11:1461.

54. Kaye KS, Bhowmick T, Metallidis S, et al. Effect of Meropenem-Vaborbactam vs Piperacillin-Tazobactam on Clinical Cure or Improvement and Microbial Eradication in Complicated Urinary Tract Infection: The TANGO I Randomized Clinical Trial. JAMA 2018;319(8):788–99.

55. Wunderink RG, Giamarellos-Bourboulis EJ, Rahav G, et al. Effect and Safety of Meropenem–Vaborbactam versus Best-Available Therapy in Patients with Carbapenem-Resistant Enterobacteriaceae Infections: The TANGO II Randomized Clinical Trial. Infect Dis Ther 2018;7(4):439–55.

56. Karvouniaris M, Almyroudi MP, Abdul-Aziz MH, et al. Novel Antimicrobial Agents for Gram-Negative Pathogens. Antibiotics 2023;12(4).

57. Motsch J, De Oliveira CUM, Stus V, et al. RESTORE-IMI 1: A Multicenter, Randomized, Double-blind Trial Comparing Efficacy and Safety of Imipenem/Relebactam vs Colistin Plus Imipenem in Patients With Imipenem-nonsusceptible Bacterial Infections. CID 2020;70(9):1799–808.

58. Titov I, Wunderink RG, Roquilly A, et al. A Randomized, Double-blind, Multicenter Trial Comparing Efficacy and Safety of Imipenem/Cilastatin/Relebactam Versus Piperacillin/Tazobactam in Adults With Hospital-acquired or Ventilator-associated Bacterial Pneumonia (RESTORE-IMI 2 Study). CID 2021;73(11):e4539–48.

59. Kaye KS, Belley A, Barth P, et al. Effect of Cefepime/Enmetazobactam vs Piperacillin/Tazobactam on Clinical Cure and Microbiological Eradication in Patients With Complicated Urinary Tract Infection or Acute Pyelonephritis: A Randomized Clinical Trial. JAMA 2022;328(13):1304–14.

60. Beauduy CE WLG. Beta-Lactam & Other Cell Wall- & Membrane-Active Antibiotics | Basic & Clinical Pharmacology, 14e | AccessPharmacy | McGraw Hill Medical. Accessed June 12, 2023.

61. Portsmouth S, van Veenhuyzen D, Echols R, et al. Cefiderocol versus imipenem-cilastatin for the treatment of complicated urinary tract infections caused by Gram-negative uropathogens: a phase 2, randomised, double-blind, non-inferiority trial. Lancet Infect Dis 2018;18(12):1319–28.

62. Wunderink RG, Matsunaga Y, Ariyasu M, et al. Cefiderocol versus high-dose, extended-infusion meropenem for the treatment of Gram-negative nosocomial pneumonia (APEKS-NP): a randomised, double-blind, phase 3, non-inferiority trial. Lancet Infect Dis 2021;21(2):213–25.

63. Bassetti M, Echols R, Matsunaga Y, et al. Efficacy and safety of cefiderocol or best available therapy for the treatment of serious infections caused by carbapenem-resistant Gram-negative bacteria (CREDIBLE-CR): a randomised, open-label, multicentre, pathogen-focused, descriptive, phase 3 trial. Lancet Infect Dis 2021;21(2):226–40.

64. Falcone M, Tiseo G, Leonildi A, et al. Cefiderocol- Compared to Colistin-Based Regimens for the Treatment of Severe Infections Caused by Carbapenem- Resistant Acinetobacter baumannii. Antimicrob Agents Chemother 2022;66(5):e0214221.

65. Wagenlehner FME, Cloutier DJ, Komirenko AS, et al. Once-daily plazomicin for complicated urinary tract infections. Journal of Urology 2019;202(4):641–2.
66. McKinnell JA, Dwyer JP, Talbot GH, et al. Plazomicin for Infections Caused by Carbapenem-Resistant Enterobacteriaceae. NEJM 2019;380(8):791–3.
67. Scott LJ. Eravacycline: A Review in Complicated Intra-Abdominal Infections. Drugs 2019;79(3):315–24.
68. Solomkin J, Evans D, Slepavicius A, et al. Assessing the Efficacy and Safety of Eravacycline vs Ertapenem in Complicated Intra-abdominal Infections in the Investigating Gram-Negative Infections Treated With Eravacycline (IGNITE 1) Trial: A Randomized Clinical Trial. JAMA Surg 2017;152(3):224–32.
69. Solomkin JS, Gardovskis J, Lawrence K, et al. IGNITE4: Results of a Phase 3, Randomized, Multicenter, Prospective Trial of Eravacycline vs Meropenem in the Treatment of Complicated Intraabdominal Infections. CID 2019;69(6):921–9.
70. Alosaimy S, Abdul-Mutakabbir JC, Kebriaei R, et al. Evaluation of Eravacycline: A Novel Fluorocycline. Pharmacotherapy 2020;40(3):221–38.
71. Yahav D, Giske CG, Gramatniece A, et al. New beta-lactam-beta-lactamase inhibitor combinations. Clin Microbiol Rev 2020;34(1):e00115-20.
72. Sagan O, Yakaubsevitch R, Yanev K, et al. Pharmacokinetics and tolerability of intravenous sulbactam-durlobactam with imipenem-cilastatin in hospitalized adults with complicated urinary tract infections, including acute pyelonephritis. Antimicrob Agents Chemother 2020;64(3):e01506-19.
73. Kaye KS, Shorr AF, Wunderink RG, et al. Efficacy and safety of sulbactam-durlobactam versus colistin for the treatment of patients with serious infections caused by Acinetobacter baumannii-calcoaceticus complex: a multicenter, randomized, active-controlled, phase 3-non-inveriority clinical trail (ATTACK). Lancet Infect Dis 2023. S1473-3099(23)00184-6.
74. Thomas G, Henao-Martínez AF, Franco-Paredes C, Chastain DB. Treatment of osteoarticular, cardiovascular, intravascular-catheter-related and other complicated infections with dalbavancin and oritavancin: A systematic review. Int J Antimicrob Agents 2020;56(3).

Moving?

Make sure your subscription moves with you!

To notify us of your new address, find your **Clinics Account Number** (located on your mailing label above your name), and contact customer service at:

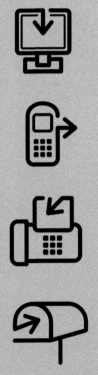

Email: journalscustomerservice-usa@elsevier.com

800-654-2452 (subscribers in the U.S. & Canada)
314-447-8871 (subscribers outside of the U.S. & Canada)

Fax number: 314-447-8029

Elsevier Health Sciences Division
Subscription Customer Service
3251 Riverport Lane
Maryland Heights, MO 63043

*To ensure uninterrupted delivery of your subscription, please notify us at least 4 weeks in advance of move.

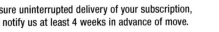

9780443130458